IF A PARTNER HAS AIDS:
GUIDE TO CLINICAL INTERVENTION
FOR RELATIONSHIPS IN CRISIS
R. Dennis Shelby, PhD

SOME ADVANCE REVIEWS

"A state-of-the-art book. This volume will be invaluable for clinicians working with male couples facing AIDS. Couples in the midst of living with AIDS are certain to find their own experiences mirrored and validated by this important and easy to read work. It is a must read for anyone wishing to understand what people with AIDS and their partners go through during the course of the illness."

Michael Shernoff, CSW, ACSW
Co-Director
Chelsea Psychotherapy Associates
New York, New York

"Shelby gives us a moving, compelling, and comprehensive account of partners facing AIDS. His balance of theory, practice, wisdom, and personal reaction is just right. This book should be on every social worker's reading list. Those involved in AIDS care will find confirmation and affirmation. Those new to the field, or uninvolved in it, will gain valuable insight into the impact of AIDS both on partners and practitioners."

Gary A. Lloyd, ACSW
Professor and Coordinator
Institute of Research and Training in HIV/AIDS Counseling
Tulane University, School of Social Work
New Orleans, Louisiana

NOTES FOR PROFESSIONAL LIBRARIANS AND LIBRARY USERS

This is an original book title published by Harrington Park Press, an imprint of The Haworth Press, Inc. Unless otherwise noted in specific chapters with attribution, materials in this book have not been previously published elsewhere in any format or language.

CONSERVATION AND PRESERVATION NOTES

If a Partner Has AIDS

Guide to Clinical Intervention for Relationships in Crisis

HAWORTH Social Work Practice
Carlton Munson, DSW, Senior Editor

If a Partner Has AIDS

Guide to Clinical Intervention for Relationships in Crisis

R. Dennis Shelby, PhD

Harrington Park Press
An Imprint of The Haworth Press, Inc.
New York • London • Norwood (Australia)

ISBN 1-56023-002-9

Published by

Harrington Park Press, an imprint of The Haworth Press, Inc., 10 Alice Street, Binghamton, NY 13904-1580

Library of Congress Cataloging-in-Publication Data

Shelby, R. Dennis.
  If a partner has AIDS : guide to clinical intervention for relationships in crisis / R. Dennis Shelby.
      p.   cm.
  Includes bibliographical references and index.
  ISBN 1-56023-002-9 (pbk.)
  1. AIDS (Disease) – Patients – Family relationships. 2. AIDS (Disease) – Patients – Coun-
seling of. I. Title.
[RC607.A26S49 1992b]
155.9'16 – dc20   91-18847
                                                                                    CIP

You get to know their lovers, and it all seems very real.

Anthony Fauci

ABOUT THE AUTHOR

R. Dennis Shelby, PhD, is currently Clinical Research Fellow at the Institute for Clinical Social Work in Chicago, Illinois, focusing on the experience of people who are seropositive for HIV antibodies. He has held a variety of clinical, supervisory, and administrative positions at Beacon Therapeutic School, a day program serving severely disordered children and their families. Dr. Shelby has treated numerous HIV-impacted men in his private practice and has presented his research and papers on the many facets of clinical intervention with HIV-related problems at state, national, and international social work and psychoanalytic conferences. The escalation of the AIDS epidemic in Chicago paralleled his doctoral studies, leading Dr. Shelby to examine the impact of AIDS in light of psychoanalytic theories. He received his doctorate from the Institute for Clinical Social Work and is a graduate of the Loyola University School of Social Work, and the social work training program of the Wexler Clinic, Psychiatric and Psychosomatic Institute, Michael Reese Hospital. Dr. Shelby's ongoing interests include a re-examination of the phenomenon of homosexuality in light of advances in clinical theory. He maintains a private practice in Chicago, Illinois.

CONTENTS

Foreword

In 1968 when I first had the opportunity to hear Heinz Kohut speak, I was mesmerized by this man who, until then, I had barely known. With great interest, sharp wit, well-reasoned arguments, and a charismatic style of speaking second-to-none, Dr. Kohut wove his tale—of how he became interested in a different way of ordering his clinical experiences, of the vital role of empathy, and of the beginning awareness of the importance of the self in the understanding of pathology. For the first time, I felt that there was a clinical theory that related directly to my clinical work.

Prior to my becoming aware of Self Psychology, I had struggled to make classical theory applicable to my work with patients. Too often what resulted was a more-or-less successful experience of being with patients followed by a theoretical construction of that work which would pass muster but would always feel forced.

In this powerful and evocative book we see demonstrated a creative application of Self Psychology that would have been enormously gratifying to Dr. Kohut. His untimely death in 1981 left much to be done in terms of the application of the theory to a variety of social problems and clinical situations; even more importantly, there have remained areas in which the theory itself has needed expansion and refinement. It was Dr. Kohut's fervent wish that those who would follow him would apply his theories in new and creative ways and would expand the theory into areas not fully mapped out by him. Dennis Shelby has written a book that moves forward in both areas.

Two basic ideas of Self Psychology are aptly demonstrated in this volume, which is the result of a prolonged immersion by the author in the lives of the research subjects. The first of these is empathy, which Kohut defined as "vicarious introspection" (Kohut, 1978). Shelby has described in great and moving detail the experiences of men whose partners have AIDS. This is not a study focused on the externals of the AIDS experience, as important as that could certainly be, but is instead an attempt to come to understand what the phases of the illness feel like to the partner. When a relationship is threatened by severe illness and death, questions about the very essence of attachment and loss are front and center. Shelby, by using his own empathic instrument in the interviewing process, has come to understand with his research subjects the meaning of their experiences. And this leads us to the second piece of Self Psychological theory that is so well applied in this study.

Kohut posited that the self of the human being is composed of its many selfobjects — those functions performed by others but experienced as parts of ourselves. The parent who joyfully mirrors the toddler's first steps is appropriately aiding the development of the child's grandiose self. In like manner, the parent who is able to soothe and comfort the irritable infant is offering him/her self as an idealizable selfobject. The third pole of development is that of the twinship selfobject in which the parent allows the child to experience him/her self as essentially like the parent in crucial ways so that the child can experience being a part of the human community.

Shelby has taken a microscope to the relationships he has studied and has given form and substance to the concept "selfobject." We read again and again of the comfort and soothing offered from one partner to another — and not only of the well partner to the sick. We also read of the strength gained by the well partner from the way in which the sick partner traverses his illness.

Most importantly, this is a book that builds upon existing concepts in Self Psychology to formulate new ones. Mourning theory is as old as Freud's *Mourning and Melancholia* (Freud 1917). In this seminal work, Freud posited that normal mourning consisted of raging at and then giving up the object, while pathological mourning involved an inability to give up the object because of its narcissistic significance. Shelby challenges current thinking, based on his research findings, and prompts us to think in new ways about anticipatory grief. He also helps us to re-think what makes for successful grieving: ". . . The mourner is not missing, yearning for, or searching for a 'lost figure,' 'object,' or representation thereof. Rather what is absent is his particular, unique experience of that individual and the shared experience—the dialogue that an intimate relationship entails" (p. 198).

There is one final thought. Shelby notes in his Acknowledgments that this book is, along with everything else, an historical document. It is entirely fitting that this is so. Heinz Kohut was profoundly interested in the humanities; he was a theoretician of his own age, concerned with the social implications of his theories. He would have been gratified to see the creative application of his ideas to one of the most confounding problems of our time.

Constance Goldberg, MS
Chicago, Illinois

BIBLIOGRAPHY

Freud, Sigmund, 1917e (1915), "Mourning and Melancholia." *Standard Edition* 14:243-58.
Kohut, Heinz. (1959), "Introspection, Empathy, and Psychoanalysis," In: *The Search for the Self*, vol. 1, ed. P. Ornstein, New York: International Universities Press, 1978, pp. 205-232.

Preface

Dennis Shelby has made a major contribution to mental health clinicians involved in AIDS care, as well as to the general population at large, in this important work, *If a Partner Has AIDS: Guide to Clinical Intervention for Relationships in Crisis.* It is sad but true that the AIDS pandemic continues to explode worldwide. In August 1990 the World Health Organization reported 266,098 AIDS cases worldwide with 133,889 cases occurring in the U.S. The scant resources that have been committed worldwide to AIDS care have understandably been largely directed to providing care and services to Persons Living With AIDS. However, as Dennis so aptly points out in this work, AIDS does not only impact the individual Person With AIDS but also impacts those in the broad and complex social milieu that surrounds the individual.

This book helps us to understand in great depth the complex and intense experience of "The AIDS Journey" within the context of the gay male couple relationship. Dennis has drawn upon his considerable talents as a clinician and a researcher in identifying the specific stages that a group of gay male couples experience when confronted with the reality of AIDS for one (and often both) members of the couple. In addition to a solid research design that helped him to identify these stages through the analysis of interview material, Dennis draws upon the useful conceptual framework of "Self Psychology" and uses a self psychologically informed lens through which one can understand the psychological meanings of the stages he has identified. This rather unique perspective of using empirical techniques in combination with a solid psychological theory base helps us to understand more fully the experience of AIDS from the partner's perspective. Such information can inform and guide the clinician in the nature and type of interventions that can be most helpful. Additionally, Dennis' work informs clinicians (and non-clinicians as well) that the feelings that well up for the partner during the AIDS journey are intense, at times may seem like they will never end, and are very frightening on many levels. However, Dennis also informs us that this intensity is expectable, is normal, has a course of its own, and indeed will not last forever. This information is quite important for clinicians to know. Additionally, Dennis' book is written in a way that is accessible to non-clinicians as well. Therefore, the information that Dennis provides us is most useful and important for the lay reader as well who is impacted by AIDS, perhaps as a partner or other significant person within the psychosocial milieu of a Person Living With AIDS.

The theory base of self psychology that Dennis draws upon is one that I feel is of special usefulness for clinicians today. It places importance on the development and sustainment of an "empathic social milieu" for the individual in order to grow psychosocially. The notion of an empathic social milieu, its fragmentation, dissolution, and the need for restoration is especially relevant when one tries to understand many aspects of the AIDS journey, and Dennis weaves the knowledge base of self psychology most skillfully when he discusses the world of the Person Living With AIDS and his partner. Dennis is able to do this because first and foremost he himself is a skilled clinician who uses his extensive capacity for empathy in all clinical work. A book such as this could only be written by someone who has extensive ability to put himself "into the shoes" of another and then use that information to further understanding. In many ways then, this book is a gift to us from a most gifted clinician.

In my work as principal organizer for the annual International Conference on Social Work and AIDS these past three years I have had the honor of hearing Dennis speak about many of the ideas he has described in this book. I agree with him that we need to further understand the world of the PWA, but we also need to understand the world of the partner and others in the psychosocial network of the PWA. Although this study was conducted with a sample of gay male couples, I suspect that many of the psychodynamics and stages which Dennis has identified for gay couples are equally true for others affected by "the changing face of AIDS." That is, although AIDS no longer is predominantly a gay disease, the partners of those affected by AIDS (be they partners in gay relationships, IV drug users, people of color, or others) will sadly continue to be impacted with issues of grief, loss, and mourning as long as AIDS continues to explode. Dennis has studied this wrenching human issue in the context of gay relationships. However, his findings will help all of us to understand aspects of this very human disease which touches all of us.

Vincent J. Lynch, DSW
Boston College
Chestnut Hill, Massachusetts

Acknowledgments

An endeavor such as this cannot be undertaken without the help, support and encouragement of many people. The Institute for Clinical Social Work proved to be an incredibly effective matrix in which to hone my clinical skills, challenge my thinking, nurture ideas, and fulfill a long-standing dream. I wish to thank the members of the faculty who served on the dissertation committee: Thomas Kenemore, PhD, who served as my advisor on this project and who gives new meaning to the word mentor; Patrick Curtis, PhD, who served as my energizer; and Constance Goldberg, MS, who refined my theoretical understanding of the results of the project. Joseph Palombo, MA, has been central in my development as a clinician and was especially integral in the theoretical formulations found in Chapter 14. Thanks also to Arnold Goldberg, Morton and Estelle Shane who shared their work with me; and to the many faculty members of the Institute whose enthusiasm along the way kept me going during all the many phases of the project and preparation of this manuscript.

An important factor in the study's success was the recruitment of participants. Thanks to Thomas Klein, MD, and Ross Slotten, MD, who have been an unwavering source of support in my clinical and research undertakings; my life-long friend Kandice Strako, MD, who also housed and fed me during the several trips to San Francisco for the study; and the staff of the Howard Brown Memorial clinic. Many friends lent their support along the way. Thanks to Bill Borden, PhD, for his periodic check-ins and helpful editorial suggestions; the guys at two steppin'; and Carl Grimm, who was a great source of comfort during the long months of writing the document. Thanks also to Sue Larmon and Ron Dorfman for their help in preparing the manuscript.

Deep gratitude is owed to the men who participated in the study. Their willingness to share their lives was the key factor in the success of this research. While the results have substantial implications for clinical theory, this work also serves as a powerful historical document. AIDS has taken an enormous toll; it has taxed human resiliency, dramatically altered the course of many lives, taken partners, sons, daughters, brothers, sisters, fathers, mothers, uncles and aunts. Examining AIDS in the context of the matrix of human relationships in which it occurs offers a powerful testimony to its impact.

This work is dedicated to the men who participated in the study and to all the gay men whose partners are ill or who have lost a partner to AIDS, especially to James, John, Tom, Wayne, Juan, Roger, Jack and Barry, participants who died during the course of, and since the study was completed. Also to my friend Russ Palmer, who, had he lived to see this work published, would surely have remarked, "'Atta boy! Go get 'em!''

Chapter I

Introduction

May 1989

In November of 1985, in the context of my clinical practice, I met Greg and Stan.[1] Stan had been diagnosed with AIDS several months earlier. Our first meeting was harrowing for all of us. On the way to his first appointment, Stan had become disoriented, parked his car, and gotten lost. He arrived at my office an hour late, sweating and terrified, clutching a slip of paper with my name and address on it. In a trembling voice he tried to explain what had happened. Yes, he said, there was someone he could call. His lover should be home from work by now. Greg arrived shortly. The two men went to find the car. We all sat down to talk later that evening.

Greg and Stan were clearly overwhelmed. Not just by the evening's events, but those of the past nine months. AIDS was rather new to Chicago then. They had encountered many losses and medical crises the last few months. Anxious uncertainty had come to dominate their lives. They wanted help, but were not quite sure what they needed. I was struck by Greg's attentiveness, his concern over the evening's events, and the non-intrusive way he deftly supplied information that Stan was having difficulty recalling. Greg operated in such a way that Stan's growing cognitive deficits were modulated, rather than accentuated. Though a good deal of complementarity was present, I also sensed considerable tension in the relationship.

The couple phrased their request for help in the form of questions regarding sources of acupuncture, meditation, massages, and other

---

1. The names of participants and clients have been changed to maintain confidentiality.

forms of alternative healing. Stan related a dream that conveyed not only his hope for such intervention, but also his conviction that he was, indeed, dying. I stated that I could not offer them alternative therapies and that I knew little about them. However, I could offer them a place to talk. I sensed that they had a great deal to talk about, but were having difficulty doing so. Stan appeared disappointed, while Greg was obviously encouraged. After some hesitation on Stan's part, an appointment was made for the following week.

Several weeks before I met Stan and Greg, my first patient with AIDS had died. It had been a draining, sometimes grueling experience for me. Tom was not only my first AIDS patient, but he had essentially a borderline personality structure. He was boarding with a man who had offered a room in his apartment to men with AIDS who had no other place to stay. Tom's family had been marginally involved, at times outright rejecting him during his illness. He was one of the first AIDS patients in the city and as such had experienced a good deal of anxiety and rejection at the hands of medical personnel.

A recovered alcoholic and polydrug abuser, Tom found a degree of comfort in his participation in several AA groups. He had also found a "home" in the support system of the Howard Brown Memorial Clinic, an agency in Chicago's gay community which provided support services for people with AIDS. Tom's experience with AIDS was characterized by being kicked out of his family or home of origin, but gradually finding other homes and relationships to help him negotiate the illness. He was enraged by the multiple rejections but relieved to find sustaining relationships. His relief and comfort were mingled with a sense of angry beholding to the people he relied upon for a sense of comfort. Tom formed an intense, but quiet, attachment to me. He experienced the relationship as tolerating the wide range of his sadness, despair, and rage that he feared might rupture his other sustaining relationships. I quickly became a central person in his experience.

In contrast to Tom, Stan had a home, an enduring relationship, and parents who were deeply concerned and who were providing funds as he awaited his disability benefits. I wanted to maximize Greg and Stan's ability to sustain each other. I decided to work with them as a couple. It would be new territory for me. There was little in the way of clinical literature on AIDS at the time, and even less on work with couples. I assumed that providing the couple a forum where they could talk about what they were experiencing would provide some relief.

The next meeting with Greg and Stan went well. I saw them separately and together. I was struck by the contrast between the two men. Alone, Greg talked freely about his fear of losing Stan to the disease, his frustration and uncertainty as to what was the best way to approach dealing with the emotional hardships they had, and were currently, encountering. Stan disavowed being terminally ill, rarely mentioned AIDS, but focused on his frustration and rage at his past employer over insurance benefits. When I saw them together, Greg appeared to actively support Stan in his disavowal. Stan remained adamant about not wanting to talk, instead wanting acupuncture. However, he slowly began to express his irritation with Greg about how they were negotiating aspects of the illness. A dialogue, moderated by myself, opened up between the two men. Both appeared relieved, and an appointment was made for the following week.

Over the next few days, Stan became ill for the second time with pneumocystis carinii pneumonia and was hospitalized. His condition quickly deteriorated and he was placed on a respirator in an intensive care unit. Greg and Stan's parents began holding a vigil at the hospital. I met with Greg and the parents several times in the ICU waiting room and in the hospital cafeteria. All were devastated. Each had sensed Stan's pain and torment since his diagnosis and urged him to seek clinical help. Stan had either become angry or not followed through on potential sources. All had unanswered questions about what Stan had been experiencing. All were hoping for a miracle. All feared that Stan was dying. There was some discussion about the issue of centrality. As next of kin, Stan's parents were signing papers, yet both viewed Greg as the central person in their son's life. Stan's mother had great difficulty with her son's being gay, and blamed herself; if he were not gay, she thought, he would not have contracted AIDS, and this would not be happening.

Stan died before a third couple session could take place. I was shocked by the suddenness of it all. One week we were establishing a treatment relationship, the second and third I was with his partner and family while Stan gradually succumbed to pneumocystis. Greg went home to be with his parents for several weeks. We planned to meet when he returned.

While Greg was away I presented the case to a supervisor. He was also profoundly moved by Greg's plight. He wondered aloud, "I mean no disrespect to the man who died, but what about his lover? What about all of the other lovers? They have to somehow manage to carry on with their lives."

Several weeks later, Greg called me from his office. It was his first day back at work. He said he was afraid he was "losing it" and began to cry on the phone. He was confused and overwhelmed, he said, and he missed Stan terribly. We met that evening and began a journey that continues to this day. I was deeply moved by Greg's pain and sadness, and the depth of the loss he was experiencing. The theme of AIDS surfaced repeatedly. Greg tested positive for the HIV virus shortly after Stan was diagnosed. For the first few months after Stan's death, Greg experienced little concern for his own health, but gradually his fear of contracting AIDS became a major source of anxiety. I began to wonder what the effects on the mourning process would be. Here was a man infected with the same virus that had killed his partner. The death of Stan from AIDS and Greg's infection with the same virus were tightly woven together. Would they ever unravel?

A psychiatric resident who knew of my work with Greg and several other men with AIDS gave me the March 1986 issue of *Psychiatric Annals*. I read through it, hoping for help with my work with Greg. There was nothing. Partners were barely mentioned, and when they were it was in reference to them leaving after their partners were diagnosed. Something in the tone of the articles bothered me. Popular opinion at the time was presenting the disease as an affliction of promiscuous, polydrug-abusing, urban gay men. The professional articles were presenting gay men with AIDS as victims—victims of AIDS anxiety, homophobia, and their lovers. But this description did not fit my experiences with Greg. It did not entirely fit my experiences with other men with AIDS. I saw men who felt stigmatized and at times victimized, but who were also making strides at adapting to the illness and the hardships it brought them. I rationalized that the clinicians who were writing these articles were just trying to get a grip on working with AIDS patients themselves, that it was still early in the course of what would be a long-term epidemic, and that research and writing on partners and the family would eventually evolve.

I kept coming across more articles, each one focusing on people with AIDS, and having little if anything to say about their partners. Physician friends told me that many of their AIDS patients had partners. The centrality and magnitude of the loss for Greg was evident. Why wasn't anyone writing about it? Why weren't people acknowledging partners?

In my academic life, the question of a dissertation was looming. I became increasingly certain that I wanted to study surviving partners. But, how, why, and what was my research question? I discussed my experience with Greg and my questions about the effects of seropositivity with the man who was to become my advisor on the project, Tom Kenemore, who encouraged me to pursue it.

* * *

In September of 1986, I went to the National Association of Social Workers convention in San Francisco. A day long symposium on AIDS had been scheduled. I hoped to get more ideas on work with partners. Instead, I was disappointed in the presentations, and resolved to proceed with this study. The one presentation that focused on established relationships was unhelpful, offering little insight into work with couples dealing with AIDS or surviving partners. A social worker spoke at length on "unusual family constellations" she had encountered in her work with AIDS patients. She had "discovered" seven "constellations," such as: married, bisexual, wife unaware of sexuality; married, bisexual, wife knows lover. At the bottom of her list of unusual constellations was: homosexual, engaged in relationship with another man. A general tendency of the symposium presenters was to say very little about the people with AIDS they worked with. Very little was said about clinical intervention or clinical understanding of what people with AIDS encounter. Rather, speakers focused on policy, or outlined over and over again the hardships facing AIDS patients. Very little in a daylong symposium matched my experience with Greg or the men with AIDS that I had encountered.

On the way back to Chicago, no doubt somewhere over Kansas, I decided that I wanted to study what men who had lost partners were going through, and the effects of seropositivity on the mourning process. But how to do both? Three hours after my plane landed I was in Tom Kenemore's office complaining about the symposium, the lack of interest in partners, and the people who seemingly did not want to get to know their AIDS patients (or perhaps had difficulty conveying just how well they had come to know their patients), let alone talk about the myriad of clinical issues involved in working with AIDS. I was not sure how I could look at both what surviving partners were experiencing and the effects of seropositivity on the mourning process. I was directed to Glaser and Strauss and their Grounded Theory methodology.

An obvious question when putting together a research proposal is how many people are affected by the problem under study. I called AIDS support agencies in New York, Washington, Denver, Chicago and San Francisco. Not one agency kept statistics on the partner status of the clients. The information was buried in their clients' files, not readily available, especially to an unknown doctoral student. In any application for agency services in the general community, the third or fourth question is marital status. I thought, "Are we as a community buying into a belief that gay men do not form relationships? Why isn't anyone asking about partners?"

I enlisted two physician friends to help me get at least a cursory idea of how many gay men with AIDS were partnered. For six months, one physician in San Francisco and the other in Chicago kept track of the partner status of their current and new AIDS patients. Both physicians' practices were composed predominantly of white, middle to upper-middle class gay men. But at least their records would give me an idea of the potential number of men with partners. Kandice Strako found that 58% of her patients were partnered, and Tom Klein found that 60% of the patients in his practice were partnered. I was surprised by the similarity and the actual numbers. I had expected around 30%. What myths had I subscribed to? Did I too want to think that nice people did not get AIDS? Had I constructed a myth to assure myself that AIDS would stay away from me? At any rate, I was convinced that the study was important and sorely needed.

Greg was giving me copies of a journal he had been keeping. Following the method of Glaser and Strauss, I began coding his entries. Several other men who had lost partners were referred to my clinical practice. I began to notice that they all started at the beginning: talking and writing about the early signs that something was wrong, their concern that it might be AIDS, and the confirmation that it was AIDS. True, this reconstruction of the experience could be understood as part of the mourning process, but I realized that I was asking the wrong question. The question, "What are the experiences of gay men whose partners die from AIDS?" was too narrow. A great deal appeared to happen before the actual death of the partner. The question was changed to, "What are the experiences of gay men whose partners *contract* AIDS?"

During a visit to Chicago, my physician friend from San Francisco told me she was following many of the partners of her AIDS patients. Repeatedly, she had encountered surviving partners who became preoccupied with their health status four to six months after the death of the partner. We both wondered, "Why then, why four to six months, what could be happening in the mourning process that the partner's status would become a focus of concern?" A sense of excitement came to dominate the rainy afternoon as we discussed her experiences with partners and the patterns that I was beginning to see in my patients and study participants. Several hours later she convinced me to come to San Francisco. She would recruit participants from among her patients. Tom Klein was equally excited, and offered to refer from his practice.

An article about the study in one of the gay community newspapers (Burks 1987) brought good response. Men who called about the study were appropriately suspicious. They all asked me why I was doing this. I replied that I felt that partners were being neglected, that no one was writing about what they experienced, and that I thought partners had their own unique experience. All who called agreed to come in and tell their stories.

This study has been quite a journey for me. I am afraid to, or just do not care to, count the tapes that fill two shoe boxes that now sit on a shelf. They represent interviews with well partners, surviving partners, partners with AIDS, physicians, nurses, social workers and support group leaders from Chicago, San Francisco, rural Minnesota, and Boston. The experiences related to me by these people were in sharp contrast to the articles and presentations that originally irritated me. Their experience was rich, sad, painful, resilient, and, at times triumphant. Very early in the study, I found myself idealizing the well partners. They kept plugging away, doing their best to care for and sustain their ill partners. "What keeps them going?" was a central question that became more refined as the study progressed. At first each interview generated more questions. Gradually the questions were answered.

One of the hardest parts of the study came from getting to know the participants. During the study, three men died. I found myself "crossing fingers" during hospital stays and when survivors went to be tested. I came to recognize the particular sense of resignation in a well partner's voice as he realizes that the end of his partner's life is near. I cheered on survivors who were taking off in new directions with renewed confidence, and I was profoundly saddened by the experiences of seropositive and symptomatic surviving partners. I found myself in their homes, offices, and hospital rooms, learning to negotiate San Francisco by car, and two-steppin' with a participant in a country/western dance bar. I also found myself feeling guilty. I could listen to their experiences, be moved to tears as I coded them, be amazed at their resiliency and often be overwhelmed by the amount of work that the study required. But, while I participated in their experience to a degree, ultimately, I could leave it. I could go home at night. I only had to listen and write about it. I did not have to experience it myself.

As the study progressed, so did AIDS. Greg's T-cell count declined to the 250 range, then went up into the low three hundreds. His count declined again to 200 and he began taking AZT. He has endured a long and painful bout with shingles, and periodically hairy leukoplakia appears on his tongue. The last few months have been difficult for him, but he continues to strive to make the most of his life. When I first began working on the project in 1986, there were less than 20,000 cases of AIDS nationwide. Now, in June of 1989, the total is over 90,000. Eighty thousand new cases are projected for 1992 (Perreten 1989). AIDS has also encroached into my social network. Several friends have tested positive, several more have developed AIDS, and several have died. In finishing this project, I recently stumbled on a secret hope: that the study would be more or less obsolete by the time it was finished. Obviously it is not.

Of the 39,000 new cases of AIDS projected for 1989, 56% or 21,000 were gay/bisexual men (Perreten 1989). Sixty percent (the potential number of partnered AIDS patients) of that number is 12,600. Assuming the partnership rates of the two physicians' practices were a reasonable reflection, it is conceivable that in 1989 alone, approximately 12,600 partnered gay men will contract AIDS. That figure is more than the total number of cases reported nationwide in 1985, the year Greg and Stan first walked into my office.

September 1990

It will soon be six years since I worked with my first client with AIDS. The number of reported AIDS cases nationwide is now over 140,000. Men who are seropositive, but have not developed AIDS, now comprise the majority of men in my clinical practice who are impacted by HIV. As the epidemic progresses, I have become acutely aware of the integral role relationships play in the experience of HIV infection. Many of these seropositive men entered treatment after the loss of a relationship or relationships to AIDS disrupted their attempts to negotiate life with the knowledge that they too were infected with the HIV virus. Following a period of depression and disorganization after being informed that they tested positive, they had adopted an optimistic, if not fighting attitude towards the infection. However, after a loss or several losses, their experience shifted to one of defeat, depression, anxiety, and the often terrifying sense of rapidly approaching death — often despite the lack of acute medical symptoms.

While most of this book focuses on the impact of AIDS on long-term relationships, men who are coupled, or in the terminology of the study, partners, in the broadest sense, it is also a study of the powerful influence that relationships play in an individual's experience of HIV infection and AIDS. This may seem like an obvious point. Community based AIDS/HIV support organizations provide their clients with case managers, "buddies" and groups. HIV impacted people often form intense and sustaining relationships with their physicians, social workers, psychotherapists, friends and family members who they experience as interested in their welfare and willing to help. As one works with and listens to HIV impacted people, it is clear these relationships offer sustaining power well beyond medical care, the assessment for and provision of concrete services, helping hands, or shoulders to lean and often cry on. Yet the HIV-related clinical literature rarely addresses the meaning of these relationships, why they are so sustaining, and why their disruption or loss is often felt so acutely.

As will be further discussed in Chapter 14, we as human beings, from birth onwards, strive to organize or give meaning to our experiences. Other human beings, beginning with our parents and/or primary caretakers, and relationships we encounter continuing on through life, serve crucial roles in the ongoing process of understanding and integrating our experiences. When a person is impacted by HIV, his experience of himself and consequently the world is often radically altered. Varying degrees of confusion, anxiety, sadness and panic are often encountered as the individual attempts to make sense of the possibility of severe illness and death, when he is accustomed to the bedrock assumption that life is ongoing and evolving. Just as HIV and the threat of death disrupt the individual's experience of himself and often threaten to rob life of its meaning, relationships serve to help restore meaning to life. They serve crucial roles in helping the impacted individual negotiate his experience of HIV infection, or in the case of surviving partners, help them to integrate the meaning of their tragic loss.

One of the benefits of the methodology used in this study is that it enables a multidimensional view of the particular phenomenon being explored. Consequently, the results of the study are at once a historical account of the experiences of partnered gay men in the face of AIDS; a documentation of the validity and sustaining power of gay relationships; a clinical study of the impact of AIDS on the dialogue of established relationships, and the mourning process in particular; and a study of the well partner's experience of terminal illness, death, and mourning in general. This book is intended to be read by both clinicians and partners who have been impacted by

AIDS or people attempting to understand the experience of their son, brother or friend.

As the results of the study were written, drafts were given to participants to review to help ensure that I had accurately reconstructed their experience. Many of the men found that reading the drafts was a profoundly moving and helpful encounter. A frequent response was, "this is my life." Several men reported that they became absorbed in the document, reliving their own particular experience as they read, their own memories and feelings being evoked and intermingled with the accounts of others who had experienced the illness and deaths of their partners. Some men had questions answered and laid to rest. In general, the response was that it was a healing encounter, one that served to organize, to help them understand the enormity of their experience as a well and surviving partner.

I hope men who are facing the illness and/or death of their partner will read this book and find it helpful. This chapter and Chapters 4 through 14 will probably be the most meaningful for nonclinicians in that they address the experience itself, rather than the theoretical perspectives and implications of the experience. Negotiating life as a gay man in our society is difficult enough and often dramatically impacts on the experience of self. AIDS has added a great burden to your life. Hopefully, reading the accounts of others who have also encountered AIDS in the context of an ongoing relationship will serve to lessen the burden by validating and giving meaning to your loss and efforts to heal the pain of your loss.

For students and clinicians, this book offers a general frame of reference for which to view the particular experience of your clients or patients. Unlike a case study approach which essentially presents a series of accounts, this methodology breaks the experience down into its components and more importantly the relationships between the components of the larger experience. In so doing, the affective enormity of the experience is conveyed, but also conveyed are implications for understanding and intervening with clients who may be experiencing difficulty as they face AIDS as a couple, or mourn the loss of a partner. One of the strong points of this approach to clinical research is that it mirrors human experience and consequently the clinical encounter. As clinicians, we are attempting to organize into a meaningful whole various communications from our clients, be they an association, an account of a recent experience, a memory, dream, facial expression or our own empathic resonance. Invariably our understanding in the therapeutic relationship arises from the relationships of various forms of communication.

Just as biomedical research with HIV has resulted in considerable advances in the area of virology and immunology in general, the clinical study of the experience of HIV and AIDS offers the potential for advances in the behavioral sciences. The results of this study indicated phenomenon not previously addressed in the psychoanalytic literature on mourning, i.e., the central role other people play in the mourning process. Advances in psychoanalytic theory, specifically the psychology of the self, and the integration of linguistic and cognitive theories into clinical theory, coupled with the results of this study, enabled the beginning reformulation of mourning theory presented in Chapter 14. After some deliberation, I decided not to alter the literature review presented in Chapter 2 as it represents what was available at the time of the formulation, research and write-up of the study. The central literature presented in Chapter 14 became available only months before the manuscript was submitted and became the final theoretical framework for viewing the study as well as the basis for the reformulation of mourning theory. I realize that only the basic themes of current literature are presented. Clinicians who are not familiar with these theorists may want to read the referenced works in their entirety.

Chapter 15 addresses clinical work with AIDS and HIV impacted individuals in general, and with seropositive surviving partners and seropositive men whose efforts at managing the impact of infection were disrupted by the loss of a central relationship(s). As the epidemic progresses, prior loss and losses to AIDS will most likely influence the experience of the HIV impacted clients that come to us for treatment. In a 1985 study, Martin (1988) found that 27% of his sample of gay men had experienced the death of a lover or close friend to AIDS, one third of whom had experienced multiple losses. Further data analysis indicated that direct correlations were found between the number of losses and symptoms of traumatic stress response, sleep problems, sedative use and the use of psychological services because of AIDS-related concerns.

As the epidemic continues, it is reasonable to assume that the percentages of men who have lost relationships to AIDS is even higher. As medical intervention continues to prolong the lives of AIDS patients and slow the progression of HIV infection in its earlier stages, and testing for HIV antibodies becomes more encouraged if not commonplace, we must become increasingly familiar with the long-term psychological impact of HIV infection. Martin's (1988) quantitative approach to the impact of loss on psychological functioning indicates that there is a population of gay men at risk for considerable mental health problems. This qualitative approach attempts to account for the meaning of the loss of a relationship and to provide a framework for clinical intervention.

The psychological impact of AIDS and HIV infection spreads well beyond the infected individuals. We all live in a matrix of love, family, friend and collegial relationships. Hence the loss or illness of one person will be experienced differently and with varying impact by a wide range of people. As clinicians we are potentially faced with a variety of clients who have lost relationships to AIDS. While this book focuses on the surviving partner and to a lessor degree seropositive men who have experienced a loss due to AIDS, it also has implications for work with others who have lost relationships through death. Hopefully this work will prove to be a valuable tool for clinically understanding this painful aspect of not only AIDS, but the experience of being human.

Chapter II

Literature Review

The experience of a partner contracting Acquired Immune Deficiency Syndrome — wondering if the partner is contracting AIDS, the formal diagnosis, caring for the partner during his illness, the death of the partner, and the mourning process — occurs over a several year period and encompasses a broad range of clinical phenomena. Relevant literature includes: clinical literature on AIDS as it pertains to the diagnosed individual and the partner, clinical literature on anticipatory mourning and grief, clinical literature on mourning and grief in general, and the existing clinical literature on mourning as it pertains to gay men and lesbian women. The results of the study will be discussed in the theoretical framework of self psychology. Hence, an outline of relevant concepts from the theory, namely, the self, the selfobject functions, and narcissistic injury, will be presented.

CLINICAL LITERATURE
ON ACQUIRED IMMUNE DEFICIENCY SYNDROME

A small but growing body of clinical literature on AIDS has developed over the past few years. The representative works address psychodynamic and psychosocial aspects of being afflicted with AIDS, or being in an established relationship with someone who has contracted AIDS. Earlier works make only fleeting references to the problems encountered by partners or the effects of AIDS on established relationships. While references to the impact of AIDS on relationships and the particular needs of the well or surviving partner are beginning to appear in the literature, to date no major work focusing on the partner or established relationships has been published.

Examples of papers focusing on clinical descriptions of the emotional impact of AIDS and potential treatment interventions include papers by Dilley (1984), Barbutto (1984), and Nichols (1983, 1984, 1986).

Nichols' (1986) is a thorough work that includes behavioral and psychodynamic descriptions of persons with AIDS, a model for assessment, a discussion of transference and countertransference issues, the role of psychotherapy, treatment of people experiencing anxiety related to the threat of AIDS, and a discussion of bereavement. The paper includes this four-stage model describing the emotional reactions as the person with AIDS experiences and hopefully adapts to the illness:

The Initial Crisis; characterized by a crisis state, emotional numbness, at times periods of nonchalance with cognitive and affective denial alternating with periods of overwhelming anxiety.

Early Adjustment; a transitional stage that is turbulent secondary to intense anxiety, anger, guilt, self-pity, and emotional lability that often is seen throughout the illness.

Stage of Acceptance; individuals who are able to reach this stage achieve a new sense of equilibrium, find meaning in their lives, have shifted their focus from dying to living, accepting their lives, not their illness.

Preparation for Death; often characterized by the patient's innate knowledge, acceptance of, and preparation for their approaching death. (Nichols adds that this stage is often marked by a quiet withdrawal from important relationships and the need for significant people to appreciate and tolerate the retreat.)

While this model reflects the experience of the person with AIDS, anyone in an intimate, ongoing relationship with the individual, such as a partner, will surely be affected by the fluctuations in the emotional state of the individual as he struggles to accept the diagnosis. A particularly poignant account of this is in Ferrara (1984, p. 1285)

> . . . Wanting to protect him not only from the possibilities of contracting the disease himself, but also the difficulties I knew were ahead of me, I asked him to leave me. He refused, reminding me that we were in this together . . . Michael cried, I guess, for about six weeks . . . eventually we were able to cry together.

Nichols' discussion of bereavement is very broad and includes friends, families and spouses. But his discussion of bereavement as it pertains to spouses tends to be so vague that it is difficult to discern that he is indeed addressing mourning as it pertains to the surviving partner of a relationship between two gay men. The same problem occurs in Nichols' (1983) paper, in which he addresses clinical work with people directly affected by the illness or loss of an individual due to AIDS—friends and families—but he does not specifically discuss the surviving partner.

Two papers on AIDS representing psychosocial descriptions of the effects of the disease are those by Siegel (1986) and Christ et al. (1986). Noticeably lacking in each paper is an adequate discussion of the impact on the well partner and the impact on the relationship. Siegel's 1986 work is a broad outline of the "social issues" involved for people diagnosed with AIDS. Her only reference to the partners of individuals with AIDS is that "the lovers and gay friends of some PWAs (People With AIDS) have dissolved relationships when the diagnosis is made" (Siegel 1986, p. 171). Christ et al., in their 1986 paper "Psychosocial Issues in AIDS," similarly neglect the well or surviving partner. In a section entitled "Special Problems of Patients and Families," the authors point out that of the patients in their pilot study (data from these patients formed the basis of the paper), "almost three quarters lived alone." The authors do not account for the living arrangements of the other patients. The authors go on to state: "in many cases the families of AIDS patients are in need of supportive care." One could initially assume that "families" includes the partner when AIDS patients are coupled. However, the authors make a clear distinction between "family" and "partner" when they state " . . . the family may get into conflict with the patient's lover or friends because they are perceived as having more control in vital treatment decisions. Finally, the family must cope with the patient's death and the many unresolved emotional and social issues" (Christ et al. 1986, p. 176). Why the authors failed to address the needs of the partners of their AIDS patients is unclear. What is clear is that, for the authors, "lovers" or partners are a foreign entity in relation to their concept of "family."

Morin and Batchelor (1984, p. 6) discuss the psychological aspects of AIDS using accounts of personal experiences as a guide. Their discussion of the impact on partners includes personal accounts by a surviving partner describing the day his partner died, and by an individual diagnosed with AIDS describing his and his partner's struggle to reconcile themselves to the diagnosis. In sharp contrast to the previously reviewed literature, the authors state:

> The mental health aspects of the AIDS crisis affects not only those with AIDS, but the people in their lives. Lovers (partners), friends and family are all likely to experience significant distress . . . . Because AIDS is a mysterious and stigmatizing illness, the psychosocial issues for significant others may be more complicated than those for other life threatening illnesses . . . . Unfortunately, lovers (partners) of people with AIDS have more reasons for developing emotional problems than concerns over their own health: they are almost certain to face self righteousness, fear and legal impediments as they help their lover (partner) through the last months or years of his life. These are psychological demands that pile atop existing grief and health worries, and they suggest the need for mental health and support services.

Further evidence of the impact of AIDS on existing relationships is seen in the authors' observation that in 1983 the Shanti Project in San Francisco provided individual counseling to twice as many friends, families and partners as they did to people who actually had AIDS. The authors describe this aspect of the AIDS crisis:

> Thus, each new case of AIDS has a ripple effect, increasing the need for mental health services. To our knowledge, no data have yet been gathered about the impact of AIDS on the demand for mental health services in either the public or private sectors, but it is clear that mental health services that are AIDS related are needed in cities that have a large number of people with AIDS. (Morin and Batchelor 1984, p. 8)

Working With AIDS (Helquist 1987) contains two brief presentations that address existing relationships and surviving partners. Helquist (1987) identifies the need for partners to achieve a balance between dependence and independence when one or both partners has contracted AIDS; the need to enlist friends to help care for the ill partner; and the role of denial, both as a potential problem and as an aid, to the couple's adjustment. Shearer and McKusick (1987) focus their discussion on survivors, addressing the needs of both family and partners.

Their discussion of surviving partners is based on clinical work with six such men. The authors identify several characteristics of surviving partners: (1) the fear of contracting AIDS that was suspended during the period of caring for the partner resurfaces in an often intense manner, often accompanied by anxiety attacks; (2) a sense of stigmatization; (3) guilt over possibly having transmitted the disease to the now dead partner; (4) men who were able to deny a causal link between their partner's death and their own susceptibility adapted more quickly than those who anticipated the same fate; (5) men who were responsible for the day to day care of their partners had a more difficult time following the death, particularly if there were conflicts with the family during the period of illness; (6) a rigid idealization of the dead partner may occur precluding the establishment of new relationships, while (they experience) an intense longing for the closeness and support that they gave their dying partners; (7) and the need to regain the autonomy suspended in order to care for their partner during his illness.

A frequent and often devastating manifestation of the disease process is AIDS dementia. Buckingham and Van Gorp (1988, p. 114) estimate that "more than half of the persons diagnosed with AIDS at some time will present with central nervous system dysfunction resulting from the HIV virus infiltration of brain structures." Symptoms of AIDS dementia include: difficulty concentrating, impaired recent memory, slowing of mentation and movement, visual spatial impairment, and affective disturbance (depression). The onset is often insidious, progressing slowly, but may also rapidly progress into severe impairment. Regarding the caretakers of such impaired individuals, the authors point out that the partners and families are "invisible patients who may need a great deal of support and attention as their level of responsibility in caring for their loved one increases. The coexistence of AIDS and dementia creates a substantial need for sustained physical, emotional and financial assistance."

Based on a community sample of 745 gay men in New York City conducted in 1985, Martin (1988) found that bereavement (the loss of a lover or close friend to AIDS) was experienced by 27% of the sample, one third of whom had experienced multiple losses. A direct relation was found between the number of bereavements and symptoms of traumatic stress response, demoralization, sleep problems, sedative use and the use of psychological services because of AIDS-related concerns. Geis et al. (1986) in a rather cursory study of nine surviving partners concluded that: ". . . the lovers of AIDS victims constitute a population at risk." In their sample the authors found: stress responses, feelings of stigmatization, frustration in negotiating the medical community, and a sense of painful isolation secondary to the ambivalent responses of biological families (pp. 43-53).

The preceding literature review indicates that clinical attention to the needs and experiences of the well or surviving partner has been inconsistent. The data specifically regarding partners and extrapolations from the difficulties faced by the person with AIDS indicates that the experience of the partner is rich, highly evocative, and has its own characteristics, problems and pitfalls. Still lacking is a thorough accounting of the partners' experience throughout the course of the disease and the process of mourning following the death of the ill partner.

ANTICIPATORY MOURNING AND GRIEF

The unique aspects of AIDS aside, several authors have addressed the impact of caring for a chronically or terminally ill spouse or family member. Studies by Zarit et al. (1980) and Rabins et al. (1982) indicate that family members of adults with dementing illness commonly experience symptoms of depression, anxiety, fatigue, and depletion as well as feelings of helplessness and hopelessness. In addition to the strain of caring for a chronically or terminally ill relative, additional elements in the experience are anticipatory mourning and anticipatory grief.

Lebow (1976) defines anticipatory mourning as " the total set of cognitive, affective, cultural, and social reactions to expected death felt by the patient and the family." Lebow distinguishes anticipatory mourning from anticipatory grief in that anticipatory grief refers to the affective components of the experience, whereas anticipatory mourning refers to the process. In describing the central aspects of anticipatory grief Lebow states: "the element of uncertainty is an inherent factor, grief increases over time, and is time limited because it ends with the death of the patient" (p. 459). Aldrich (1974) defines anticipatory grief as "any grief occurring prior to a loss as distinguished from grief which occurs after or at the time of the loss" (p. 4). Aldrich further distinguishes anticipatory grief as being " . . . experienced (or denied) simultaneously by both the patient and his family, while conventional grief is experienced only by the survivors" (p. 4).

Lebow (1976) identifies several elements in the experience of anticipatory mourning: a series of emotional struggles to accept the death; grieving the day-to-day sufferings; changes and physical separations; the mutual denial between patient and family that may create a distance in the relationships; giving up plans and dreams for the future that included the patient; apprehension about uncertainties of the illness; unpredictability of the course of physical deterioration of the patient; anxiety inherent in the adjustment of roles; and the stress of making treatment and care decisions (p. 459). Barton (1977, p. 59) identifies the adaptive tasks required of families during the dying process:

While providing care for the dying person and being immersed
in the context of death, the family must continue to meet its
member's needs, function as a unit in society and provide a
structure for the growth and development of its members. The
family must adapt to the many changes resulting from the
dying person's illness, maintain its identity and begin to provide for the adaptation to the ultimate loss of the person by
reorganizing to continue its function after the member's death
. . . . All of these activities are accomplished against a background of pervasive sense of loss and transition which in itself
is stressful and disruptive to the integrity of the family's structure and function.

Clearly the process of anticipatory mourning is highly complicated, involving adjustment to considerable changes in relationships and the very organization of daily life as the death of the
family member approaches. The choice of the term "anticipatory
grief" implies that the central dynamic is the threatened loss of the
spouse or family member. As the authors describe the phenomenon,
one could assume that for well partners there will be a co-mingling
of affects associated with mourning the actual day to day losses and
the strain of caring for a terminally ill spouse or partner, with the
affects accompanying the anticipated loss of the partner, and the
survivor's possible potential infection with the HIV virus.

MOURNING

The clinical literature on mourning, or the series of experiential,
intrapsychic, and behavioral reactions of individuals in response to
the loss through death of a significant relationship has evolved considerably since the publication of Freud's "On Mourning and Melancholia" (1917). While that work is often cited as the paper in
which subsequent theorizing on the intrapsychic nature of mourning
has evolved, a more basic statement of the nature of mourning was
established in Freud's 1912-1913 work *Totem and Taboo*:

. . . Mourning has a quite specific psychical task to perform: its function is to detach the survivor's memories and hopes from the dead. When this has been achieved the pain grows less, and with it the remorse and self-reproach. (p. 843)

With this statement, Freud set the framework for conceptualizing mourning, regardless of theoretical framework, that has continued to this day. The two interrelated and enduring elements are: (1) mourning concerns two central figures, the mourner and the deceased (more specifically, the memories, hopes and affects – essentially, the meaning system connected to the deceased) and (2) mourning is a process that (in an undistorted form) consists of a movement of the memories, hopes, etc., from a central, painful, if not overwhelming aspect of the survivor's life to a less central, less affectively charged position.

Bowlby (1961, 1980) states that from the publication of "On Mourning and Melancholia" until the 1960s, the few psychoanalytic authors who discussed the phenomenon of mourning did so within Freud's original proposition – that much psychiatric illness is an expression of pathological mourning – rather than discuss mourning per se. In keeping with the psychoanalytic tradition of viewing adult psychopathology as being the result of childhood experience (and a tendency to generate broad theory based on experience with a few people, usually patients in treatment), writers such as Jacobsen (1943, 46), (as quoted in Bowlby, 1980) discussed adult depression in terms of the child's reactions to a separation from its mother. Klein, (1935, 1940) (as quoted in Bowlby, 1980) discussed mourning in children more directly in terms of their "pining for the lost object" and emphasizing the first year of life and the centrality of the feeding and weaning process as being a critical time in the development of adult pathology. Bowlby (1980) asserts that what authors such as Jacobsen were really talking about was childhood grief and mourning, though they did not label it as such. The one exception to the lack of direct attention to the mourning process of adults is Lindeman (1965) who studied 101 people including: psychoneurotic patients who lost a relative during the course of treatment, the bereaved relatives of patients who died in the hospital, bereaved disaster victims (of the Coconut Grove fire in

Boston) and their close relatives, and relatives of members of the armed forces (p. 7-8). Lindeman's goal in his study of acute grief was to gather data on "symptoms reported and of the changes in mental status observed progressively through a series of interviews." Lindeman subsequently developed a descriptive account of the behavior associated with acute grief: (1) somatic distress, (2) preoccupation with the image of the deceased, (3) guilt, (4) hostile reactions, and (5) loss of patterns of conduct.

In the early 1960s, mourning in adults as a process in its own right began to be addressed within the context of both intrapsychic and descriptive paradigms. Examples of intrapsychic approaches are Pollock (1961), who discusses the process of mourning in the context of an ego-analytic framework; and Palombo (1981, 1982), who discusses the topic within a self psychology framework. Descriptive approaches are represented by Parkes and Bowlby.

Descriptive approaches to the phenomenon have utilized interviews with surviving spouses, and then organized the data into behavioral and experiential stages of the mourning process. Examples of this approach are Parkes (1972) and an aspect of Bowlby (1980). Though descriptive and intrapsychic approaches utilize different paradigms, each provides us with useful frameworks for understanding the various aspects of the experience of mourning. Two of the previously cited authors, Bowlby (1980) and Pollock (1961), incorporated both descriptive paradigms of behavioral and experiential stages in the process and intrapsychic paradigms.

Descriptive approaches to mourning have utilized interviews of surviving marital partners, and organized the data into behavioral and experiential stages of the mourning process and are represented by the works of Parkes (1972) and Bowlby (1980). Parkes (1972) interviewed 22 widows at 1, 3, 6, 9, and 12 1/2 month intervals following the deaths of their husbands. Based on the data gleaned from the interviews, he conceptualized the process of mourning as consisting of five experiential phases: alarm, searching, mitigation, anger and guilt, and gaining a new identity. Bowlby (1980), in reviewing nine studies of surviving marital partners that also utilized interviews and/or questionnaires over time since the partners' deaths (including Parkes 1972), conceptualized the mourning process as consisting of four stages:

1. Phase of numbing that usually lasts from a few hours to a week, and may be interrupted by outbursts of extremely intense distress and/or anger.
2. Phase of yearning and searching for the lost figure, lasting some months and sometimes for years.
3. Phase of disorganization and despair.
4. Phase of greater or less degree of reorganization. (Bowlby 1980, p. 85)

In reference to intrapsychic approaches, Bowlby (1980) points out:

> . . . authors regardless of theoretical framework agree that the process of healthy mourning involves to varying degrees the withdrawal of investment in the lost person and that (it) may prepare the way for making a relationship with a new one. How we conceive of their making this change, however, depends on how we conceptualize affectional bonds. (p. 25)

In this context, Pollock (1961) discusses mourning using the language of ego-psychology, hence his conception of affectional bonds is described in terms of self representations, object representations, and the decathexis of the object representation. For Pollock, mourning consists of the decathexis of the object representation of the deceased individual, and the gradual incorporation into the psyche of the reality of the death and subsequent irrevocable loss; essentially, a realignment and modification of the self representation of the surviving individual and the object representation of the deceased individual. The ability of the individual in mourning to recall memories of the deceased, and acknowledge the accompanying pain, is an integral aspect of the process. Eventually the object representation is modified into sets of memories. The hallmark of ego-analytic thought on the mourning process is the assertion that the ability to work through ambivalent feelings towards the deceased is crucial for the transformation of the object representation into a set of memories and the subsequent availability of energy to invest in new attachments. Though not explicitly stated, inherent in this model is the position that to adequately mourn, the individual must have reached the oedipal level of development and consequent intrapsychic structure. This effectively precludes the use of this theory in understanding mourning as it pertains to gay men as in psychoanalytic theory; homosexual men have not achieved the Oedipal stage of development (Lewes 1988), hence, are (theoretically) unable to successfully mourn the loss of their partner.

Palombo (1981, 1982) discusses mourning using a self psychology paradigm. In this framework, the central aspect is the loss of the selfobject functions that were provided by the deceased. Palombo (1981) states: "Mourning is not simply the work associated with the detachment from and dissolution of the object representation, it must also include those reactions associated with the loss as a loss of a selfobject which brings about an imbalance in self-esteem" (p. 12). For Palombo, the intensity of, and particular response to, the death is dependent on the particular selfobject functions and the degree to which the surviving partner relied upon them to maintain a narcissistic equilibrium. Hence, in the self psychology model, the selfobject functions, as well as the attachment to the object, are integral aspects of the phenomenon of mourning. Grief is the psychic pain the individual experiences due to the loss of the selfobject functions, while an integral aspect of mourning is the restoration of the resulting disequilibrium brought about by the loss.

An extension of the framework proposed by Palombo is the role played by individuals with whom the mourner has an established relationship. Shane and Shane (1990) discuss the role of the selfobject matrix necessary for mourning. The authors assert that for mourning to take place, the remaining significant people in the mourner's life must validate the depth of the loss and sustain the mourner through the experience of his or her pain. Though the authors discuss this in relation to childhood and adolescent mourning, one can assume parallels to adulthood experiences of the loss of significant relationships.

CENTRAL CONCEPTS OF SELF PSYCHOLOGY

Both intrapsychic and descriptive approaches to mourning provide useful frameworks for understanding the phenomenon. The self psychology model will be employed in that it: (1) provides a framework from which the entire experience under study can be viewed — namely the loss and alteration of selfobject functions, and (2) it does not by default place the subjects of the study in a less capable, if not pathological, position.

In self psychology, the concept of the self, its development and functioning is the central aspect of the theory. Kohut (1977) defined the self as "the center of the individual's psychological universe." Baker and Baker (1987) add:

> It is what "I" refers to when we say: "I feel such and such and I do so and so." We may describe the nature of what the self experiences and the actions that the self undertakes as a consequence of those experiences. (p. 5)

The self is also the embodiment of self esteem or "normal narcissism" and develops through interactions with selfobjects. Kohut and Wolfe (1978) state:

> Depending on the quality of the interactions between the self and its selfobjects in childhood, the self will emerge either as a firm and healthy structure or as a more or less seriously damaged one. The adult self may thus exist in states of varying degrees of coherence, from cohesion to fragmentation; in states of varying degrees of vitality from vigor to enfeeblement; in states of varying degrees of functional harmony from order to chaos. (p. 3)

The self evolves in the direction of an entity that is able to internally regulate self esteem, calm and soothe the self and set appropriate but challenging goals. Kohut maintained that the child is born with a relatively cohesive if archaic sense of self. Eventually, through interaction with selfobjects, the self matures into a tripolar structure.

Selfobject functions are psychological functions, with which people are not born, but which are experienced as a part of, or within the self, aspects of which are eventually internalized into the matrix of the self as structures. These structures within the self represent enduring functions that accrue to the self as a result of the internalizations of experiences with significant others. The awareness of these functions is generally absent, except when not present,

at which point the experience of the absence is felt as an injury to
the self (Palombo 1989). In an attempt to further define selfobject
functions, Stolorow et al. (1987) state, "Selfobject functions pertain fundamentally to the integration of affect into the evolving organization of self experience" (p. 86).

The three central selfobject needs of the archaic self which eventually develop into the three poles are: idealizing, which forms the
idealized parental imago; mirroring, which forms the grandiose
self; and twinship/alter ego, which enhances the actualization of the
pole of talents and skills. Baker and Baker (1987) elaborate on the
selfobject functions:

> *Idealizing* . . . our need to merge with, or be close to, someone
> who we believe will make us safe, comfortable and calm
> . . . An external object serves an internal function – calming
> and comforting and so functions as a selfobject for the child.
> . . . Initially there is a wish to merge with the idealized paren-
> tal imago; then there is the wish to be very near a source of
> such power; eventually the mature person is satisfied knowing
> that friends and family are available during times of distress.
> (p. 4)
>
> *Mirroring* . . .The delighted response of the parents to the
> child – the gleam in the mother's eye – is essential to the
> child's development. This response mirrors back to the child a
> sense of self worth and value, creating internal self respect.
> . . .In the context of a generally responsive environment, the
> intensity of the grandiose self is diminished, but not destroyed.
> (p. 3)
>
> *Twinship/alter ego* . . . the need to feel a degree of alikeness
> with other people. The small boy may stand by his father when
> he shaves, The son also "shaves" using a bladeless razor.
> These sort of experiences lead to a feeling of being like others,
> of being a part of and connected to the human community
> . . . . (pp. 4,5)

Through a combination of empathic meeting of selfobject needs,
optimum frustrations of needs, and the transmuting internalization
of the selfobject functions of caretakers, the child's self acquires

permanent structures that regulate self-esteem, tension, and the ability to pursue goals consistent with skills and talents (Freinhar, 1987).

Self psychology holds that psychopathology in adulthood is ultimately derived from deficits in the overall structure of the self or from distortions of the self (Muslin 1985). As stated earlier, adult selves exist in varying degrees of coherence, vitality, and harmony. Consequently, selves vary in their degree of vulnerability to narcissistic injury or the loss or failure in a self-selfobject relationship and the consequent fragmentation of the self that occurs. Fragmentation is the experience of the breakdown of the self. Fragmentation states can be either ubiquitous, of minor degree and short duration, or chronic, protracted and intense.

Regarding minor fragmentation experiences, Kohut and Wolfe (1978) state:

> Occasionally occurring fragmentation states of minor degree and short duration are ubiquitous. They occur in all of us when our self-esteem has been taxed for prolonged periods and when no replenishing sustenance has presented itself. We all may walk home after a day in which we suffered a series of self-esteem-shaking failures, feeling at sixes and sevens with ourselves. Our gait and posture will be clumsy, and even our mental functions will show signs of discoordination. (p. 13)

In sharp contrast, a more severe and intense fragmentation state is described as:

> . . . ushered in by a massive loss of self-esteem, followed immediately by the advent of the global anxiety referred to as disintegration anxiety (the terrifying fear of the loss of humanness). Directly after the advent of disintegration anxiety, the self is experienced as losing its cohesiveness, with the usual experience of splitting or fragmentation of the self functions and self perception, including reality testing, memory, and orientation in space and time. There is also the loss of the intact experience of self observing; the various experiences of the different organs previously coalesced together in the intact experience of the total bodyself are now experienced as sepa-

rate and become the focus for enhanced attention and even
preoccupation (hypochondria). In addition the patient is in
the throes of a separation reaction, with its attendant features
of loss of vigor, esteem and meaning in life. (Muslin 1985,
pp. 211-212)

Selfobject failures (the absence, withdrawal or alteration of
selfobject functions) or events that distress the self and result in
varying degrees of fragmentation are referred to as narcissistic injuries. As indicated above, the self may respond to perceived or
actual threats with a wide spectrum of experiences ranging from
"such trivial occurrences as a fleeting annoyance when someone
fails to reciprocate our greeting or respond to our joke to such ominous derangements as the furor of the catatonic and the grudges of
the paranoiac" (Kohut 1972, p. 379). Narcissisticly vulnerable
selves respond with the more intense manifestations of actual or
anticipated narcissistic injury with either "shamefaced withdrawal
(flight) or with narcissistic rage (fight)" (Kohut 1972, p. 379).
Hence, the self may become acutely enraged or acutely depleted.
   Muslin (1985) states:

. . . episodic fragmentations or near fragmentations or simple
instances of loss of self-esteem or threatened loss of worth are
part of one's modal reactions to a complex world of victories,
near misses and failures. In a more or less cohesive self the
repair in most instances will be effected by a mature self-
selfobject encounter. In those instances where the demands for
cohesion are intense, the previously cohesive self will frag-
ment, albeit temporarily and seek out an archaic self-selfobject
encounter in which a merger will be effected. (p. 214)

To illustrate this process, Muslin offers an example highly relevant
to the experience of a partner contracting AIDS:

. . . in the case of a person who has just been informed that his
or her longstanding state of weakness is due to a malignancy in
the colon, the psychological reactions are frequently the self
experience of fragmentation. This distress, one hopes, will be
followed by the self-selfobject merger effected with a trusted

caretaker or relative. In such situations, if empathic caretakers recognize the manifestations of the fragmentation and respond appropriately with a dose of mirroring or allow themselves to become the target for idealization, the fragmentation experiences will be short-lived. (p. 214)

For the purpose of this study, the conceptualization of human bonds, or the relationship between the well and ill partner, will be that proposed by Stolorow et al. (1987). That is, it will be viewed as a multidimensional, complex object relationship. In this framework, the term selfobject, ". . . refer[s] to a class of psychological functions, a dimension of experiencing an object." Though proposed for the psychoanalytic setting, the authors conceptualization provides a framework with which to view the well partner's experience of his ill partner throughout the course of the larger experience under study.

Our listening perspective becomes thereby focused on the complex *figure-ground relationships* among the selfobject and other dimensions of experiencing another person. . . . We are suggesting that a multiplicity of such dimensions coexist in any complex object relationship, with certain meanings and functions occupying the experiential foreground, and others occupying the background, depending on the subject's motivational priorities at any given moment. Furthermore, the figure-ground relationships among these multiple dimensions of experience may significantly shift, corresponding to shifts in the subject's psychological organization and motivational hierarchy, often in response to alterations or disturbances in the tie to the object. (Stolorow et al. 1987, pp. 25-26)

MOURNING IN THE CONTEXT OF GAY AND LESBIAN RELATIONSHIPS

The clinical literature on grief and mourning as it pertains to gay men and lesbian women is sparse. A thorough search resulted in one paper devoted to the topic, the use of a case treatment/history to illustrate a concept in another paper, and a work from the popular media. As the publication dates indicate, all were written before AIDS began to profoundly impact the lives of gay men.

Though not a clinical work, *The Mendola Report* (Mendola 1980) uses transcribed interviews with gay and lesbian couples who describe their experiences in homosexual relationships. In a chapter addressing the surviving member's experience of the death of a partner, the author provides several interviews with surviving partners of long-term relationships. The interviews illustrate the marked similarities with heterosexual individuals following the death of a spouse, but also the potential problems posed by the lack of social and legal sanction despite the longevity of the relationship.

Siegal and Hoeffer (1981) represents the one contribution to the literature specifically addressing mourning and bereavement as it pertains to gay individuals. The authors discuss stages in the grieving process and the stigma attached to individuals who have lost spouses [as identified by Parkes (1972)]. The authors also discuss the potential problems posed by the "lack of societal mechanisms, sanctions and resources to aid the bereavement process of gay individuals." In a statement that recalls the previously discussed inadequate representation of the surviving partner of AIDS-related fatalities, the authors assert: "the social environment may not be supportive of persons engaging in same sex relationships and ignores gay people when a death occurs" (Siegal and Hoeffer 1981, p. 523). The crux of the paper is that the social ostracism and consequent need of many gay people to conceal their sexual identity and the central role the relationship played in their life, may serve to intensify the isolation and depression experienced by surviving members of relationships. In addition, the lack of social sanction and support may serve to deprive surviving partners of important roles in rituals designed to comfort and acknowledge the depth of the loss.

In a paper, "The Use of Diagnostic Concepts in Working With Gay and Lesbian Populations," Gonsiorek (1982) discusses the case of a severely depressed older lesbian woman. The patient and her partner of many years lived in a rural area, isolated from other people as well as other lesbians. The author identified the isolation and lack of acknowledgment of the patient's loss as integral factors in her depression, and asserted that validating the depth of her loss and subsequent disruption were integral aspects of a successful treatment outcome.

SUMMARY

This literature review provides several contexts in which to view the well and surviving partner's experience. The clinical literature on AIDS indicates the potential stressors placed upon the well partner: concern for his own health, negotiating medical personnel, negotiating potentially ambivalent, if not hostile, families, caring for his ill partner, and potentially experiencing stigmatization due to the considerable anxiety that surrounds the disease. The literature on anticipatory grief and mourning indicates the considerable losses that the significant people caring for a terminally ill family member encounter: the loss of plans and dreams for the future, alteration in roles, the uncertainty of the disease course, the experience of considerable affect secondary to these multiple losses, and anticipated final loss of the relationship. The literature on mourning serves as a reference for the individual intrapsychic experience that follows the death of a loved one. The literature on mourning in the context of lesbian and gay relationships indicates that validation of the centrality of the relationship may be lacking for the surviving partners of homosexual relationships. Also indicated is the potential role that validation plays in fueling the process of mourning. Again, this study covers an experience that encompasses several years of a person's life, and a wide range of clinical phenomena necessitating a wide ranging literature review. However, by focusing on the selfobject functions that each man provides the other, and the alteration and loss of those functions, one can track a potentially account for the private or internal experience of the well and surviving partner.

Chapter III

Methodology

RESEARCH STRATEGY

The question for study, " What are the experiences of gay men whose partners contract Acquired Immune Deficiency Syndrome?" lends itself to the research goals and strategies of Clinical Ethnography. Curtis (1988) defines Clinical Ethnography as:

> . . . the empirical study of psychotherapy or other related clinical areas. (1) Using research methods derived from anthropology and qualitative sociology such as participant observation and key informant interviewing. (2) employing systematic methods of data collection and qualitative data analysis such as the Constant Comparative Method associated with Grounded Theory.

Schwartz and Jacobs (1979, p. 37) state the philosophical base of Qualitative Sociological research as follows:

> A tacit assumption of any and all such methods is that some sort of consensus or common knowledge exists in groups and is sustained over time by social processes.

Schwartz and Jacobs maintain that the goal of sociological research is "to gain access to the member's point of view'" (Schwartz and Jacobs 1979, p. 37) or "gaining access to the life world of other individuals, or reconstructing . . . the reality of a social scene" (Schwartz and Jacobs 1979, p. 4). Once one has devised an appropriate way of gaining access to the "point of view" or experiences of individuals, the task then becomes a ". . . systematic generating of theory from data, that itself is systematically obtained from social research'' (Glaser and Strauss 1967, p. 2).

The principles for obtaining data on the experience of the well and surviving partners of men who contracted Acquired Immune Deficiency Syndrome were participant observation and interviewing. Schwartz and Jacobs (1979, p. 37) describe these two strategies as

> . . . for the most part variants and extensions of the practical methods any intelligent lay person would use to get at the consensual meanings of a group of people with whom he is not familiar.

While interviews are the main source of data, participant observation refers to the particular stance of the researcher during data collection. The underlying assumption of the concept of participant observation is that the researcher cannot help but participate to varying degrees in the reality of the group or member under study, as they are being interviewed and/or observed. Schwartz and Jacobs discuss the problem of maintaining the balance between involvement that allows access to the ''insider's perspective'' while not becoming so involved that the researchers' objectivity is compromised. Schwartz and Jacobs (1979, p. 57) offer several possibilities for the degree of participant observation:

1. The investigator is known to others as a social scientist and confines his activities while among them to gathering information and observing.
2. The social scientist makes his identity known to all from the outset. However he adopts the role of a bona fide member.
3. The researcher conceals his identity but adopts a social role which is naturally defined by the group as someone who gathers information.
4. Unknown to others as a social scientist, the researcher adopts some role such as a factory worker and simply lives the life of that worker.

The stance taken by myself during this study was that of ''The investigator who is known to others as a social scientist and confines his activities while among them to gathering information and observing'' (Schwartz and Jacobs 1979, p. 56). I presented myself to prospective and actual participants as a clinician and researcher interested in what they were experiencing as partners of a man who had contracted or died of AIDS.

Consistent with field study methodology, data were also gleaned (when available) from personal journals and the researcher's case notes. Health care and social service personnel who routinely encounter well and surviving partners were also interviewed. The use of multiple sources of data within a particular field study is a characteristic of qualitative investigation which distinguishes it from experimental investigation. The field method is described as:

> . . . not an exclusive method in the same sense, say, that experimentation is. Field method is more like an umbrella of activity beneath which any technique may be used for gaining the desired information, and for processes of thinking about this information. Though each technique has its own logic, and can be used exclusively, there is no rule which forbids using a mixture of them in field work. (Schatzman and Strauss 1973, p. 14)

Consistent with the goals and strategies of Clinical Ethnography and its roots in Qualitative Sociology, the design of this study was for the researcher, as participant observer, to interview gay men whose partners were currently ill with or who had died from complications of Acquired Immune Deficiency Syndrome, examine their personal journals (when available), interview individuals who routinely encounter well or surviving partners, and incorporate case notes from the psychotherapeutic treatment of well and surviving partners. The obtained data was then used to reconstruct the reality of the experience of men whose partners have contracted AIDS and to generate a theory that accounts for the experience, its thematic progression, and variations.

The combination of the clinical perspective of the researcher, the broad range of data sources, and the specificity that one is able to achieve with the constant comparative method, yielded a rich and detailed accounting of the partner's perspective or experience. Human experience is rich, varied, and comprised of many interrelated components. The theory includes interactions between the "well" and "ill" partner, interactions between the "well" partner and his social and family matrix, and the internal or "private" experience of the well partner.

The theory developed as a result of this study is substantive in nature. That is, it pertains to a specific, substantive area of inquiry: the experiences of gay men whose partners have contracted AIDS. It does not purport to be on the level of formal theory with its degrees of specificity and inclusivity that allow for broad application. Glaser and Strauss distinguish between substantive and formal theories:

> By substantive theory, we mean that developed for a substantive or empirical area of sociological inquiry, such as patient care, race relations, professional education, delinquency, or research organization. By formal theory, we mean that developed for a formal, or conceptual, area of sociological inquiry, such as stigma, deviant behavior, formal organization, socialization, status incongruency, authority and power, reward systems, or social mobility. (1967, p. 33)

Thus, the substantive theory generated by this study pertains to the experience of a partner contracting and dying from AIDS, not the broader experiences of caretaking for a terminally ill spouse and the mourning process following the spouse's death. Clearly, while the results or generated theory have implications for formal theories in the areas of anticipatory grief and mourning, they are only implications. The goal of the study was not to test or elucidate established theory, rather to reconstruct the experience of the well and surviving partner.

SETTING

Interviews with participating partners and professionals were conducted in Chicago, Illinois and San Francisco, California. The interviews and participant review of drafts occurred between September, 1987 and March, 1989. The majority of participants resided in the metropolitan areas of these two cities. One participant resided in Boston, another in rural Minnesota. The actual interviews were conducted in a variety of settings: the researcher's private office, his home or the homes of participating partners. In the case of the Minnesota participant, the interview was conducted by phone. Interviews with professionals were conducted at their work stations or at pre-arranged locations.

CHARACTERISTICS OF PARTICIPATING PARTNERS

A total of 32 men participated in the study. Each defined himself as either: a gay man who is the partner of a gay man with AIDS; a gay man with AIDS who was partnered to one of the other men participating in the study; or the surviving partner of a relationship with another man who died of AIDS. At the time they entered the study, 11 men were surviving partners—their partners having died of AIDS two weeks to three years prior to the first interview, nine men had partners who were ill with AIDS, and 12 men were the ill partners of men in the study. (Couples where both men were ill were counted as ill partners.) During the course of the study, three ill partners died. Consequently, three men made the transition to surviving partner. The men in the study considered themselves partnered from 2 to 13 years prior to the diagnosis. The majority of the relationships were from 4 to 7 years in duration. Ages of the men in the study ranged from 23 to 52 years. The majority of participants were in their thirties.

Professionals who routinely encounter gay men with AIDS and their partners were also interviewed. These participants consisted of physicians, nurses, social workers and support group leaders. Professional participants worked in the Chicago and San Francisco metropolitan areas. Interview data from professionals was used primarily to compare with my observations of participating partners, and to develop questions regarding areas of experience for investigation.

RECRUITMENT OF PARTICIPANTS

Participants were recruited through a variety of means. Chicago participants responded to an article on the study in *OUTLINES* (Burks 1987), one of the gay community newspapers; were advised of the study by one of two private physicians; or were advised of the study by the leaders of support groups for partners at the Howard Brown Memorial Clinic (an agency providing AIDS support services). Several participants recruited friends for the study. The San Francisco participants were recruited from the practice of a physician and a contact in the nursing profession. The Boston participant read about the study while visiting Chicago. The Minnesota participant learned of the study via a friend who returned to that state with a copy of the newspaper article.

DATA COLLECTION METHODS AND INSTRUMENTS

Interviews with participants were tape recorded. To ensure accuracy, quotes for data analysis were taken directly from the recorded interview. Data gleaned from personal journals was taken directly from the text. Data from the researcher's private practice was taken from case notes written following the session. The interviews were semi-structured. The basic questions for the interviews were, "What has been your experience as the partner of a person with AIDS, or a person who has died from AIDS?" Additional questions and subsequent interviews were recursive (Schwartz and Jacobs 1979), that is, further questioning was derived from the content and questions of previous interviews. Data obtained from the observations and experiences of professional/volunteer individuals who encounter the partners of men with AIDS also served as a source for interview questions.

Participants were asked to contract for three interviews. The majority of participants remained in the study for the three interview span. In order to capture transitions and progression in the experience, the majority of interviews occurred over a six to eight month period, with several men being followed for well over one year. During the course of the study three men withdrew and or moved, which prevented further contact. When the participant was the partner of a man currently ill with AIDS, at least one conjoint interview was attempted. Several couples in the study chose to be interviewed conjointly throughout the process of data collection.

DATA ANALYSIS

Data was collected, organized, and analyzed according to the methodology for qualitative social research "Grounded Theory" detailed in Glaser and Strauss (1967) and Glaser (1978). The goal of this methodology is to construct theory that is grounded in observed data. In accordance with the Grounded Theory method, data collection, organization and analysis occurred simultaneously. The methodology incorporates the Constant Comparative Method (Glaser and Strauss 1967, p. 105). According to the method, quotes from interviews or journals were coded according to categories, a category representing a conceptual idea. Quotes were constantly compared with previous quotes (p. 106). During the process of coding, theoretical ideas were placed in theoretical memos. Theoretical memos are the theorizing write-up of ideas about categories and their relationships as they strike the analyst while coding (Glaser 1978). The memos became the basis for delimiting the theory (Glaser and Strauss 1967, p. 109). As data collection, organization, and analysis continued, categories became refined, the theory (reconstructed experience) developed and coded quotes then became the tools for illustrating the theory (Glaser and Strauss 1967, p. 110).

SOURCES OF ERROR

Two potential sources of error are myself and the partners participating in the study.

The first source of error involves my observing, recording and interpreting the experiences of the partners. For the past eight years, I have maintained a private clinical practice designed to meet the needs of gay men. In the context of private practice, I have treated a number of gay men with AIDS or AIDS-related problems in individual and couples therapy, as well as several surviving partners. Given my prior experience of treating surviving partners, I most likely had, on some level, preconceived ideas as to what these men experience. I am also a member of the gay community. This places the researcher as a member of one of the highest risk group for developing AIDS. The centrality of my position as a member of a high risk group may have served to enhance my ability to enlist partners for participation in the study, and to empathically communicate with the participating partner, but may also have served to bias my observations and interpretation of the data.

The second potential source of error involves the partners' ability and willingness to accurately relate their experiences and perceptions, as well as the type of person who would volunteer for such a study. In the researcher's clinical practice with partners, he has observed the intense and at times volatile affects that accompany the illness and loss of a partner to AIDS. In clinical practice the researcher has observed that partners enlist a great deal of energy in containing and suppressing these affects; hence, for a variety of reasons, participating partners may have been hesitant to convey the depth of their affective experience.

An additional potential source of error concerns the racial, socioeconomic, and regional backgrounds of the participants. The majority of the participants were from solid middle class socioeconomic strata. The majority were college educated, many had professional careers and all but three were white. While their lives had been substantially disrupted by the disease, none of the participants was in dire financial circumstances. All had been able to manage on savings accounts and disability policies. As participation in the study was voluntary, potentially only a certain segment of partners were attracted to, and willing to participate in, the process of relating their experience to an unknown researcher.

Data collection methods and analytic strategies took into account these identified sources of error. The researcher recorded the interviews to ensure accuracy of the descriptions made by the partners and in-depth interviews occurred with all participants. The strategy for data analysis utilized in the study involved a process of repeated comparison of concepts and categories between diverse cases. Hence, the method of data collection and the strategy for data analysis are designed to ensure the development of a theory grounded in the data regarding the experience of the partners. The data obtained from health care and social service workers provided an additional set of observations and experiences other than those of the researcher. Additionally, a strategy termed "membership checking" (Lincoln and Guba 1985) was employed. Several participants representing surviving partners, well partners, and ill partners reviewed the generated theory and commented on the accuracy with which it conveys their experience. The comments and observations of these participants were then integrated into the final text, as were several revisions based on participant feedback. As a further aid to objectivity, an activity termed "debriefing" (Glaser and Strauss 1967), a process of reviewing the organization and analysis of the data with an objective individual, was incorporated, with the researcher's advisor, an individual experienced in this methodology, serving in that role.

LIMITATIONS AND GENERALIZABILITY

There are several possible limitations to the results of the study. The 32 participants reflect only a small number of the thousands of partnered men with AIDS and partners of gay men who are ill with, or who have died from, AIDS. The study was primarily conducted in the Chicago and San Francisco metropolitan areas, hence, rural areas were represented by only one participant. One could also argue that the theory or results are the reconstruction of the experiences of the 32 men who participated in the study. A method of counteracting these potential limitations is theoretical saturation, which Glaser and Strauss (1967, p. 61) define:

> . . . no additional data are being found whereby the sociologist can develop properties of a category. As he sees similar instances happening over and over again, the researcher becomes empirically confident that a category is saturated.

Glaser and Strauss (1967, pp. 3-4) describe the approach to the study as:

> . . . an initial, systematic discovery of the theory from the data of social research. Then one can be relatively sure that the theory will fit and work. And since the categories are discovered by examination of the data, laymen involved in the area to

which the theory applies will usually be able to understand it, while sociologists who work in other areas will recognize and understand theory linked with the data of a given area.

Theory based on data can usually not be replaced by more data or another theory. Since it is too intimately linked to data, it is destined to last despite its inevitable modification and reformation.

Thus, while the number of participants in the study is relatively small and represents a limited geographical area, the methodology employed in the study will help to ensure the development of a theory that by virtue of its thoroughness and closeness to the data is readily applicable with possible modifications to men in a similar position or in other locations. The extent to which the theory will be generalizable to other gay men in similar positions, or to men in lower socio-economic strata or racial groups will remain largely unknown and will depend on future explorations of other researchers. The only difference in the experience of the rural participant appeared to be the longer distances that had to be traveled to obtain medical and psychological support, the consideration of rural isolation, and planning for the care of the partner during the region's severe winters.

An additional area of limitation concerns the number of participants who had reached the later areas of the mourning process. The majority of participants joined the study during the illness of their partner or within one year of their partner's death. The mourning process for the participants tended to proceed at a slower pace than the span of time allotted for the interview phase of the study. Consequently, the number of participants who were experiencing, or had experienced, the later areas of the experience was considerably lower than in the earlier areas. Additional participants were recruited in an effort to saturate the last area, *"Back into the World."* However, the numbers of participants in that area totaled 6, as compared to previous areas, most of which the entire sample had experienced. Potentially seropositive/symptomatic partners mourn at a slower pace given the more complicated nature of the process. Clearly the experiences of these men is a future study unto itself.

The extent to which the theory can be generalized to other segments of the population (such as married heterosexuals who experience the illness and death of their spouse) will be subject to judgments of clinicians regarding the utility of the conceptualizations (Kennedy 1979). The issue of generalizability for this particular research project serves to point out a key aspect of clinical work with a gay/lesbian population: for much of our clinical work, clinicians must generalize from theories developed regarding heterosexual development and experience. Whether the population of the study precludes generalization to other populations will again be a source of potential future exploration.

Chapter IV

Introduction to the Results

When a gay man's partner contracts AIDS, he enters an experience that will actively occupy the very center of his existence for several years. The memories and potential repercussions of the experience will most likely continue to influence the surviving partner's experience of himself and the world for the rest of his life. In the words of one partner, "It was an immense journey." It is a journey that takes two men from initial concerns that something may be wrong, to the expected or unexpected confirmation of AIDS, to the uncertainty of life during the partner's illness, to the physical decline and death of the ill partner. With the death of the ill partner, the well partner, now a surviving partner, must continue on the journey alone as he mourns the loss of the central person in his life. The infectious nature of AIDS adds a powerful dimension to the mourning process of the surviving partner, one that will profoundly influence its outcome.

The experience of a partner contracting AIDS consists of nine distinct areas or categories of experience. Some partners will enter the experience with a period of WONDERING if the partner is becoming ill with AIDS. Others will enter with an unexpected CONFIRMATION of the diagnosis. Partners then encounter THE LONG HAUL, the period of the partner's illness. The next area of experience, FEVER PITCH, encompasses the period immediately preceding the death of the ill partner. It is followed by CALM AND PEACE, during which the ill partner succumbs to the disease. The areas of experience that encompass the illness and death of the partner are sequential in nature and largely dictated by the disease course.

The journey becomes a solitary one as the well partner makes the transition to surviving partner when he experiences CHAOS, the realization that the partner is indeed dead, and he is alone. In RE-TREAT, the surviving partner enters into an intense dialogue with his deceased partner.

EXPLORATION is a period of decreased preoccupation with the deceased partner and the surviving partner's ventures into the world of the living. The final area of experience, BACK INTO THE WORLD, is ongoing and encompasses the surviving partner finding new meaning in life without his deceased partner. In contrast to the earlier areas of experience, those that encompass the mourning experience have more fluid boundaries and are not as sequential in nature. CHAOS returns repeatedly throughout RETREAT. During EARLY EXPLORATION, the frequency and intensity of CHAOS declines considerably, but is easily activated. Similarly, the partner may experience RETREAT as he moves out into the world in EARLY EXPLORATION.

Within this framework, there are variations in length of the time periods, and in the intensity of affects associated with each area of experience. Each area or category of experience is comprised of several distinct properties. Properties are component aspects of experience that together give each category its unique characteristics. This theory is primarily drawn from the viewpoint of the well or surviving partner. Initially, the experience occurs in the context of a relationship. With the death of the ill partner it becomes the experience of one man. Areas of experience that occur while both partners are living include properties that address the interactions between the two men; between the two men and their families, friends, and professionals; and the private experience of the well partner. Quotes from ill partners are sometimes used to illustrate processes that influence the experience of the well partner. Areas of experience after the death of the ill partner consist of interactions of the surviving partner with families, friends, professionals, and again, his private experience.

Variations in WONDERING, CONFIRMATION, THE LONG HAUL and FEVER PITCH are attributed to the variable nature of the disease course, to when the HIV infection is identified, to the personality characteristics of the men involved in the relationship, and to the characteristics of the relationship itself. The knowledge of the presence or absence of HIV infection in the well partner imparts its own special meaning. For many partners, it comes to symbolize whether the well partner will be spared or follow the same course as the ill partner. Variations in the length and intensity of affects associated with CHAOS, RETREAT, EARLY EXPLO-RATION and BACK INTO THE WORLD are accounted for in the characteristics of the relationship, the personality characteristics of the surviving partner, the supportive or non-supportive relation-ships that he has at his disposal, and, most significantly, the pres-ence or absence of HIV infection.

Throughout the Results, the term "Dialogue" is employed. Dia-logue refers to the area of shared experience and its many com-ponents that exists between two people in an ongoing intimate and sexual relationship. As each relationship is comprised of two unique individuals, each relationship will have its own unique dia-logue. Some aspects of the dialogue may change and evolve over the course of the relationship, others will endure throughout the lives of the individuals and their shared experience. The compo-nents include the object relationship in particular, the selfobject functions each partner experiences, and the collective and individ-ual hopes, dreams, fears, triumphs and frustrations encountered in an ongoing relationship. Ultimately, the dialogue is the sense that another person is an integral part of one's daily experience, that two people are participating in life together.

Partners enter the experience either at WONDERING (a period of time when one or both partners wonder if one of them is about to become ill, collect evidence and hope against all hope that AIDS is not about to enter the relationship), or CONFIRMATION (the ini-tial shock, emotional upheaval and intensive medical intervention that initially accompanies an AIDS diagnosis). The variation in en-try is accounted for by several factors. One factor is the time of the onset of the disease. Several of the partners in this study were diag-nosed early in the epidemic when AIDS was not so prevalent, the medical and gay community were not as familiar with early signs and symptoms, and testing for the HIV antibody was not developed or as common as it is currently. A second factor is the highly vari-able nature of the onset of the disease. A third factor is insulation, the feeling that may evolve when men are partnered over a long period of time that AIDS is outside of the sphere of the relationship.

The long latency period of the HIV virus (now believed to average ten years) creates one of the cruelest factors in the context of a long term relationship. One or both of the men may have been exposed to the virus before meeting the other, or may have been exposed during a sexual encounter outside of the relationship and may transmit the virus to the partner. As the relationship grows, commitments to each other are solidified and an assumption of longevity evolves. Dreams and plans for the future become an integral aspect of the dialogue between the two men. Then, AIDS and the threat of death creeps in or suddenly enters the relationship and hence the dialogue. The assumption of longevity is shaken, hopes and dreams for the future are shattered, and the two men find themselves on a journey that they may have contemplated only in their darkest fantasies.

Chapter V

Wondering

All of the signs I saw in my two friends were there. I was now seeing them in my lover.

WONDERING is characterized by increasing anxiety and a growing sense of doom, a sense that something is terribly wrong, that one of the partners may indeed be developing AIDS, that the relationship and the lives of one, probably both, of the partners is in danger. One or both of the men may be struggling with this fear. One may have gathered more evidence than the other. They may or may not be talking about it. No one wants AIDS to be real. The powerful, underlying fear, for many couples, is that talking about the evidence and subsequent concerns will make it all too real. The properties of WONDERING are: *Gathering Evidence*, the process of noticing symptoms that could indicate HIV infection; *Restless Nights*, the well partner's growing anxiety as evidence continues to mount; *Hot Potato,* the efforts of the partners to talk about their concerns; and a variation, *Waiting for the Bomb to Drop*, seen when the HIV infection has been identified, and labeled, but symptoms do not yet indicate an AIDS diagnosis.

GATHERING EVIDENCE

It started in February when he had a severe bout of the flu. He kept going to the doctor, but nothing was definite. I kept wondering if he was coming down with AIDS or cancer. He never really recovered. By summer I was quite worried; his clothes were hanging on him and he was missing days from work. I knew something was terribly wrong.

When partners enter the experience at WONDERING, they do so by *Gathering Evidence*, noticing symptoms and physical changes and comparing what they observe in their partner with what they have seen in friends who contracted AIDS, or what they have read or heard about the disease in the media: "He had fevers, he had night sweats, he had diarrhea, and he had lost a lot of weight." "We heard that a former boyfriend of his had been diagnosed, meantime his cough was getting worse." At this point the partners may or may not be talking about the evidence or sharing their concerns with each other. One partner may have collected more evidence than the other. Anxiety starts to mount, and the process of the partners being identified as the "ill one" and the "well one" begins. Some well partners, in retrospect, are surprised when they think back and realize just how much evidence existed before the diagnosis. "It started so slowly we didn't even notice it. He lost weight and then the fevers began." However, partners rarely forget the first realization that the evidence may indicate AIDS, "I will never forget that night in February when in my mind it all added up to AIDS." "I remember his first night sweat. I was terrified, thinking that it might be AIDS. I kept thinking, please God, please, don't let it be AIDS."

The terror that accompanies AIDS is seen in an aspect of evidence gathering. Partners may gather evidence and weigh it on the "AIDS side" and the "other side." The other side often includes diseases such as tuberculosis or cancer. Each piece of evidence is weighed. When evidence comes along that can be placed on the "other side" it is welcomed. When evidence falls on the " AIDS side," anxiety mounts. "Looking back, I can't believe we were doing that: hoping that he had cancer or TB, anything but AIDS." The well partner may go along with the ill partner's hopes in order to soothe him. " He was putting a lot of energy into thinking it was TB." "I thought it was AIDS all along, but I went along with it."

Partners may try to minimize or ignore the evidence they observe, but as they try to minimize their fears, new evidence may emerge. "In the back of my mind there was a nagging suspicion. Things did not seem right—that we were moving in that direction. At first I would just push it out of my mind, but things kept happening."

The process of evidence gathering is complicated by the high degree of AIDS anxiety that exists for many men in the gay community. The fear of contracting the disease is often great, and it is not unusual for men to go through periods when they are convinced that they are becoming ill. For some it will be a false alarm, for others it will be an indicator of things to come. The less anxious partner may try to soothe his partner's fears. "He was a self-admitted hypochondriac. He was always worrying about AIDS, I was always trying to calm him down and reassure him that he was OK." "I kept saying, 'Mike, I think something is wrong, I wish you would go to the doctor,' he kept saying that I was being hysterical — again." The anxiously expressed fear of contracting AIDS may have an unhinging effect on partners. "One day I lost it and yelled that he wouldn't be satisfied until he did come down with AIDS. When he was diagnosed, I was devastated." The fear may be written off by one of the partners as AIDS anxiety: "Jim kept saying he was coming down with AIDS, I just thought he was somatizing. He took out mortgage and disability insurance, I thought he was being kind of outrageous, but then he did get sick." The characteristics of the relationship — which partner tends to bring up problems for discussion, which partner tends to deny problems, and how much the couple talks about anxiety-provoking topics — are all factors that determine who acknowledges symptoms first, who talks about their concerns, and how concerns are expressed, if at all.

The well partner may feel he is the first to know, having weighed the evidence and resigned himself to what may lie ahead. Though "hard" evidence, such as that provided by medical monitoring, may be lacking, or the ill partner may not be sharing the knowledge conveyed by his physician, the well partner may have a "gut sense" that his partner is progressing toward an AIDS diagnosis. "I felt like I knew long before he was diagnosed that he had AIDS. I felt in January, when he first had symptoms, that I knew what was going on." The well partner's position as an observer rather than the person in the process of becoming sick may enable this more objective view. Yet it is a perspective that carries with it its own brand of fear.

RESTLESS NIGHTS

When he first started having the night sweats I would lay awake at night praying that it was not what I had feared.

As he wonders if his partner is becoming ill and the evidence continues to mount, the well partner experiences *Restless Nights*. The fear of losing the partner to AIDS becomes all the more real as the evidence grows. The future begins to feel more and more frightening and less optimistic. The well partner may begin to wonder what life would be like alone. "Sometimes I would lay awake, watch him sleep, and wonder what is going to happen to him, what will become of us?" Partners rarely feel they can share their concerns with others. "I didn't want to frighten anybody," "I did not want it going around that Nick was coming down with AIDS." It is often a private fear, the fear that comes with a growing sense of certainty that the central person in the well partner's life is in the process of developing a terminal illness, not cancer or TB, but AIDS. That what may have happened to friends, or perhaps is known from the media, is about to occur in their home. That the relationship, the sense of togetherness and belonging, the hopes and dreams for the future-all components of the dialogue, will end with the death of the partner. "I was terrified for a good year and a half."

For some men who have experienced the illness and deaths of friends to AIDS, the threat of AIDS entering the relationship may represent a convergence of losses. For these men, restless nights may become restless days and weeks. "I began having trouble sleeping at night. My friends had just died and then Jim started getting sick and I was not feeling well either. I was more worried than he was. Jim never complained, even though he was feeling worse and worse. I finally was so distressed that I went to see a therapist."

HOT POTATO

We would talk about the symptoms he was having and he would say, "Oh my god, I hope it is not AIDS." I think he sort of knew, too, that was what it was going to be.

The growing evidence and the fear of AIDS coming directly into their lives may become a *Hot Potato* for the partners as they try to find a way to talk about, or forget about, their concerns. "He really was not feeling well, dragging around, trying to get through a day's work. I figured the last thing he needed to hear was that I was scared shitless." "Because he was so afraid of AIDS, I pooh-poohed everything he said about it." During conjoint interviews, several couples were surprised at just how much evidence each partner had collected, and the extent of their fears, prior to the diagnosis.

Couples often have difficulty discussing issues that they perceive as threatening to the bond of the relationship. Rather than risk losing the relationship, they remain silent. "How do you tell someone you love that you are worried that they are coming down with AIDS?" AIDS represents a very real threat to the relationship, and both partners may try to make it a less real possibility. "The lesions were there, I could see them, but I chose to deny there was anything wrong." "Mike had this real macho style but he was really a little boy inside. He hated doctors and being sick. I knew something was wrong, but when I said he should go to the doctor, he would just write it off, so I let it slide until I was so worried I got mad." When couples have difficulty talking about issues, partners may end up feeling that the facts were hidden from them. "To this day, I still wonder how long he knew he was sick. John was not much of a talker, especially when it came to anything regarding his past sexual adventures. He had linked AIDS up as some kind of revenge for his past exploits. Even after the diagnosis, he would not talk to me about it."

No one wants the man he loves to contract AIDS. Partners, in their despair, may wish they could trade places, so that their partner might live. "We would talk about AIDS and our fear of it, of one of us coming down with it. I said if one of us would come down with it, it would be me. Ken said, 'No!, its going to be me.' " "When Brad was diagnosed with ARC, I went down to be tested, somehow I came up negative. I was furious. He was ecstatic. If I could trade places I would, I'm older, I have lived longer, it just isn't fair that he should be the one sick and me somehow be spared."

Partners may struggle to maintain the hope that it is not AIDS. The "ill partner" may ask the "well partner" to back off. "I kept fretting and fretting. Each visit to the doctor was non-conclusive.

One day he said, 'Please, let me have my own little dream.' I knew
then that he was just as worried as I.''

An integral aspect of *Hot Potato* is that in wondering if his partner is becoming ill with AIDS, the "well partner" also implicates
himself. "I figured that if he was getting sick, then I was also exposed to the virus." Each piece of evidence also indicates that the
well partner may also be in danger. If antibody statuses are unknown, the well partner assumes he is seropositive. However, the
implications are experienced as so powerful, that well partners often prefer to keep it as an assumption. "I was terrified for him and
me." The potential infection and illness of the well partner imparts
an additional dimension to the experience. The fear is not so much
that AIDS is in him, but that AIDS is inside the relationship; AIDS
is inside "us." The "ill one" and the "well one" is a delineation
in roles only. "I assumed I was positive, and consequently felt ill
also. He happened to be sicker than I was."

The well partner may become preoccupied with his own health.
"Every little thing that came along caused me to worry that I was
getting ill too." "Every cough, every rash sent me through the
ceiling." As anxiety producing as the assumption of infection can
be, well partners choose to test the assumption at different points in
the experience. There are different reasons and meanings behind the
decision, depending on when it occurs. Well partners often feel that
assuming positivity, but banking on the chance that they are negative, gives them an edge in managing the illness of the partner. "At
least by not knowing, I have that little bit of hope. If I found out I
was positive, I would have nothing."

WAITING FOR THE BOMB TO DROP

*He was in a study and found out that he was positive, plus his
T-cells were low. We watched his T-cells go down for 2 years.
It was a constant worry. We knew it was coming.*

Waiting For The Bomb To Drop is a variation in WONDERING
observed when the partner is aware of his antibody status, is being
monitored medically, has declining T-cell counts, symptoms that
indicate depressed immune system functioning, or symptoms so ad-

vanced as to warrant a diagnosis of AIDS-Related Complex. In this variation, the concerns have been confirmed as valid and labeled. "I was having what I thought was an infection of some sort in my mouth so I went to the dentist. He sent me to the university medical center. The doctor said I had thrush, and since I was a gay man, I probably had ARC. I freaked. My brother linked me up with Dr. S. All the tests came back positive, some other things come along and she also felt I had ARC." In this situation, the symptoms have been labelled and made explicit. The fear of the partners then becomes the development of full blown AIDS.[1]

NOTE

1. In relationships where one or both of the men have been diagnosed with ARC, or are aware of declining T-Cell counts, one observes processes similar to those that will be elaborated in THE LONG HAUL when one of the partners has been diagnosed with AIDS. While there are parallels, the difference is significant. With ARC or low lab counts, the fear is of the partner contracting AIDS, and eventually dying. With AIDS, the fear is for the death of the partner.

> Initially, We did not want to be away from each other for a second. We became a lot closer. Emotionally, it took us about a month or two to stop crying. If something good happened, we would cry. If something bad happened, we would cry. At some point it just stopped, and we began to enjoy things. We want to live a good life as long as it lasts.

With the labeling of the symptoms as ARC, the processes observed in these couples are similar to those that will be discussed in the future areas of CONFIRMATION and THE LONG HAUL. As the above quote indicates, the partners initially *Close Ranks*, mourn the loss of hopes and dreams for the future, feel the *Slap in the Face*, and may wonder if the diagnosis is real. "Initially all the work we were doing on the house came to a stop." They must decide to whom they will *Reveal* the diagnosis: "At first we kept it to ourselves, then I started noticing that other couples had the same medications on their counters. Now, we know a lot of couples in the same situation. We do a lot of talking about what it is like." A *Game Plan* evolves: "I am on AZT, I eat right and get plenty of rest, actually, I don't have any choice but to get plenty of rest." "I get furious at him if he forgets to take his pills." The partners must *Balance* the stress, alteration of their lifestyle and potential loss of the partner that the disease entails. "I can't do as much as I used to, I get tired out easily." "Sometimes I get irritated when he nods off in the middle of something, then I feel horrible." Couples may also experience *Renewal* in the relationship. "It really has brought us a lot closer, I really don't feel alone with it. It's our disease, our situation, not just my disease." *Waiting for the Bomb to Drop* may become the dominant experience of partners in the future as antibody testing, and medical monitoring of presymptomatic, seropositive men becomes more routine.

Chapter VI

Confirmation

I thought it was walking pneumonia, but then he was in the hospital. A day later, they did a biopsy and diagnosed him. We were feeling so numb those first couple of weeks.

CONFIRMATION encompasses the initial diagnosis of AIDS and the emotional upheaval that follows. For some partners, the diagnosis was completely unexpected. For others, it was a confirmation of their worst fears that had come all too soon. For all, it was a shock, an insult to their relationship, a sudden destruction of plans, hopes and dreams for the future. Assumptions of longevity, of the partner always being there, of growing old together, are dashed and replaced by uncertainty, the fear of what the disease may bring, and of being alone.

CONFIRMATION is a period of great emotional upheaval for both partners. Often the ill partner is hospitalized, with the resulting disruption in daily routine. Anxiety and fear run high. A profound sense of numbness and unreality initially pervade both partners' experience. The diagnosed partner may be very ill, depressed, desperately needing the presence of his well partner, and on some level, fearing his partner will leave him. The well partner is experiencing his own fear and sadness and attempting to make sense of the diagnosis and its implications for his partner, the relationship, and himself. He is also attempting to "be there" for his partner and holding down his job, where he may or may not feel comfortable informing his employer or co-workers why he is looking so harried or taking time off. Household pets and routines must also be tended. If the antibody status of the well partner is unknown, both partners may be worrying that he too is infected. Well partners tend to assume they are positive, regardless of test results. Some partners will test the assumption in the wake of CONFIRMATION. Others will wait until a later point in the experience.

Often, the well partner hides the depth of his despair from his partner, saving it for time alone. His overriding concern is being there for the ill partner. At first, life may seem meaningless for the well partner, but gradually, as CONFIRMATION comes to a close, a new purpose in life evolves; the hope of sustaining his partner until a cure is found.

The properties of CONFIRMATION are: *Slap In The Face*, the initial shock and insult that follows the confirmation of AIDS; *Profound Sorrow*, the well partner's despair as he struggles with the evidence that the relationship will one day end with the death of his partner; *Closing Ranks*, the partners being drawn closely together by the impending loss; *Automatic Pilot*, the well partner's efforts to keep his feelings at bay in order to attend to the needs of his partner; and *Is This Real?*, the sense of disbelief in the reality of the diagnosis, the hope that it is only a bad dream.

SLAP IN THE FACE

The diagnosis was a real slap in the face: Too close to home.

For some partners, the diagnosis is unexpected. "It never occurred to us that it could be AIDS, he had the test six months earlier and it was negative." "I knew something was seriously wrong, but I did not think it was AIDS." "It all happened so suddenly. I came home from work one day and he had a temperature of 104 degrees, then the doctor's office, then the hospital, and then the doc said it was AIDS." Several of the partners of men in this study were diagnosed when AIDS was not as prevalent in the gay community. This, coupled with a feeling of insulation that several couples related, may account for the lack of wondering if AIDS was a possibility: "We did not know that much about it. None of our friends had gotten sick." "Since we had been monogamous for the two years we were together, we really thought it would pass us by." "Its like, if it is not happening to you, its not really happening." "We were hearing more and more about AIDS and were talking about doing some volunteer work. Then he was diagnosed." If the partner had not been tested or been followed medically, evidence that something was wrong may have been lacking. "I was shocked, I hadn't noticed anything, no signs or symptoms. One day he was sick. The next week, he had AIDS."

For men who entered the experience at WONDERING, the diagnosis and the events leading up to it are a confirmation of their worst fears: " I came home from a trip. He was still running a fever. He told me that the antibiotics he had been taking weren't helping and the doctor wanted him to go to the hospital. I just knew it was the beginning of the end." "For six months we had been hoping that it was not AIDS, but then the biopsy came back positive." Despite months of wondering and gathering evidence, partners may continue to hope for another diagnosis. "Even though I knew it had to be AIDS, when I called the hospital for his biopsy results, I kept hoping in the back of my mind that it was not pneumocystis. I did not want to believe that it was finally happening."

When men have been diagnosed with ARC, have other symptoms, or have been aware of declining T-Cell counts, their partners are anxiously following developments as well. For these men, the diagnosis is still experienced as a shock: "We had been watching his T-Cells go down for several years, but when it was officially declared AIDS, it was still a tremendous shock, as if we had not been anticipating it all along." "It came too soon, much too soon."

The partners in the study were informed of the diagnosis in a variety of ways. Many learned of the diagnosis together: "The doc came in and said, 'the biopsy showed pneumocystis.'" In other cases, the ill partner had to do the informing: "I came out of the doctors' office. Ken was in the car waiting. It took me a few minutes before I could speak." The ill partner may not be able to immediately inform his partner of the diagnosis: "He had been sick and to the doctor a few times. He was in a gloomy mood all week. I asked him what was bugging him so. He said, 'sit down.' I will never forget the way he said 'sit down.' I knew something awful was up."

Sometimes the well partner must inform his ill partner: "I am still pissed about the way it happened. I was in the hospital room and the doctor called up, and said the biopsy was positive, and that

it was AIDS. That left me to tell Stan." Sometimes the well partner
may decide to hold back the information. "We knew his T-Cells
were low. He had been having skin problems and just not feeling
well. We went to Mexico. I think we both knew it would be our last
real vacation. While we were there, I noticed lesions on his back. I
did not say anything. I wanted him — and us — to have one last vacation. When we got home, he noticed them in the mirror and called
out for me. We just held each other and cried."

Regardless of who does the informing, the diagnosis is experienced as a tremendous blow. "We were in shock." "It was as if
someone reached down my throat and yanked my heart out." "It
was like somebody kicked me in the stomach." Both men are now
faced with integrating the reality of AIDS into their lives. Not the
joint business venture, new home, dream vacation, or the daily irritations with each other. "We were both going to quit our jobs and
go to cooking school. We wanted to open a restaurant or inn someday." "We were saving to buy a house, now we are going to take
the money and go to Europe." They must now reconcile themselves
to the uncertainty of the disease course, potential disruptions in lifestyle, financial pressures, the possibility of the well partner also
being in danger and the very real threat of the loss of their dialogue
through death.

The bonds that hold relationships together are mysterious and
powerful. AIDS in a relationship is often experienced as an insult,
the antithesis to the bond — something dirty, vile and evil that has
entered into sacred territory. An integral aspect of any slap in the
face is insult, and rage. "It was a dirty trick that mother nature
played on us." "I was furious. He is such a good person. I hated it
when anything bad happened to him, and I really hated it when he
was diagnosed. He just does not deserve to have anything bad happen to him." "The rage was there all right. But what do you do
with it? Who do you get angry at? God? nature? the virus? the
medical community for not having a cure?" A profound sense of
injustice is often felt by one or both men. "I am 26 years old. I
should not have to be thinking about death." Those whose message
may be viewed as moralizing on the topic of AIDS and transmission
become an easy target for the partner's rage. "The Surgeon General's pamphlet and AIDS posters on buses these days all imply that

one catches AIDS by being promiscuous. They are saying we had a promiscuous relationship. We did not have a promiscuous relationship."

PROFOUND SORROW

The most despairing time was when he was first diagnosed and I knew that he was going to die because of AIDS. That yes, he was going to die. It was going to happen some day.

Partners are left trying to reconcile what they have heard about AIDS in the media with its presence on home turf. What they soon discover is that AIDS, in the context of a relationship, carries very different meanings from those popularly ascribed to it. "We loved each other so much. His diagnosis with AIDS just seemed incomprehensible." For some partners, the antithesis of the disease and their bond is brought home by the timing of the diagnosis. "We had our seventh anniversary and his diagnosis at the same time. It was pretty dreadful."

The well partner experiences *Profound Sorrow* as he attempts to integrate perhaps the most devastating implication and threat of the diagnosis: that the dialogue with his partner will someday be lost through death. "It was a hard, hard two weeks." As in *Restless Nights*, it is often a private sorrow. " I would come home from the hospital, sit in the dark and cry." The well partner senses his need for support, but may not know where to turn. In the past he may have turned to his partner, but with his partner ill, he does not want to overburden him. "Ken was so sick, I could not let him see just how devastated I was." Friends may be available and supportive, but partners may not feel comfortable sharing the depth of their sorrow: "It was nice of people to have me stop by for dinner on the way home from the hospital, but what really felt good was to go home and cry." Employers or colleagues may sense that something is wrong. If the well partner feels he must hide the truth, then the sense of sorrow and aloneness may be enhanced. "I had left work in a hurry to come home and call for his biopsy results. Right after I found out that he had pneumocystis, my boss called thinking that something had happened at work to upset me. I said no, that I just had something at home to deal with. I hung up the phone and started to cry. Being so distraught, but not being able to take advantage of the opportunity for support devastated me."

Part of the profound sorrow is the helplessness that partners often feel. "I just felt helpless, like there was not much I could do but weather the storm." In the past, when problematic issues between the two men interrupted the dialogue of the relationship, they could discuss it, fight about it or act it out, essentially to find a way to resolve the problem or reduce the tension in a more or less satisfactory way, and resume the dialogue in its familiar manner. AIDS represents the first unresolvable issue. There is no compromise, no reconciliation, no sense of boundless continuation of the relationship. "It felt like God stepped in and said, 'Stan is going to die and there is not a damn thing you can do about it.'"

CLOSING RANKS

Richard: "The afternoon I received my diagnosis, I was overwhelmed and numb at the same time. That evening, the numbness wore off and the reality hit me. Ken was with me that afternoon and evening. He was like a promontory of rock in the midst of a raging sea that I desperately needed to cling to so I would not drown."

Ken: "I felt so helpless. He was so upset and crying. All I could do was hold him and listen."

Richard: "But that is exactly what I needed. I needed him to be there."

The threat of the loss of the dialogue brings with it a sadness that only the two men involved can fully understand. While it may be one man's life and terminal diagnosis, it is the two men's relationship. The diagnosis and subsequent threat draws the two men together, often more intensely together than they have been at any other point in the relationship. "Right after his diagnosis, I hated to go to work. I hated to leave him." "He would get upset if I was the least bit late getting to the hospital." Each partner needs the other. In being there for his ill partner, the well partner feels less helpless.

With his well partner at his side, the ill partner feels less afraid and more grounded in a world that may no longer make sense. "Right after the diagnosis, I don't know how I would have managed on my own. I think I would have gone right over the edge." "I felt my place was at his bedside." The shared sense of sorrow provides the partners with the most comfort they can obtain. What they both want is no longer a possibility. The two men cannot make AIDS go away. "What I wanted more than anything was to wake up from a very bad dream."

Depending on the relationship, closing ranks may be characterized by a great deal of talking, sharing of feelings, concerns, and fears, or it may be a quiet vigilance. Initially the two partners may be the only ones in their friendship and family systems to know of the diagnosis. The partners must begin to decide to whom they will reveal the diagnosis. "Who we should tell and not tell felt like an enormously important decision. It felt like so much was already at stake. We did not want to make any wrong moves." Keeping the diagnosis secret may initially feel fine, but later in the experience it may become a burden. Some couples immediately inform their close circle of friends. Rules begin to be laid down for how the diagnosis is to be handled between the two men. Often it is the ill partner who makes the rules that the well partner is expected to follow. "Mike just would not talk about it much. I think he was afraid I would break down if he did. He would get irritated every time I started to cry." "John would not talk to me about having AIDS. We both knew it was AIDS but he would not talk." "I was expected to inform all of our friends for Jim."

A central aspect of *Closing Ranks* is the consolidation of the "ill one, well one" delineation. The well partner takes his role of the "well one" quite seriously. The sense of an important job to do cuts into the profound helplessness that the well partner may feel in the wake of the diagnosis. "I wanted to get him home from the hospital. I thought I could take better care of him." Elements of the *Game Plan*, how the well partner plans on taking care of his partner, begin to evolve and will crystallize in the next area, THE LONG HAUL. The sense of a job to be done may give partners who

experienced difficulty with self definition a stronger and more secure sense of themselves. "For so long, I struggled with who I am
in relation to Mark, who am I at work. Now I know who I am and
what my role is in this relationship."

Each partner may be wondering where the disease came from.
They may or may not be talking about it, but often each is silently
blaming himself. "Before I met Stan, I lived in San Francisco. I
assumed I picked it up out there, long before anyone knew what
was happening." A tremendous amount of guilt may be associated
with being the "transmitter." "If it could ever be proven that I
gave AIDS to Mike, I could never forgive myself." Rarely does the
issue of transmission become an arena for conflict. The relationship
is already facing the threat of loss. Open conflict over whose fault it
was would only increase the disruption. While individually each
man may be wondering and blaming himself, together the partners
often decide to let the issue pass. "What difference does it make
where it came from? Gary is sick, and I am positive, we could have
picked it up before we met, or while on one of the occasional
'flings' we both had after we were together."

The Well Partner's Status

> *I feel like I do not deserve to have AIDS, nor do I deserve not
> to have it, either.*

The diagnosis serves to add further weight to the well partner's
assumption that he, too, is infected. Often the assumption of being
HIV-positive is experienced as considerably less dangerous than
having the assumption confirmed. The well partners in this study
tended to have themselves tested at one of three points: in the wake
of the emotional upheaval and numbness of CONFIRMATION,
during the future areas of THE LONG HAUL, or during the mourning process in the later part of EXPLORATION. The partners who
tested in the wake of CONFIRMATION felt it was a mistake, and
that they did not fully consider the implications. "Stan was just
diagnosed, and the doctor said I should be tested. I really was not
thinking clearly at the time and just went along with it. I should
have given it more thought, and he should have talked to me about

the potential stress [that] knowing I was positive, with Stan sick, would cause." When the well partner tests positive, there is a sense of both being in the same boat, but also sadness that both men may experience the same fate. "It really has brought both of us together." "I was really hoping John would turn up negative. One of us is enough." The well partner, as does his ill partner, often harbors the hope that he will be negative. "I guess there was one little hope, one tiny ray of hope that I would be negative." The well partner testing negative serves to reassure that the "well one" will remain well and be able to care for the ill partner. "At least we knew that Ray would not get sick also; one sick person is enough." When the well partner tests positive, often the ill partner experiences his own version of profound sorrow. "I assumed he would be positive, but I kept hoping, praying for that slim chance. When he came home from his appointment, I could tell by the look in his eyes. Since that day, it has felt like we are both in a 'dance of death.' I may be ill and diagnosed, but it is a dance that we are both in." "It is impossible to describe the depth of the feelings that go along with knowing you are positive. It eats away at the very core of your being."

When the well partner tests positive, he experiences the emotional upheaval that comes with confirmation of his status, but his concern is often tabled in lieu of caring for his partner. "We were both pretty upset when I tested positive, but I just pushed it to the back of my mind. I had too much to worry about. Jim had to come first." "I knew I was positive through Stan's illness, but somehow I did not think much about it, I was too busy worrying about Stan." In comparison to men who are not partnered and test positive, the responses of the well partner are often less intense. "I find myself checking lymph nodes and wondering if each cold or rash is it, but I would quickly forget about it." Having the ill partner to organize around provides a buffer for the well partner who is positive. However, later in the experience, during the mourning process, the surviving partner will experience a surge in his anxiety over contracting the illness himself.

Partners have distinct reactions to the "well one" testing negative. On one hand there is relief in knowing that the well partner will remain well and be able to care for the ill partner. The ill partner may gain a sense of comfort in knowing that they have someone to leave a legacy to, that one of them will survive. On the other hand well partners may not at first believe they are negative, and fight against their status. "The doctor told me I was negative. I really do not believe him. Maybe it was just a false test result." "When he told me I was negative, I said there has to be some mistake." The ill partner may be overjoyed, while the well partner is angry. "Rick was furious. I was so happy for him. I had to tone it down for a while though, because he would start to get mad if I showed how happy I was."

Some well partners may feel pressured by physicians and friends to have themselves tested. "His doctor said I should be tested. Every time I tell one of our friends about the diagnosis, they all ask me about my test results. That is something I am not ready to deal with yet. I feel pressured and find myself getting angry when people treat it so lightly. I have enough to think about now as it is."

AUTOMATIC PILOT

I tried not to think of the future aspects of it. I tried to just concentrate on getting through that particular time. Deal with the future later, first get him back on his feet and back to work. It was sort of like running on automatic pilot.

In the wake of the diagnosis, the fear, sorrow, numbness and the often myriad tasks that need to be tended to, the well partner may feel that he is running on *Automatic Pilot.* While he is feeling a wide variety of emotions, tending to the needs of his partner, his job and their home, a sense of not really being connected to the world may evolve. In between periods of connection to his partner, he may feel a certain detachment which, while perhaps disturbing, may also seem like a blessing. "I just kind of turned off the emotion and dealt with what had to be dealt with, helping him out the best I could." "I felt if I started to let myself really feel what was going on inside me that I would surely lose it. It worked. Somehow I made it through those first few weeks."

Being on *Automatic Pilot* does not negate the feelings and experiences described by the earlier properties. They occur side by side. While men report the sense of being on automatic, it is clear that all of the other feelings are occurring as well. In the wake of the disruption of the dialogue, with so much to integrate, the self provides a buffer. Though it may leave well partners not quite feeling real, they are able to get through the initial chaos of the partner's diagnosis, while tending to his needs and the needs of others. "I found myself thinking that I would sort out all that I was feeling later, once things settled down."

Partners running on automatic are models of efficiency. In retrospect they are amazed at how much they were able to accomplish. "When he was in the hospital, I would get up at five, go to the gym, go to work and then spend the evening at the hospital. On my days off, I would get up, and in three hours, cook all my food for the next week so I would not be at the mercy of hospital food." "I divided my life like pieces of pie. When I was at work, I did not think about George, I could not think about him and get anything accomplished. When I was at the hospital, I was at the hospital. When I was home in bed, I was home." *Automatic Pilot* will return again in the future during the periodic crises of THE LONG HAUL and again in the midst of FEVER PITCH.

The well partner running on automatic often feels quite satisfied with all the tasks he is able to accomplish and often feels "high, on some kind of buzz." However, colleagues, friends and ill partners often notice the change in his usual style of relating to people and tasks. People observing rather than experiencing automatic pilot often become concerned. "When he is running on auto, I get worried, because I know he is not letting a whole lot of stuff in or really processing what is happening emotionally." Well partners are often puzzled by expressed concern. "I don't know why you are worried, I really do feel fine." "It is a drive to keep going, to keep everything in the best order as possible." For some partners, the observation of auto pilot by colleagues may threaten to give away their secret. "Every now and then someone at work would ask me if everything was okay. I would get nervous and make up some excuse." For some men, denying the extent of what they are dealing with carried with it a sense of sadness. "There were times when I wanted so badly to tell some of my closer colleagues, but I just felt it was too risky.''

IS THIS REAL?

The first few weeks after he was home from the hospital were kind of a lull in the storm. He was looking better, and had more energy every day. Even though I was continuing to set things up, looking into what groups he could go to—in the back of my mind I kept wondering if this really was happening.

CONFIRMATION comes to a close with a growing sense of the emergency having passed. The ill partner may be looking and feeling better. If he was hospitalized, he is now home. The initial infection that led to the AIDS diagnosis is either abated or under control. The ill partner may have returned to or be planning his return to work. The dialogue between the two men that was disrupted by acute illness and any physical separation, such as a hospital stay, may feel as though it is returning to its familiar state. This sense of life returning to normal may cause one or both partners to wonder, ''Is this real?'' and to hope that it was only a bad dream.

Having weathered the initial storm, partners may either plunge back into old routines or seek a change of pace. ''After his diagnosis, we went to my sister's place in Florida, just to get into a different environment.'' ''He could not wait to get back to work. I think he really wanted to prove that he could still hack it.'' Both partners have reason to wish that life would get back to normal, and that AIDS would be behind them. Men often experience the diagnosis as a crushing blow to their self esteem. They may hope that getting back to work will help restore their sense of worth. The ill partner's life is at stake and the well partner's relationship to the ill partner is at stake. Both partners may participate to varying degrees in promoting the belief that all of this is not real. For some men, this hope runs parallel to their efforts on behalf of their partner's new status and potential needs as a person with AIDS. For some couples, the hope may manifest itself in not following through on referral suggestions or in more effort at ''getting him back on his feet'' than integrating the reality of the diagnosis. However, in the next area of experience, THE LONG HAUL, this hope will be shattered. Medical problems will arise again, and the dialogue cannot quite return to its familiar state. Uncertainty is now present at some level in the dialogue, the uncertainty that stems from the threat of the loss of the relationship through death.

Chapter VII

The Long Haul

It was an immense journey. Though it lasted only six months, it felt years long.

THE LONG HAUL covers the period of time between the decline of the initial shock of the diagnosis and the approaching death of the partner. Depending on the disease course, THE LONG HAUL can last several weeks, months, or years. Most of the partners of the men in this study were ill for six months to two years. During THE LONG HAUL, the ill partner may experience long periods of relatively good health, contrasted by periods of acute illness. The ill partner may also develop AIDS dementia which can subtly or dramatically impair cognitive and emotional functioning.

A chronic, powerful, and anxious sense of uncertainty ebbs and flows, at times pervading both partner's experience during this period. "It was like walking on a tightrope. The feeling of uncertainty was always there, even in the calm periods." While the partner is in periods of good health a sense of optimism often develops, yet the knowledge of the terminal nature of the disease lurks in the background. Although both partners are highly aware of the possibility of death, concrete evidence is often lacking; the ill partner may look well and feel well. Holidays and vacations may be greatly appreciated, but at the same time, a sadness periodically surfaces as both partners wonder if this will be their last one together.

The occurrence of yet another bout of pneumonia, other medical problems, or hospitalization often brings discouragement, and is a reminder of the tenuous nature of the situation. With acute illness and/or hospitalization, the sense of crisis that accompanied the confirmation of the diagnosis returns, and the well partner may again find himself running on *Automatic Pilot*. During THE LONG HAUL, both partners' main concerns are keeping the ill partner healthy, prolonging his life as long as possible, and continuing the dialogue of the relationship—the sense of shared experience that has come to dominate the two men's experience of each other.

The properties of THE LONG HAUL are: *This Is Real*, the well partner's realization that the diagnosis is a reality and that their lives have been fundamentally changed; *The Game Plan*, how the partner and the couple plan to manage the illness; *Revelation/Negotiation*, informing family and friends of the diagnosis and the negotiation of these relationships; *Balancing*, the most intricate and important property that involves the balancing of ever-increasing responsibilities, stresses, and loneliness in the face of the decline of the ill partner's physical and often mental status, essentially balancing on a tightrope of hope while trying not to fall into despair. *Fever Pitch*, periods of acute medical crisis; *Renewal*, periods of renewed connection and deepening of the relationship; and *Derailment*, events that severely diminish the dialogue between the ill and well partner, or that place added burdens on the well partner.

THIS IS REAL

I still was not understanding, not believing it was happening until a few months after they first said it was AIDS. A few months after his first hospitalization, he got very sick, and I had to take him back to the hospital. When he was being admitted, his name came up on the computer screen and under diagnosis it said 'AIDS.' I thought, "This is real! This is real!"

Initially, following the diagnosis, there is a hope of life getting back to normal. Both partners may welcome evidence that sustains this hope. CONFIRMATION tends to come to a close with wondering *Is This Real?* The well partner may be aware of his hope that life will return to normal, that perhaps the diagnosis is "only a bad dream," even as he goes about setting up support groups, gathering information and other elements of his *Game Plan.* "There I was on the phone, talking to all of these different agencies, while in the back of my mind, I kept thinking that we really were not going to need all of this."

Often, there is evidence that life is getting back to normal. The ill partner may be feeling better, returning to work, the sense of emergency is passed. However, evidence continues to mount that life is not returning to normal. There are pills to take, doctor appointments to keep, support groups to attend, and diminished physical capacity. A medical or emotional crisis often is the signal that the evidence adds up, that the diagnosis is real, and that life will be radically altered. "After he came home from his first bout of pneumocystis, I thought we could settle down, but two days later, his temperature shot up and his doc said to get him to the hospital. It hit me then, things were not going to get back to normal. It felt like at any time we were going to have to cart him off to the hospital." "Things were going pretty smoothly. I was starting to relax. Then he called his mother and told her about the diagnosis. After he talked to her, he became really depressed. I began to sense just what life was going to be like from now on."

Partners often become aware of a chronic air of uncertainty as to what each day will bring in terms of emotional states, energy, or a potential new infection. However, the basic reason for life not returning to normal is that now there exists the very real threat of the loss of the partner through death. Where before there was certainty and continuity in the relationship, now there is the potential, at some unpredictable time, for the loss of the partner, the relationship, and hence the dialogue. "Things were never quite the same again. Always in the back of my mind was the thought that there was an end in sight. Holidays, even on vacation, I would find myself wondering if this would be our last." The unpredictability of the ill partner's medical status enhances the uncertainty. The realization that life is not going to return to normal is often very discouraging and devastating for the well partner. "I very quickly realized that no, life was never going to be the same again."

THE GAME PLAN

I thought if I do everything just right, he won't die. But it was like trying to save a man falling over a cliff.

With the realization that the diagnosis is indeed real, the partner steps up his efforts at assembling *The Game Plan* and ensuring that his partner follows the rules. Before, he may have tried to disbelieve the diagnosis. As the reality becomes evident, he comes to believe in his Plan.

Many elements go into the formulation of the Plan. It is based on what the ill partner has told his well partner that he needs from him during the initial shock of CONFIRMATION: "I need you to be strong"; the particular beliefs of the well partner regarding vitamins, healthy food, exercise; information gleaned from the so-called "underground" healthcare systems: "I subscribed to a newsletter about alternative treatments"; information gleaned from traditional medical sources: "I would sneak into the medical school library and read journals"; the needs of the well partner: "When he is feeling good and looking good I feel better"; needs of the ill partner: "He gets so depressed, I try and cheer him up or give him a push"; and the particular ways the relationship functioned prior to the diagnosis: "I learned a long time ago, I can't force or push anything on him, he has to think it was his idea." The Plan tends to emerge quickly, within hours or days of the diagnosis, and may be altered as the partner acquires new information regarding treatment possibilities.

While there are common elements, the details of *The Game Plan* vary with the relationship. Each relationship is a unique entity comprising two unique individuals. Since the Plan is based on intimate knowledge of the partner, how the two men function as a couple, and the particular beliefs of the well partner, it will vary among couples. The common elements are that the well partner (1) devises a regimen for his ill partner; (2) determines how he is going to conduct himself; and (3) has underlying hope for his Plan.

Often the plan for the ill partner centers around food and exercise. "I put him on an exercise regimen. I set up a small gym in the basement." Gaining back lost weight or keeping up the weight of the ill partner is a common focus. "I make him a protein drink. He just hates it, and I often have to make him drink it, but he gained his weight back." The partner may also attempt to change longstanding habits. "He was the worst eater in the world. He would almost faint at the sight of fresh vegetables. Well, I thought, enough of this. He is going to learn to eat his veggies."

The emotional needs of the partner are addressed as well. "I keep pumping him to have a positive approach to all of this." During the often long periods of relative good health following diagnosis, the well partner may see to it that dream vacations are planned and executed. "We drove from Vancouver all of the way to Baja." "We just got back from Spain." The partner may go to considerable effort to insure his partner's access to support services. "We had a farm that was ninety miles from the nearest city that had a support group, plus he was in a drug study and his physician was in the university hospital. He got so much out of the group, I did everything I could to see that he got there. At first he would take the bus. But when he started getting sicker, I would drive him. I was augmenting our income with some consulting work at the time. Eventually, I packed up the computer and we took a small apartment in the city." He may also see to it that friends and family are engaged in supportive ways. "If he is down, I will call up a couple of his friends and tell them he needs a phone call." The partner makes sure that the couple enjoys life while the opportunities exist. "Several weeks after his diagnosis, I said, 'Don, we can't just sit around here and mope, waiting for you to get sick. We have a lot of living to do yet, and we are going to do it.'"

Another element is how the well partner is going to conduct himself. The well partner takes his plan and the centrality of his role in his partner's life quite seriously. "It was an intense personal responsibility." "I went to every medical appointment with him." Often there is the sense that if anyone can see his partner through this it is he. "I could not wait to get him home from the hospital, I felt I could take better care of him." "I knew what we were up against. It was up to me to see us through this." Partners may be affronted by precautions taken by medical personnel and decide that they will never treat their partner as "though he were diseased." "I refused to wear gloves or a mask when I was around him." How the partner plans on handling his feelings about the situation is included as well. "I kept up a pretty stoic stance." As in CONFIRMATION, the partner may attempt to keep his sadness away from his partner. "I would not let him see me cry." As the ill partner faces the disease, the well partner is often determined that he will have all of the support and care that he needs. "I wanted him to have the best, and he did."

In describing their *Game Plans*, the most frequent word participants used was "push." "I push him to eat." "I have to push him." "I pushed him to go to a group or a shrink." "If he was

feeling sorry for himself I would give him a push." The well partner comes to view himself as the energizer for the ill partner. "I felt
that I was his coach and his cheering section." The well partner
may also protect his own health so that he can continue in his efforts. "Knowing that he was ill, I did my best to keep myself as
healthy as possible. I ate well, got plenty of rest, exercised and I
stopped drinking."

The third and bedrock element of *The Game Plan* is the hope
that, by following the rules, the well partner will be able to sustain
the ill partner until a cure is found. "I really thought he could beat
this disease if I could just keep him alive long enough until a cure is
found." "I thought he would be the first one that made it." This
hope may be at the foreground of the well partner's consciousness
or in the background, and may rise and fall during the course of
THE LONG HAUL, yet it is always there in some shape or form.

The Plan can come to have great, if not magical, power for the
well partner. Invariably, the boundaries between life enhancing and
life saving become blurred. Partners staunchly guard against inter-
ferences with the Plan, and at times, following the rules can have a
desperate, if not obsessional quality. A great deal of energy goes
into carrying out the Plan, with the well partner going to great
lengths to insure that the plan is followed, often at considerable
emotional, physical, and psychological sacrifice to himself.

The ill partner is often highly aware and appreciative of his partner's efforts, acknowledging that he may well have died long before
if it were not for the hovering attention, force feedings, and psychological sustenance that these activities engender. "David keeps me
going. He reminds me to eat, to take my meds. My body is weakened. I am just not as strong as him. He looks after things. I cannot
imagine being here all alone, without someone to make me eat. I
probably would have died several times before if he was not here."
"Do not get AIDS without having a boyfriend around. I would have
kicked off long ago if it was not for him."

Conflicts arise and may be accompanied by considerable anger
when the ill partner is not following the Plan. "It was a constant
battle to get him to do the things he should do." For the well partner, the stakes are high: life or death. The ill partner may have quite
different needs—proving he is still capable of functioning in his
career, not feeling able to eat the meal his partner prepared, or

wanting to experience the pleasure of old habits. Well partners often experience intense panic when they fear that their partners are "giving up" or placing their health at risk. Anger at the partner is often mingled with anger at themselves for either not choosing the right plan, not following the rules correctly or not being a good enough coach. "I felt that I could not let myself mess up." For many well partners, sustaining their ill partners becomes their mission, their meaning in life. The well partner is faced not only with a potential failure in his mission, but also with the loss of meaning in a life that has come to feel all too precarious. "I do not want to lose him."

One of the most common medical problems encountered in AIDS and treatment of the subsequent infections is loss of appetite. Food and making sure his partner eats can become an obsession for the well partner, and may become a source of conflict. "You read everywhere how important it is to keep up their weight, so I am constantly trying to get food into him." For the well partner, the ill partner's lack of appetite and disinterest in food may come to symbolize giving up and giving in to the disease, and hence, to death. For the ill partner, the lack of appetite represents an agonizing revulsion towards food. "When your appetite goes, it's just gone. Not only do you not care about food, the thought of it is just repulsive. I can hear Doug out there in the kitchen cooking up something that he thinks will tempt me and I'll begin to dread it. You just take a small bit of something solid, wash it down with a big drink of liquid and hope it stays down. I know he sometimes takes it personally, but when you are that sick, you are just that sick."

Conflicts around food can reach intense proportions. "It got to the point where if one more person called and asked me what I had to eat that day I was going to scream!" When eating becomes a battleground, both men end up feeling bad, the well partner because he must not be doing something right, and the ill partner because he senses not only the well partner's anger, but the efforts behind the push. "I take it personally when he gets so angry at me because I do not want to eat. I have to stand back and say that it is not my fault, and it is not his fault either." Well partners become very tuned to their partner's emotional state. Panic, and renewed efforts at the Plan ensue if he senses that his partner is "giving in." "Your body gets worn down and you get to the point where you don't want to fight any more. Just too tired." "I can sense it. He gets so frightened that I am going to die. It is like overkill nursing. It is real sweet, but when you are that sick, you are just that sick."

Reluctance or refusals to seek medical or psychological attention, going on long business trips when ill — essentially anything that the well partner perceives as placing his partner at risk — may be met with consternation if not anger or rage. " He insisted on going on an overseas business trip. I was so angry with him, but I could not convince him to cancel it." "I would get so furious, he would do anything to not eat vegetables. I am from California, so I think of vegetables as very important. I'd also get mad at his Doc. He would say 'whatever Will wants . . . .' So there he was chain smoking and eating chips and dip for dinner!"

Often an element of the Plan is to defer to the ill partner when it comes to discussing issues related to the disease, death and dying, or any conflicts that may be brewing in the relationship. While both partners may be thinking about the same issues, the well partner adopts the stance that issues should be discussed on the ill partner's time table. "There were a lot of things I wanted to talk about, but I just felt they should wait until he indicated that he was ready." Ill partners may resent this, feeling the burden is placed upon their shoulders and wish that their partner would initiate discussions. The extension of this dynamic is that it is often the ill partner who expresses anger for the relationship. Often it is he who gets frustrated and asks the partner why he sticks around, tells him to go and find someone else, or to "fuck off and quit bothering me." "He went through a really rough period were he would tell me to leave him and find someone else, or that he wanted to sleep alone that night. It really hurt and pissed me off, but I just quietly endured it. I wonder what would have happened if I had yelled back?" The well partner can feel deeply wounded and resentful when the ill partner lashes out. Often, he learns to either respond in such a way that the anger is contained or to distance himself. "It used to really get to me, but now I realize he has a right to get mad. I either let him stew, or tell him that I am in this thing also, and he needs to treat me better."

The Game Plan serves both the ill partner and the well partner. It provides the ill partner with life sustaining and enhancing attention when he is unable to care for himself and with the knowledge that someone cares deeply for him. It also insures access to the support of friends, relatives, and medical attention. The Plan serves the well partner in that it gives him a desperately needed map to follow during the uncertainty of the disease course, while providing him with a sense that he is doing something to help his partner. The initial helplessness experienced by well partners during the diagnosis is gradually replaced by their Plan and its execution. By tending to the ill partner's physical and psychological needs, the well partner is enhancing the ill partner's ability to remain emotionally available. The sense of "we are in this together" helps to keep at bay the feelings of loneliness and isolation that emerge when one partner is in the world of the living and healthy while the other is in the world of the sick and dying. "Looking back, there really was a gap between us, at times a chasm. Try as I did, it just could not be bridged."

The cruel twist to *The Game Plan* is that it inevitably fails. Despite the heroic efforts of partners and medicine, the body eventually succumbs to the disease process. Well partners who had great hope in their Plan are left following the death of the partner with a deep sense of failure. In the face of such high stakes, the boundaries between life enhancing, life sustaining and life saving become blurred. Following the death of their partner, some surviving partners have a great deal of difficulty acknowledging the great amount of love, devotion and giving that went into caring for their ill partner. Instead, they are plagued by what they perceive as the failure of their *Game Plan*.

REVELATION/NEGOTIATION

How do you tell someone you love that you are dying?

Revelation is a category that flows throughout the entire experience. During THE LONG HAUL, it involves the informing of relatives, friends, and perhaps employers of the diagnosis. Both partners need to reveal the diagnosis at different points and for different reasons. The process of revelation is often a painful one and can involve an elaborate plan worked out between the partners concerning whom to tell, whom not to tell, when to tell and how to tell. As the above quote indicates, *REVELATION* often involves the conveying to close and special people the painful news that one has contracted a terminal disease. And not only a terminal illness but AIDS, the disease that has caused so much panic, anxiety and has become inextricably linked with homosexual activity. Often the revelation is a double or triple revelation. For the ill partner who has hidden his sexuality and the relationship from his family, he must reveal that he has AIDS, that he is gay and that he has a partner. The well partner must then negotiate the ill partner's family through the course of the illness, and often after his partner's death. At first, the task of revelation may feel quite onerous. "It felt like such an important decision. We did not want to make any mistakes."

The well partner may not feel as strong a sense of duty or need to inform his family of his partner's condition, doing so more out of a wish for support than a sense of duty. "I went home a few months after his diagnosis. One night, after the others had gone to bed, I told my mother and broke down crying. I just laid there crying in her lap. I guess there is nothing like mother's comfort." The response of the well partner's family often focuses on their concern for their son's health. Well partners may find this burdensome, especially if they too are concerned about their health. "Sometimes I wish I had not told them. Whenever I call, the first words out of their mouths are not 'How is Steve?' but, 'How is your health?'" The revelation of the illness may also be a multiple revelation for the well partner. "They always thought of us as friends. I guess I did not mind them thinking that way. It gradually became clear to them that we were much, much more than friends."

In anticipating disclosure to individuals who do not know explicitly of one's sexual orientation, anxiety regarding the revelation of one's homosexuality becomes entwined with the anxiety over one's illness, or partner's diagnosis of AIDS. While fear of rejection is a factor, the fear of being treated differently is the overriding concern. The ill and well partner both want friends and relatives to be steady. "My mother gets so anxious as it is, I did not want to have to deal with her stuff on top of everything else I was dealing with." Part of the concern is the fear that friends or family will be so devastated that they will have to be taken care of by the partners rather than be a source of support. "They really do not need something else to worry about." Another prominent fear is that the diagnosis will be experienced as such a burden that friends or family retreat from the relationship. "On one hand, I wanted everyone to know and to stick with me. On the other hand, the idea of someone pulling away was just too devastating."

Relationships with friends and relatives are potential sources of a great deal of support. However, the initial sadness or shock of an informed individual also brings home the reality of the situation. "When I told my best friend, he broke down and cried. There I was, feeling guilty that I had upset him so." A sense of shared sadness however, may be experienced as comforting. "We just held on to each other and cried."

"Checking in" by friends and families may be experienced as either supportive or an irritating reminder of the illness. "I appreciate it but sometimes it gets to be a bit much. It is not like I am always on the verge of death." "I like the phone calls, but frankly, I get tired of giving medical updates. I want to hear what is going on in other peoples lives." If the partner with AIDS has lost weight or does not look well, he may see this reflected in the expressions of informed friends, a reflection that he may not want to see. "I finally got him to go to a party for the first time since his diagnosis. He had gained a lot of weight back, but he still was thin. He was very concerned about being with people. He said he did not need any reminders about how sick he had been."

An AIDS diagnosis is often accompanied by a massive loss of self-esteem for both partners. "We felt embarrassed and ashamed, like we were icky, tainted, spoiled." Men whose experience is that of fighting a long battle to win their parents respect as gay men and recognition of the validity of their relationship are often faced with a sense of potential loss of that respect. "It has not been all that long since she finally began to ask about Terry." Often the parents are in their mid to later years, and may be in frail health. The ill partner may fear sending them to an earlier grave, or adding an unfair burden to their lives. "I would not be a bit surprised if one of them had a coronary or a stroke."

The underlying fear often is that the ill partner feels that he will deeply disappoint his parents. The more the ill partner feels is at stake, the more overwhelming the task of *REVELATION* will be.

"When I was growing up, my brother was the one showered with attention. Well, he has turned out to be a massive disappointment to them. My father and I have developed a great deal of respect for each other over the past few years. They are proud of me and what I have achieved, essentially on my own. I know it would be devastating for him to find out I was gay, let alone that I had AIDS." The more vulnerable the ill partner feels because of shaken self-esteem, the more he dreads anything but an immediate acceptance of himself, his plight, and his partner.

The well partner often receives more support when informing his family than the ill partner does when informing his. "It was very painful. We sat here in the kitchen and I held him while he talked to his parents. Several times he started to cry so hard that I took over and talked to them for a while until he was able to continue. I told my mother a few weeks later." Families invariably respond in a manner consistent with their previous style of functioning. Families that are acquainted with the partner and who have integrated him into the family system more readily rally to their son and his relationship. "His mother called me and told me that she was counting on me, since she lived so far away." The process for an otherwise accepting family may be a bit slower when they are forced to integrate the reality of the diagnosis, their son's sexuality, and his partner at the same time. "We hit her [mother] with a lot at once, but we all hung in there. In the long run, she was a tremendous person."

The well partner may be greatly relieved when the ill partner informs his parents, especially if he has been delaying the revelation. "I was so relieved when he finally told them. I did not have to be the one to do it, especially if he was very sick." The ill partner may also be relieved once the revelation has been made, especially if the family turns out to be supportive. "After he told them, it was like a burden had been lifted off his chest. They have been tremendously supportive."

A family that has maintained a distant relationship with their son may maintain their distance or may want to become closely involved. "They sent him cards and letters, but never came to visit, even though they lived only 60 miles away." "After so many years of having minimal contact with him, and certainly not any with me, they showed up, wanted to know everything and to call the shots." At the minimum, the family must integrate the reality that their son's partner is the central person in his life. Families may have understood the relationship as being more like friends than spouses, but over the course of THE LONG HAUL the centrality of the bond becomes evident. Some families may fight against this, attempting to dictate treatment decisions or aftercare plans. "Thank God we had the power of attorney drawn up and we had a doctor who knew I had been designated to make decisions. I had to show it to them. He was too out of it. Things were tense for awhile, but once they settled down we got to know each other." Some families may come to greatly appreciate their sons' partner and take comfort that their sons are in such good hands. "His mother called me and told me how grateful she was that I was there, also that she was counting on me, since she lived so far away."

The crises of the diagnosis and acute illnesses can create difficulties for families and partners as all parties attempt to realize that the centrality of family relationships that existed in childhood have altered considerably over the years. The threat of the loss of a son may prompt a regression on the family's part and they may attempt to re-establish or assume the primary relations of childhood, not the secondary status that evolves as adult love relationships are established. "I wanted to say, 'For Christsakes, he is not eight years old, he is a grown up man, and I am his lover.'"

Well partners may be very impatient with family members' expression of ambivalent feelings regarding homosexuality and may attempt to shield their partners from any negative feelings or reactions. Families often confuse any inherent sense of "wrongness" about homosexuality with the "wrongness" of their son facing a terminal illness. "I spent a lot of time with her [mother] just talking about it and answering questions. Sometimes I had to try very hard to be patient with her, but I did not want Stan to have to listen to her homophobic stuff." "It was pretty hard to sit there while she blamed herself for doing something wrong, and that if he was not gay, he would not have this disease." Just as men with AIDS and their partners may feel tainted and stigmatized, so may their families. "She was afraid to tell her neighbors what was really going on."

If their partners are very ill, some well partners are faced with meeting and negotiating families on their own. "She [mother] knew me and that we had lived together for ten years, but he had never sat down and said we were lovers. They did not think he was going to make it out of the hospital with his first bout of pneumocystis, so there I was on the phone telling her that he was gay, that I was his partner, that he had AIDS, that the doctor thought he was not going to make it, and to get out here as soon as possible."

Partners who have planned ahead will have legal documents to fall back on. However, this serves to only partially mitigate the burden of an angry, hostile family. Often the partner becomes viewed as the "symbolic transmitter" of the disease. The family can either contain this fantasy and attempt to balance it out against the care they observe the well partner giving or they can act it out, convinced that this would not have happened "if it were not for that man." "It was awful, I was walking down the hospital hallway and his mother appeared and started screaming 'Get out of here! Get out! You snippy! You are the one who gave this to him!' They were so hostile and started so many yelling matches that the staff threatened to bar them from the hospital. The social worker negotiated separate visiting hours so we would not run into each other."

In sharp contrast, other families establish deep ties with their son's partner along with the sense that they are all helping to take care of him. These relationships often endure after the death of the partner, organized around the shared sense of loss. "I really did not know them all that well. I had met them a few times and spoken to them on the phone, but I really learned to respect and enjoy them." In the long run, both partners benefit from the establishment of a harmonious network. "It was great knowing that there were not going to be any problems with his family. His mother told me that she considered me his spouse and that she would go along with whatever I decided." In the case of a conflictual relationship with the family, the well partner may have to endure it long after his partner's death, in the form of lawsuits or less formal but equally burdensome interactions. "There was kind of a truce right after he died. They even invited me over to their house after the funeral. But a few days later they started in again, wanting into the apartment and wanting the name of his lawyer."

Many of the same factors come into play when informing friends. The overriding concern is to gain support, not to be treated differently or feel that their friends' distress is an added burden. "The most helpful friends are the ones who do not treat me any differently." Again the revelation may be a double or triple one, especially if one or both of the partners has a large number of heterosexual friends or colleagues who do not know of their orientation or the relationship. "I have always kept my personal and private lives separate." Some partners deprive themselves of potential support because the process of informing people of their diagnosis, orientation and partner status may feel too messy, when what they desire is unconditional support. "A woman that I worked with went through her husband dying of cancer the same time Jim was sick. I could see by the look in her eyes that she was going through the same things I was. I would have loved to talk to her about it, but it just felt too risky."

The well partner may go against his partner's wishes and inform family or friends. "He did not want his family to know, but during his second hospitalization, he was so sick I went ahead and told them." The partner may inform others in the face of a medical emergency, or in the service of added support for the well partner. "He did not want anyone to know. He said he did not want their sympathy or to be treated any different. His birthday was coming up and I wanted to have a surprise party for him. I stuck my neck out and told our close circle of friends. The party came off without a hitch. Afterwards he said, 'They know, don't they?', I took a deep breath and said yes, that I had told them. He was not angry at all." Once informed, friends often become an extensive support system for the relationship and the hardships the partners face. "Subsequently they have just been great."

Often during THE LONG HAUL a "special relationship" develops with a member of the ill partner's family, usually a sibling or at times one or both of the partner's parents, most often his mother. Ties that develop with the partner's siblings are very important. "His sister had visited a few times and I really liked her. After he became ill, we developed a very close relationship." The partner and sib are often closer in age, and the quality of the loss is more similar. It is not the impending loss of a child, and the two individuals feel more of a sense of equality. The sib may become invaluable in helping the partner negotiate the other members of the family and when necessary, mediating conflicts. "Later on she told me that she had answered some of their parent's pretty basic questions. I don't think I would have had the patience to endure that." When sibs are not available or not as involved as the parents, strong ties may develop with the mother or father. Often there is a sense of being "adopted" by the family. "His mom said as far as she was concerned I was part of the family." The central factor again revolves around the shared understanding of the pain involved with the terminal illness of someone all parties love in their own ways.

Some men will have to inform their employers. "He was very apprehensive about telling his company. He works for a very conservative financial firm. They were wonderful. He did not know it, but he was scheduled to be laid off. When he told them what was going on, they kept him on at full salary until he had to go on disability." "My company has been great. Out here, any major corporation has had plenty of experience in dealing with employees with AIDS." Other men may opt for saying they are ill but with another disease. "I told them it was cancer."

Individuals whom one or both of the partners experience as being exceptionally sustaining become helpers. Helpers can be friends, professionals performing a specific function, or family members, especially the sib with whom the well partner has developed a "special relationship." Regardless of relationship or function, helpers are experienced by the partners as people who can be relied upon emotionally or physically, or who steer the way through difficult tasks such as negotiating disability procedures or obtaining support services. The ill partner's physician becomes a central figure in his life and an intense sustaining bond often develops. "I really trust him. I know he is going to do his best for me." Well partners often benefit from knowing and trusting the ill partner's physician and are highly aware of and comforted by their ill partner's alliance. "He keeps talking about how wonderful she is, I am going to go down and meet her next time he goes in." The more confident and comfortable the well partner is with the physician, the less likely conflicts are to develop, especially the difficult situation of the physician being targeted as not doing all he can in behalf of the ill partner. "It was really comforting having Dr. S. as his physician."

People who have helped "steer the way" through bureaucratic tasks or have provided help during acute illnesses or the emotional roller coaster that both partners experience are often highly regarded during THE LONG HAUL. "It was by accident that we found him. He is a social worker at the hospital and knew how to do just about everything: disability, support services, you name it, he seemed to be able to make it happen." Later, they are remembered fondly by the surviving partner. Helpers, be they friends, relatives or professionals, form a supportive network, each contributing in their own way to the sustenance of the individual men and the relationship.

FEVER PITCH

We were lying in bed, watching TV. He had a cat scan the day before. The doctor called and said that we had better get him to the hospital right away. They had found a tumor in his brain stem and were afraid that his respiratory system would shut down.

For many partners, THE LONG HAUL will consist of periods of relatively good health contrasted by periods of acute illness. "In between his hospitalizations, we had some very good quality time. But the times he was really sick were just hell." When the partner is acutely ill and/or hospitalized, the well partner often experiences the return of *Automatic Pilot.* As in confirmation, the well partner is often attempting to manage his career and the couple's home, negotiate parents, and be with his partner as much as possible.

Periods of acute illness add to the sense of uncertainty that the partners experience. Each episode may bring with it discouragement and a reminder of just how tenuous life has become. "I am discouraged. I thought the aerosol pentamadine would control the PCP, but it didn't." "Whenever he is sick I start dwelling on the mortality. That is when it really slaps you in the face." Acute illness may strike when the well partner is unavailable to care for his partner. "I was out of town. My father had been hospitalized and was very ill himself. I called home to check on Jim. He was totally confused. He could not find his shoes. He did not know what day it was. I was panic stricken. I had to call some friends to go over there and stay with him until I could get back."

Both partners may experience relief when the emergency passes and the partner again returns home. Yet each may wonder what will come next. "After each hospitalization he seems to have lost a little more ground. It takes him longer to bounce back." "I did not think this was going to be the last round. But, I did think that we were farther along in the battle than I ever thought would happen."

BALANCING

When your partner has AIDS, it is like you have it too.

The most complicated and necessary category of THE LONG HAUL is *Balancing.* Essentially it is an ongoing, evolving, and difficult attempt throughout THE LONG HAUL to balance on a tightrope of hope and not fall into despair. Hope stems from the dialogue between the partners — the sense of togetherness, that each one is there for the other — and from the sustenance derived from the support of friends, family, professionals and support groups. Despair stems from a disruption in the dialogue and the sense of aloneness that accompanies the disruption.

Illness and depression are the central causes of disruption in the dialogue. Since illness and depression due to the multiple losses that both partners encounter are central to the experience of THE LONG HAUL, the need for a balance is acutely necessary to prevent the well partner from falling into despair. Integral components of *Balancing* are the *Game Plan*, the sustenance derived from supportive relationships with "helpers" and other individuals to whom the diagnosis has been revealed, and the dialogue between the partners. *Balancing* is essentially the private experience of the well partner.

Individually and collectively, each partner faces stresses that threaten to tax him to the point of being overwhelmed and falling into despair. The ill partner is faced with the knowledge of his terminal illness, the stigma and anxiety associated with AIDS, the multiple losses incurred throughout the illness: individual dreams, career goals, financial problems, identity, physical decline, in many cases cognitive impairment and the daily grind of feeling more or less ill. The well partner is faced with the knowledge of his partner's terminal illness and the subsequent threat of his loss through death. Additionally, he must physically care for his partner through the periods of illness, be with his partner through his losses, experience the partner's depression and anxiety, and negotiate his partner's family. As the ill partner becomes increasingly disabled and the well partner's responsibilities increase, a growing sense of aloneness often comes over the well partner as the dialogue decreases and he anticipates life without his partner. Collectively, the partners face the loss of their dreams and goals for the relationship and the threat of the loss of each other through death—the ultimate disruption in the dialogue.

Balancing is an individual and collective need, hence there are individual and collective aspects to this property. The aim of *Balancing* is to maintain the dialogue between the partners in the face of potential and actual disruptions. A variety of experiences go into helping each partner maintain his and their balance. The central need is for sustaining human relationships and experiences in the face of the multiple stresses incurred with the disease process. Individually, the support of family and friends, the "special relationship," and professionals help each partner fight off despair and maintain the dialogue. Collectively, one can observe adjustments in the relationship which also serve this function.

When the partners enter the experience, either at WONDERING or CONFIRMATION, the partners begin to identify themselves as the "well one" and the "ill one." The diagnosis of the ill partner serves to set the two men apart; one is now ill, the other is well. If both men develop AIDS, the partners tend to keep elements of the original "ill one/well one" constellation. While the diagnosis sets the two men apart, the well one/ill one delineation and other elements of *The Game Plan* serve to bring them together. Each partner has a role to follow, a role that ultimately serves to preserve and maintain the dialogue. Yet these roles have their own pitfalls and need for balancing. In the course of negotiating the relationship prior to the diagnosis, a process has gradually occurred where each man has become the central figure in the other's life. The diagnosis of AIDS, while setting them apart, also thrusts each man into an even more central role.

In the midst of THE LONG HAUL, partners are often acutely aware of how their lives have changed. "There have been a lot of changes in the past two years. It is amazing the amount of changes one, two I guess, can endure." The well partner is often acutely aware of his partner's losses, reactions to the losses, and efforts to keep going in the face of the illness. "He was never able to return to work. He was very disappointed by that." "His energy level is so poor. He is going to work, but that is about all he is doing. All his energy is going into being able to get through a day's work." The well partner is also acutely aware of how both their lives have changed. "I feel like it has totally disrupted our lives. We still socialize with people, but all of the people we socialize with have AIDS, or are somehow involved with it." Partners whose social networks have been hit hard by the epidemic face the loss of friends to the same disease. "You are confronted on a daily basis with people who are not there anymore. It is hard to keep up positive energy when, little by little, people are being whittled away, right out of your life." But partners are also aware of the people who have been helpful. "It has been real neat to see all of the people who come around and check on us, all of the people who have helped out, all of the people who have been there, instead of 'cut and run.'"

In the face of so many changes and losses, the ill partner may experience a profound loss of meaning in life. "After I was diagnosed, I would sit and wonder, 'Why am I going on?'" The answer is often easier for the well partner. "I am going on to keep him going on." The well partner takes his role as the "well one/strong one" quite seriously. At first, the well partner may question his capacity to endure the hardships, but often it is an automatic decision to stick by his partner. Later, during THE LONG HAUL, well partners may come to realize just how strong they are. "You come across a lot of inner strength that you may not have known was there before it was put to the test."

In relationships that have endured over time and are based on a solid sense of connection and togetherness, partners have undoubtedly experienced periods of disruption in the dialogue, times where their partner was more or less depressed, preoccupied, or ambivalent and consequently more or less available. However, the partner eventually pulled out of his depression, or resolved his ambivalence and once again the dialogue was established. Hence the partners know that while a disruption in the dialogue can be painful, the dialogue can be re-established.

The fuel for the well partner's dedication appears to be the hope of the re-established dialogue, and the knowledge of the strength of the attachment between the two men. The threat of the loss of the partner versus the intimate knowledge of the strength of their attachment, the comfort, and the hope that come from a dialogue with their partner forms a "tension" that serves to fuel the well partner's efforts to sustain his partner as long as possible, hopefully until a cure is found. "I go on as if there is no end to this whole thing. I just try to make sure that we live our lives as normally as possible."

Impact of the Ill Partner's Emotional Status

For several months after my diagnosis and going on disability, I was a couch potato. I just laid around all day, nothing interested me. I was very negative. I just did not see any point in going on. But my friends and Jeff kept plugging away, trying to cheer me up. I don't think it was any one thing, rather it was an accumulation. We kept coming across people who really cared. One day I realized the reason to go on was to keep living the best my body would allow and that was reason enough. I have been a very negative person all of my life – but now I think I am more positive than I ever have been. I get up, go to my doctor and chemotherapy appointments, and I am gradually painting my house. If I get half a door done, one wall or a whole room in a day, it is all fine.

Often men go through a several month period of depression following the diagnosis of AIDS, and the dialogue may be diminished. Essentially, the well partner is not experiencing the same quality of connection as before, while he is also faced with the knowledge of the terminal condition of his partner. "It was very difficult to come home from work and find him curled up on the couch in front of the

TV. He was not watching TV, he was just sitting there and hiber-
nating.'' A highly consistent process is observed in men following
an AIDS diagnosis. Concurrent with the initial depression and anxiety another process is occurring. The ill partner is gradually informing others of his diagnosis, establishing or strengthening the alliance with his physician, and becoming involved in support groups
or individual therapy. The men who make the best adaptation to the
illness appear to be those who do not have a prior history of severe
depression or anxiety, have experienced support in the past from a
variety of relationships and whose financial status is not in acute
danger. Gradually, the experience of supportive, caring and helpful
people interested in the ill partner's welfare reaches a "critical
mass" and the partner finds his depression lifting and a renewed
interest in life.

Initially, the well partner is often depressed also and both men
may experience the other as "pulling back." "You keep saying
that I was depressed and withdrawn. You were pretty withdrawn
yourself." The hope of restoring the dialogue serves to fuel *The
Game Plan*, and the partner's continued attentiveness. Throughout
THE LONG HAUL the well partner often is giving a great deal but
not getting a great deal back. As mentioned before, depression,
anxiety and illness all serve to interrupt the dialogue. Yet the well
partner continues to give. "I kept pushing him, trying to get him
interested in something."

To fuel his efforts, the well partner needs his own sources of
support. If the initial desire of the ill partner is to not reveal the
diagnosis to friends, the well partner may find himself feeling quite
isolated in the face of his partner's depression and the lack of
sources of support. "I was beginning to feel cut off from my friends
and all alone." Some men may go against their partner's wishes in
order to obtain support from their friends. "I was over at John's
house one afternoon a month or so after the diagnosis. He is like an
older gay brother to me. I was moping around, he asked if Jim and I
had a fight or something. I just broke down and told him everything. He held me and I cried for a good half hour." Some men will
join a support group for partners and gain a great deal of sustenance. "I go to a support group for significant others. It has been
great. I have established some good friendships." Other men will

rely on the informed circle of friends and their careers. "I keep busy with my professional activities. That helps balance against my constant preoccupation with his illness and my potential illness."

Well partners are often greatly relieved to see their partner's depression lifting. "I do not know whether it is the spring weather or what, but he has just been in a super mood lately. Before, I could not get him out. Now, I cannot keep him home." Partners are especially relieved to see a growing determination to keep fighting the disease. "He comes back from his group and says, 'You would not believe those people. So much strength and energy'. I say, 'yeah, I bet they are saying the same thing about you.' It rejuvenates him, gives him that extra will to keep going." A strong "fighting spirit" often evolves within individuals diagnosed with AIDS. They become determined to fight the disease and continue on with life as best they can. "You have to be a fighter with this disease or else it will overtake you. I think that is why we have lasted so long, we are both fighters. There are a lot of things we want to do yet."

A great deal of sustenance is gained by fighting the disease in accordance with the individual's and couple's Plan. This also serves as a powerful balance against despair, fueling the fight to go on. At times this can reach the degree of men striving to be the "best AIDS patient" or an "AIDS poster boy." The well partner may also push this spirit as it is a reassurance that his partner is not giving up. A potential problem is that this stance is easier to maintain when one is feeling well. It is considerably more difficult to maintain during periods of illness or in the wake of a major loss, such as the need to retire from one's employment and go on disability insurance. At times, a balance must also be struck between the need to fight and have a positive outlook and the need to mourn a loss, which requires the validation of depressed affect.

An integral component of the experience of AIDS is the series of losses that the individual encounters. Each loss is experienced, mourned, perhaps raged against, and hopefully integrated and adapted to by the partner. This process takes time and each loss may be accompanied by a disruption in the dialogue. Thus each loss of the ill partner is potentially also a loss for the well partner. "It was a hard few weeks after he went on disability. He was really depressed. He can be pretty unbearable when he is down and grouchy. But gradually, he settled into a routine and perked up again.''

Often the couple's sexual relationship is lost for at least part of THE LONG HAUL. "After he became ill, the sex just went away completely. He just was not interested.'' The ill partner may lose his desire for sex, knowing that he contracted the disease through a sexual encounter. "I know how I got this disease and I am trying really hard to work my way back into having sex again.'' When people are ill and/or stressed, the desire for sexual experiences may be greatly diminished. "Who wants to have sex when you have a 101 degree temperature?''

Some couples will try to make an effort to reestablish the sexual relationship. "He will go along with it, but I know he is just doing it for me, not because he is into it.'' Fear of transmission may also be a factor, and early attempts to reintroduce sexual encounters may be anxiety-ridden. "It was really awkward at first, gradually we got back into it, though it was never the same.'' Often it is the ill partner who is more concerned with this despite precautions taken in the service of "safe sex.'' "He keeps saying that he is worried about giving it to me. We do safe sex, but he is still anxious.'' The loss of the sexual component of the dialogue is often hardest on the well partner. His desire is often not as affected as his partner's and he may yearn for the intimacy of the sexual encounter. "It wasn't so much that I was horny as much as I just wanted to feel close to him.''

THE LONG HAUL is often experienced as a series of highs and lows, of calm periods and medical or emotional crises. The well partner may find himself burning out, or fearing that he will burn out. Often there is the feeling that AIDS is creeping into every aspect of their lives. "It was getting pretty intense for awhile. With the support groups and all, gradually all the important people in our lives either had AIDS or their lover had AIDS.'' Seeking extra support from friends or renewing interest in religious or metaphysical pursuits all serve to balance the well partner's feeling that the illness is threatening to become consuming. These outside supports and interests enable him to maintain his efforts on behalf of his partner and restore the dialogue as much as possible. Ultimately they are a significant factor in the well partner's adaptation to the gradual diminishing of the dialogue over the course of the illness, and a buffer against falling into despair. "We went down to the beach for the Harmonic Convergence. There was a wonderful energy there. I am sure there were other people with AIDS, but the energy felt so different, so peaceful and exciting, so removed from AIDS and what it brings."

The Well Partner's Antibody Status

> *I assumed I was positive also. The day I found out my test result was an emotional rollercoaster – the worst day of my life. I guess I had that hope – a tiny little hope that I would be negative.*

A tremendous amount of dedication and energy goes into being the "well one." Partners are acutely aware of the sense of burden that is now a part of their lives, yet they rarely complain. Rather, they continue to push themselves and often their partner on in an effort to adapt to the disease as well as possible. Potential threats to the partner's functioning as the well one are guarded against, often by both partners. The most common perceived threat is seropositivity and the potential illness of the well partner. "I was so afraid that I would get sick while Jim was ill. I needed to stay well so I could take care of him."

THE LONG HAUL proved to be the second point at which the well partners in the study chose to have themselves tested. Well partners often fear that finding out they are positive will plunge them into despair, and drastically interfere with their ability to carry out the Plan. "There was just too much to worry about already. I do not think I could handle the emotional upheaval I have seen other people go through and manage all that I am having to manage now." The assumption of being HIV-positive which began during WONDERING or CONFIRMATION continues for men who have chosen not to test their assumption. "I have not been tested, nor do I intend to be tested. But there is no doubt in my mind that I have the virus also."

Generally, the decision to have oneself tested is made in terms of balancing the anxiety of knowing with the anxiety of not knowing. Men who decide to test during THE LONG HAUL are usually feeling quite stressed, if not depleted, over the amount of energy expended on their partners' behalf. They may have physical symptoms that suggest immune impairment, and are experiencing a good deal of anxiety over the possibility that they, too, will contract the disease. "The anxiety that I was experiencing was getting out of hand. I had a rash, and it came to the point where it was making me so nuts that I had to find out if it was related to being HIV positive." Testing at this point is approached with considerable apprehension. "The day before, I thought about cancelling, but I said, enough. I am going to go ahead and do this." A positive test and the potential for emotional distress threatens to disrupt the role of the "strong one." A negative test releases them from the fear of AIDS, but also sets them apart from their partner.

If the partner tests negative, he is greatly relieved. "I was negative. I cannot describe how relieved I am." He may at first not believe the results. "I am going to be tested again in a few months, then I will be certain." With the negative results, the partner is spared the guilt of possible transmission. "I felt wonderful knowing that I had not passed it on to him." He may also find that he has acquired added energy to put into helping his partner through the illness. "Now that I do not have to use the energy worrying about being positive, all of my energy goes into taking care of him."

The ill partner is often relieved as well. "It is great knowing that we are not going to have two sick people in the house." Some ill partners are less demonstrative of their relief than others. "He did not really react, but I know he felt good about it." Some well partners feel an enormous pressure to test their status. Physicians may recommend it, friends often inquire when they are informed of the ill partner's diagnosis and parents worry. Well partners may come to resent this feeling that they are being pressured into something that carries great consequences that they may feel only they fully understand. "The fact is that I do not want to know, not now anyway. A couple of friends had me believing that there was something wrong with me for not wanting to find out for sure."

Some men come to view testing during THE LONG HAUL as potentially providing them with an alternative to the illness of their partner. "After so many months of struggling, I realized that I wanted to live, not follow Martin. If I test positive, and go on AZT and that gives me a few more years, then that is fine." Earlier in the experience, the partner may have felt his own desire to live was somehow disloyal to his partner. But as the experience continues, and he encounters data regarding early intervention, he may begin to view himself in terms other than his partner.

In couples where both men have developed AIDS, the partner who is the second to be diagnosed tends to hold on to his status as the "well one." "I guess I still think of myself as the well one. I tend to look at John as being the one who is slightly more frail. He tires easily. I will be the one who takes on the physically demanding tasks." When the previously well partner is diagnosed, both men have to make adjustments. "I found myself kind of resenting it. Hey, I am the one who is supposed to be sick! I have to admit I enjoy being taken care of. Seriously though, it was very disconcerting, having to worry about both of us being sick at the same time."

There may actually be periods when both men are sick. "I was two weeks into a bout of pneumocystis and Don started getting sick. The more it looked like he was coming down with it also, the more I panicked. I knew I just did not have the energy yet to be able to take care of him the way he would need." During periods of mutual illness, the partners will have to rely on support services. "They were great, we would not have gotten through it if it was not for the help we received. As soon as I was back on my feet, I could manage for both of us."

The diagnosis of the "well" partner may also be experienced as a different kind of loss for the ill partner. "I was really getting a lot of comfort out of thinking that he would survive me well into the future. I really do not have any close family, and I wanted to leave my estate to him, sort of a legacy. My dream was that he could take the money left over and use it to build a new life for himself once I am gone." A strong sense of "being in this together" develops in couples when both have AIDS. However, a fear lurks that both men will be sick at the same time. "That is our biggest fear. That one time when there was an overlap, between my being fully recovered and his coming down was a real nightmare. But, other than that, we are making the best of it."

Falling into Despair

*One day I was coming home from work. It had been a rough
week. Stan had been very depressed and withdrawn. He had not
been sleeping well, so neither was I. I found myself furious and
thinking "Why doesn't he hurry up and die." I was devastated
when I realized what I was thinking.*

Perhaps the most painful experience for the well partner during
THE LONG HAUL is becoming enraged with his partner. The well
partner may find himself wishing for a quick end to the situation,
that his partner would hurry up and die. In a milder form, he may
become preoccupied with his own life, worried about his health and
his future or discouraged by the lack of joy in his current existence.
"A couple of times I found myself sitting in a chair across the room
from Don, watching him sleep, and daydreaming about what I
would do when this was all over." The well partner is often
shocked and feels horribly guilty when he finds himself wishing for
an end or preoccupied with his own status. It is experienced as an
affront to the *Plan* and his role as the "well one" whose job is to
look after and care for his partner. Often, this experience comes
back to haunt him after the partner's death in the form of guilty
ruminations. Not only has his *Game Plan* failed, but he lives with
the knowledge that he had sometimes wished his partner dead. This
often appears at a point in the mourning process of intense missing
of the partner, when the surviving partner would give anything to
have him back.

An integral component of the well partner's balancing is the emotional state of the ill partner. Again, depression and anxiety interfere with the dialogue and decrease the well partner's experience of
his mate being there for him. "It is hard when he gets into one of
his slumps. He just mopes around, doesn't do anything around the
house, he is grouchy, and nothing I try seems to help." The degree
to which the well partner feels burdened and overwhelmed, if not
resentful, appears directly related to the degree to which he experiences the dialogue with his partner. The well partner's falling into
despair and wishing for an end, or preoccupation with his own un-
met needs or uncertain future, is triggered by a disruption in the

dialogue. It may come in reaction to a protracted withdrawal or verbal lashing out by the ill partner. "For one and a half weeks he moped around, and laid on the sofa. I got frustrated and said, 'Damn it get up and do something.' As soon as I had said it I felt horrible." "When he gets into a mood it can be pretty awful. I got so pissed the other night, I had to go out for a walk and cool down." While the scales may be greatly tipped in the direction of giving to the ill partner, the well partner is able to keep giving and not fall into despair as long as he experiences some sense of dialogue with his partner. "I need his stability, his love. There is so much that he gives me. I love to watch him sleep just to know that he is there."

Some partners will find themselves becoming purely overwhelmed in the face of extended periods of caring for their partner during acute illness. "I hit the lowest point during the whole year and a half after I was up all night trying to get him settled. He was so miserable, could not sleep, and could not stop the sweating. I had worked all day before and had several crucial meetings the next day. Around seven a.m. he finally dozed off. I laid down beside him and just started to bawl. I cried and cried."

Disruptions in the dialogue occur from time to time in all relationships. When they occur in a relationship where AIDS is a factor, they are experienced more intensely. The stakes feel higher, stresses are greater and the despair is deeper. Partners function as each other's "rock in the raging sea." Each needs the other to be there, in his own way. Well partners may forget that they have needs as well, as they pour energy into caring for their partners. Each man is bound to become discouraged during the course of the illness. When the well partner becomes discouraged, he often feels that he has failed.

RENEWAL

It really felt wonderful. It was late. We had been out with friends. We came home and found ourselves sitting in the dark, holding hands and talking. I don't remember what exactly we talked about. I just remember how good it felt.

While partners may face a series of minor or major disruptions in the dialogue over the course of THE LONG HAUL, they often experience *Renewal* in the relationship as well. When the system of Balances is in order and physical health is good, partners find themselves in deep discussions, finding out new things about each other, experiencing renewed joy in old activities or new experiences. "The stupid things, the private moments, mean so much more, just because you are together and sharing." They may discover or rediscover the depth of their commitment and the qualities that attracted them to each other in the first place. "I always thought he was a strong, loving person. These past few months have really proved that. I have also seen a very vulnerable side of him." "It definitely has brought us closer together than ever before." Equally important may be the two men finding a way to acknowledge and share their mutual grief. "Sometimes we cry together. I do not think we feel sorry for ourselves, but we do find ourselves just holding each other and crying."

These experiences are quite meaningful for both men and are often experienced as islands of calm in the midst of a life that has become an ocean of hardships. "We went away for the weekend and declared the bed-and-breakfast an 'AIDS-Free Zone.'" Some partners may find themselves doing volunteer work with other AIDS patients, passing on the tricks of adaptation to the illness that they have discovered as a way of repaying the help they have received from others. "We both are on disability, so when we are feeling up to it, we work for a couple of agencies. People have been so kind and given so much to us, we feel that we should repay them somehow."

Couples may find themselves moving in together after maintaining separate residences over the course of a several year relationship. "This disease has cemented our relationship. We finally settled down and moved in together. Before, we were into a lot of competitive stuff. Now we are more into each other." A weekend retreat may bring a welcome respite and reconnection. "We spent the weekend downtown at a hotel. It was wonderful. No phone calls, no support groups. Just the two of us."

Several couples in the study were married during the 1987 March on Washington. "We were planning on going to the March on

Washington. A friend of mine told me about the wedding ceremony they were going to have. I thought it sounded terribly romantic. I put the bug in Dan's ear and he liked the idea also. I spent several days running around shopping for rings. Dan set limits on me, I was getting a bit extravagant. We settled on a gay jeweler who wasn't weirded out about ordering two men's wedding bands. We put the fear of God in him that they had to be ready by Thursday when we were to leave for Washington. Well, they were, and we went to the wedding. We were a little disappointed that it was so political. We were getting real tired standing through all of the speeches. But when the ceremony finally came around, it was very moving. I am really glad we did it."

DERAILMENT

I thought I was prepared for anything, but I was not prepared for him to lose his mind.

Derailment is a category that flows throughout the entire experience. *Derailment* during THE LONG HAUL results from those experiences that significantly impair the couple's ability to sustain their dialogue and/or place added stress on the well partner. During THE LONG HAUL, the most common forms of *Derailment* are: the emergence of AIDS dementia in the ill partner; parents who refuse to acknowledge the centrality of the relationship and cannot contain their anger, subsequently creating a series of conflictual interactions around their son; a disease course that progresses rapidly after CONFIRMATION; and partners who have a great deal of difficulty talking to each other about the disease and the impact on their lives.

AIDS dementia moderately to severely impairs cognitive and emotional functioning and can sharply curtail, if not cut off, the dialogue. The development of symptoms creates added anxiety for the well partner as he must become increasingly vigilant, being certain that his partner has taken his medication, remembers to eat and has not gotten lost or disoriented. The partner may also be faced with his partner not recognizing him. "The first time it happened I was shocked. He got up one morning and asked, 'Where is

Donald?' I said, 'I am Donald.' He then said, 'No, not you, Donald, my boyfriend Donald. Where has he gone? Is he coming back soon?' I just wanted to break down and cry.''

Severe forms of AIDS Dementia may require the partner to be institutionalized. "He completely lost his mind. I couldn't take care of him anymore. He got to be more than I could manage at home." When the partner must be institutionalized, the well partner is deprived not only of the emotional dialogue but his partner's physical presence as well. The well partner may feel acutely isolated and cut off. Life may feel in limbo. His partner is alive, but only a shell of his former self. Often the well partner is left with an acute sense of failure that he could not sustain his partner at home.

Parents who create conflict about the care of their son and/or refuse to acknowledge the validity of the relationship create a tremendous burden for the well partner. "I did not know that people could be so ugly." Many well partners in the study feared that their partner's parents would step in and take their partner "back home." While this did not happen to any of the men in the study, professionals who were interviewed did say that they had seen this occur with devastating effects on the partner. Some parents may threaten or raise the possibility of such action, and even if they do not follow through, it creates considerable anxiety and burden on the partner.

Some partners have to become vigilant, protecting their partner from the actions of parents that may be against the ill partner's wishes. "Walt was very specific. He did not want his parents praying or carrying on around him. It got to the point were I did not want to leave them alone with him, because his father would start trying to exorcise demons from him. A couple of times, Walt asked me to, 'get them out of here.' " The effects of burdensome parents may be greatly mitigated by the presence and support of a group of friends or by a sib of the ill partner who has formed a "special relationship" with the well partner. An added burden is created for the ill partner as well, as he is often acutely aware of the tension that exists among his caregivers.

In cases such as the one cited in *Revelation/Negotiation*, hospital personnel may intervene, affirming the partner's rights, and attempting to contain the parents' acting out. Whether conflicts with the parents are mild or severe, they create added tension for the well partner during THE LONG HAUL. After the death, the surviving partner is left with a set of unpleasant memories that color the mourning process. The deep sense of insult, if not betrayal, by the ill partner's parents leaves a good deal of rage that must be reconciled by the surviving partner as he attempts to reconcile himself to the death of his partner.

For some men the experience is that of going from CONFIRMATION to FEVER PITCH. If the ill partner's physical and emotional state decline rapidly after diagnosis, the well partner is often left confused and wondering exactly what happened. "It all happened so fast, one thing after another. It felt like from the time he was first diagnosed until he died three months later we were going from crisis to crisis." Within days or weeks of the diagnosis, a well partner may experience several months of intense caretaking followed by the death of his partner. For these couples there may not have been time to re-establish a sense of equilibrium or dialogue in the relationship. "After he was diagnosed, Jose was out of the hospital for 11 days. Then something went wrong with his pancreas and he was back in again. Then he got brain lesions. After that second hospitalization, he was never the same. He was very ill, and the next six months was spent just trying to take care of him the best I could." For these men, the *Game Plan* may be characterized as just trying to keep their partner well cared for and comfortable.

During the course of THE LONG HAUL a particular illness may leave the partner severely disabled. "He had a massive seizure. When he came out of it, he could not see, could not talk. He could hear, but that was about all." "When he lost his vision he lost hope. There was nothing I could do about it." Often in these situations the well partner is faced with long periods of caring for his partner without the sustenance that the dialogue provides. "It is like a big part of him has been killed, long before he ever dies."

If the couple has difficulty talking about the disease and their lives, the well partner may be left feeling confused, and also deprived of the dialogue and the opportunity to convey or to receive much needed explanations. The unanswered questions leave gaps in the experience that are all too easily filled with guilt. There is an insidious pain, and sometimes resentment, associated with not knowing just what the partner was thinking about or feeling. "He would never talk to me about it, he would talk to other people, but not me. I was glad he was able to talk to someone, but I was also irritated that it wasn't me."

For all of the partners in the study, there was some form of *Derailment*. The disruptions varied in degree and intensity. Some were able to be checked by renewed communication between the partners, others with the intervention of friends, family or professionals.[1] For others like those cited above, the Derailment was extreme and very little could be done to mitigate the impact on the well partner. For these men, *Derailment* became their dominant experience during the partner's illness and left them with a set of associated memories and affects as they attempted to mourn the loss of their partners.

NOTE

1. Though not observed in the partners participating in the study, in the context of clinical practice, I have since worked with several couples where, following the diagnosis, the well partner attempted to leave the relationship. Attempted, in that while the well partner experienced the basic bond of the relationship as being broken and did pull back emotionally, at times threatening to leave his partner causing considerable turmoil for the ill partner, he did not actually leave but remained very involved in the caretaking of the ill partner. All cases have had similar dynamics: (1) There was a prominent over-adequate/under-adequate constellation in the relationship, with the well partner in the under-adequate position. (2) There was considerable pre-existing conflict and tension in the relationship. (3) In the context of the dynamic constellation, the ill partner had a strong tendency to overtly undermine and undercut his partners efforts at self definition. While the well partner was highly resentful of this, his own pronounced need to idealize his mate kept him "locked" into the relationship. (4) In the wake of the diagnosis, the well partner experienced himself as doing his best to care for his partner and taking a great deal of pride in it. (5) The ill partner again began the pattern of undercutting, the well partner's idealization was shattered, and he was flooded with angry affect and his own sense of inadequacy secondary to the disruption of the idealization. (6) The well partner became in a very real sense paranoid of the inadequacy of the ill partner that the illness represents and pulled back emotionally, at times thinking about and threatening to leave. In the language of this study, restoring the dialogue for these men would have meant a return to the

original dynamics of the relationship, which the well partner resists. (7) Both men then tended to disavow that one of them had been diagnosed with a terminal illness and the old conflicts of the relationship became the dominate focus. (8) After a period of considerable turmoil, the partners I have worked with to date settled into a modified living arrangement and conceptualization of their relationship and the well partner remained very involved until his partner's death.

Chapter VIII

Fever Pitch

We have been at this such a long time, I guess I never really thought it was going to happen. But now it seems clear that after two years of fighting this disease, he really is going to die.

THE LONG HAUL comes to a close with the transition to the next area of experience, FEVER PITCH. FEVER PITCH encompasses the experiences of the well partner during the last weeks or days of his partner's life. Usually, by this time, the ill partner is gravely ill and the dialogue between the partners is substantially diminished. An increasing sense of aloneness comes to dominate the well partner's experience. The well partner is negotiating family, medical personnel, his own career, household business and the needs of his partner, all while evidence continues to mount that the end of his partner's life, and their dialogue, is near.

The properties of FEVER PITCH are: *Realization* that the end is near; the return of *Automatic Pilot* as anxiety and tasks mount; and *Calm and Peace*, periods of reconnection between the partners. FEVER PITCH is a period of sharp emotional contrasts and at times almost frenzied activity. Anxiety often runs high and sadness begins to mount, as does exhaustion. The well partner may experience a sense of detachment as automatic pilot returns. However, periods of reconnection between the two men—verbal exchanges, quiet handholding, and looking into each others eyes—bring with them a sense of calm. Well partners must balance the pain they feel with the recognition of the physical decline of their partner and the growing certainty that death and the subsequent loss of the dialogue is the only way the ill partner can be released from a life that has become a mere existence. With the partner gravely ill there are

myriad tasks that need to be accomplished, family, friends, medical
staff and other professionals to negotiate. The well partner's life
does not come to a stop. Careers often must be tended to as well. If
the well partner's employer does not know of the situation, excuses
must be made.

REALIZATION

*I knew he was sick, but I kept thinking he was going to get
better. I kept hoping for a miracle. One day, I realized that
there were not going to be any miracles.*

The transition to FEVER PITCH is signaled by the well partner's
Realization that his partner is indeed going to die. The well partner
may or may not be fully aware of the extent of his partner's physical
and psychological decline. Gradually the evidence adds up that,
indeed, the struggle against the disease is coming to a close, that the
hope for a cure will not be realized. "One day I realized that we
were at the point of no return. Even if a cure did come along, it
would be too late to help him." Some partners more readily accept
this than others. Partners who are terrified of the impending
loss may renew their efforts to save their ill partners or may get
into conflicts with medical personnel, accusing them of not doing
enough or "giving up."

Evidence comes from a variety of sources: from the well partner's own assessment, the physician's prognosis, and the responses
of friends and family. "Being with him day to day, I did not really
realize how much he had declined. When his sister came in I realized it when I saw the look on her face." Depending on the disease
course, FEVER PITCH can last from several days to several weeks.
It may be a gradual process or quite sudden. "The week before he
died, he had a surprise birthday party for me. He was fine, in a great
mood, and enjoyed himself. Three days later he was sick, and I was
trying to get him to go into the hospital." "It was a very intense
three days. He came home from the hospital on Friday. Sunday
evening he was not well at all and by Monday morning he was
having respiratory problems. That afternoon we put him on mor-
phine."

Whether gradual or sudden, the integral component of the transition is the often dramatic decline in the dialogue between the two men. In previous categories, partners felt "we are in this together." As the ill partner's health and often mental status decline, an ever-increasing sense of aloneness and isolation creeps over the well partner. At the same time, the well partner is drawn nearer to his partner's side. "The last couple of days I would not leave the hospital." "The last weeks were very lonely. He was just trying to survive, to get through the last few days he had. He just did not have the energy to talk much or to give back." The well partner is usually highly involved in, if not totally devoted to, caretaking as the partner requires ever increasing attention and monitoring. In the past, the well partner has taken comfort in the dialogue. Now he takes comfort in knowing that his partner is comfortable: "I felt like his guardian."

The physical and mental decline of the ill partner is extremely painful for the well partner. "It is so hard to see how much weight he has lost. His clothes hang on him. Just two months ago they fit. Now his arms and legs are sticks. I can see the bones in his face. He is very quiet and withdrawn now. We don't talk much. He sleeps most of the time. We will watch TV for a little while together in the evening, and I'll hold his hand or stroke his hair. He always used to like my stroking his head. He still manages to smile when I do it." The well partner becomes increasingly vigilant. Often, he is acutely aware of how the quality of both their lives has declined. The well partner may yearn for their old way of life, an evening out or some other form of respite. But he is pulled back to his partner's side, anticipating feeling guilty if he were to enjoy himself, or worried about the wellbeing of his partner if he were left to the care of others. "I was getting exhausted. I thought about going out for an evening, just to get a break. I could not bring myself to do it. I did not feel there was anyone I could trust to take care of him. Plus, how could I enjoy myself with him at home, dying?" "I would not leave except to run an errand, and then only if Pam or Terry were there with him. I felt I could trust them to take care of him."

It has now become clear that the partners live in two different worlds: the world of the living and the world of the terminally ill. "There was a chasm between us. Try as I did, it just could not be bridged." As the disparity in their respective spheres increases, so does the well partner's missing of the ill partner. There is often a sense that the ill partner is there but not there, a ghost of his former self. "I came to feel that it really was not Walt lying there. It was his body, but not the Walt that I knew." "Towards the end it began to feel that there was a soul occupying a dead body." "We would sit together and watch TV or just lay around. But, it was very different. We were together, but I still felt alone and isolated. He really was not the same person those last few months."

As the illness envelopes the ill partner, he may come to realize that death does not seem such a bad possibility: "I came the closest to dying this time that I have yet. I was surprised, that when I was so sick, I realized how painless death really is. It is a different world. I realized just how painless it would be to slip into death. It also scared me a little." As he anticipates death, he may become increasingly withdrawn. "Towards the end, friends would call on the phone and he did not want to talk to them. I am not sure exactly why, he just asked me to talk to them for him." Well partners invariably sense this acceptance and may struggle to accept it themselves, or may fight against it, attempting to push their partner, or pushing medical personnel for increased efforts on their partner's behalf. "Looking back, I can't believe that I was calling Dr. S. and asking about aerosol Pentamidine six hours before Mike died." Others, in their acceptance, attempt to prepare themselves for the approaching final loss of their partner. "Somehow, I knew when we were getting ready to take him to the hospital, that this would be the last time."

Until the emergence of FEVER PITCH, *The Game Plan* and *Closing Ranks* served to help bridge the two very different worlds that the presence of AIDS has created for the two men, the world of the living, and the world of the dying. Now the well partner comes to realize that his *Game Plan* has failed, that his partner is dying, and no cure is in sight. The intensity of connection that Closing Ranks provided is no longer possible. The well partner is not able to "be with" his ill partner the way he was following the diagnosis or during THE LONG HAUL. "He was very quiet the last few weeks, as if he were halfway between sleeping and being awake."

The "special relationship" that began to emerge during THE

LONG HAUL between the well partner and a relative of the ill
partner often solidifies during FEVER PITCH. As described earlier, the special relationship is often with a sib of the ill partner,
usually a sister. "Patty [my sister] and I became quite close during
those last few weeks. She was able to come down and literally
move in to help take care of him." "Once we got to know each
other, Betty and I became very important to each other." The similarity that the well partner and the sib experience in relation to the
impending loss appears to account for the strength of the tie. Sibs
and partners are usually closer in age than partners and parents, and
the quality of loss may feel more similar. There is a sense of equality between sibs and partners that often does not emerge between
well partners and the ill partner's parents. If sibs are not closely
involved, the ill partner's mother can become the central ally.

When the ill partner's mother is the person with whom the
relationship forms, it can be very strong and equally sustaining.
"Will's mother is a wonderful lady. We really got to know each
other while he was sick." "My parents live far away and were not
at all involved in the situation. She told me that I had become another son to her."

The special relationship serves to sustain the well partner in his
growing sense of isolation. As the dialogue declines, the special
relationship helps to fill the void by providing the well partner with
the sense that he has a strong ally in taking care of his partner.
Another person who understands the pain and sadness of the impending loss is a powerful buffer against the growing isolation.
"Pam and I felt like a team." "Having his sister there made it a lot
easier. I did not feel as alone." "I do not know how I would have
gotten through those last few days without her."

AUTOMATIC PILOT

*I do not know how I managed to get through those last few
weeks. I was running back and forth from the hospital, dealing
with his parents, keeping updated by his doc, trying to keep
the business going, keeping friends updated. All while trying
to be with him as much as I could.*

As the partner declines and requires increasing care, life can become very complicated for the well partner, and *Automatic Pilot* returns. "I was taking care of two lives, his and mine." The ill partner may be at home or hospitalized. If he is at home, a great deal of care is needed. Friends and family may be providing a great deal of assistance, or home health care personnel may be involved. The atmosphere of the home is often greatly altered. "In some ways, it did not feel like our home anymore. Between his family and our friends, it sometimes felt like Grand Central Station." If the partner is hospitalized, then the well partner is often shuttling back and forth, attempting to be with his partner as much as possible. The well partner's family often needs tending to. "They really did not know the city, so I was driving them to the hospital or I would get friends to drop them off and pick them up."

All of this occurs while the evidence continues to indicate that the end is near. Tension, anxiety, and sadness continue to mount. In the wake of so much to do and so many intense feelings, a sense of detachment may come to dominate the well partner's experience. "Looking back, a lot of the time it did not seem real. I was doing so much and dealing with so many people, trying my best to figure out what Will needed, all on four hours of sleep a night or less."

Some families are easier to negotiate than others. Conflicts that arose during THE LONG HAUL may continue, or they may settle somewhat as the partner declines. Often conflicts revolve around the centrality of the well partner in the life of the ill partner. Parents who have come to accept this over the course of THE LONG HAUL are better able to ally with the well partner. If centrality remains an issue, than the conflict may continue in a subdued form. "His mother was a real trip. She would look at me and say, 'Well, may I go visit with my son for awhile?'" If previous conflicts had been intense, then parents and the well partner may be leery of each other and a tense truce may prevail. "His mother showed up the last few days. She was being politely civil to me this time. I kept my distance. I did not trust her. I did not want a replay of her screaming at me in the hallway."

The special relationship with a sib of the partner can be invaluable in negotiating the family. "Betty was great. I think she helped them understand a lot about our relationship." "Pam was a great buffer between me and the family." Parents may complain about the way visiting hours are handled to a son or daughter before they complain to their son's partner. The ill partner's sib may help soothe parental feelings, saving the well partner an additional burden.

In contrast, deep ties and respect between parents and the well partner can develop. "I really did not know them all that well up until Stan was in the hospital for the last time. We spent many hours together in the ICU waiting room. Not the best circumstances to get to know someone, but we came away from it with a lot of respect for one another." "His mom was really great. She is a strong, loving woman." When parents and partners are able to find their common ground, a great deal of support for each other can be realized.

If the well partner chooses not to tell his employer about his partner's condition, he must either make excuses or attempt to continue with his job responsibilities as usual while caring for his partner. "John was sick back in the earliest days of the epidemic. I work for a very conservative financial firm. I did not want them to know about it. Every day I left work and ran to the hospital. It was not easy, showing up at work and pretending that nothing was wrong." "No one at work knows that I am gay or that Jim was sick. But I have enough seniority to just say, 'I can't come in, I have a family emergency.'" Having to hide the situation at work can greatly add to the burden. However, the detachment of *Automatic Pilot* serves to help mitigate the strain. Other partners are able to tell employers and receive a great deal of support. "I was pleasantly surprised. I was getting tired and just said 'enough.' I told the airline that Will was sick and was dying. They told me to take as much time off as I needed, with pay no less."

Some men prefer their ill partner to be at home until the end. Others cannot bear the thought of their partner dying in the home, or are just unable to sustain the effort that may be required in caretaking. If an extensive support system of family and friends has not been developed, the well partner can feel overburdened, exhausted, and unable to continue. "The few times he was in the hospital I could not wait to get him home. But towards the end, I prayed they would keep him there. I was just too exhausted." "It got to be more than I could handle, it was 24 hours a day.'' Partners may experience guilt when they decide they cannot handle the situation any longer. "I felt badly about doing it because I felt I was doing it for myself. The last four days he was home, I did not sleep at all. I called the doctor's office and almost begged the nurse to get him hospitalized so I could have a rest.''

The antibody status of the well partner may also emerge as an additional burden. Well partners who know they are positive are often able to push concerns for themselves aside and focus on their partner. However, the possibility that the well partner may experience the same fate can reemerge as he spends his last few days with his ill partner. "When my lover was in the hospital for the last time—his gravest moments—I felt swelling in my lymph nodes. From that point on, I assumed I was positive." The question of transmission may again arise. "Those last few days he was in the hospital, I would find myself thinking, 'Oh God, please don't let me be responsible for this.'''

While some men found the feeling of detachment somewhat disconcerting, it is clear that *Automatic Pilot* has considerable value. It enables the well partner to manage his many tasks and intense feelings without becoming overwhelmed. As in CONFIRMATION, well partners were aware of what they were feeling, but Automatic Pilot served as a powerful buffer. "I knew it was all there, but I did not want to stop and feel it. I was afraid that if I stopped, I would go right over the edge.''

CALM AND PEACE

As sick and out of it that Walt was during those last few days, he still had his lucid moments. I would live for those few minutes a day when I knew he recognized me.

Calm and Peace begins as a property of FEVER PITCH, then gradually becomes a discrete category. *Calm and Peace* is the well partner's experience of feeling re-connected to his partner, of a reestablishment of the dialogue. It may take the form of quiet conversations during lucid moments, a squeezed hand, a look of recognition and understanding in the ill partner's eyes. It may come in the very last moments of life, when he is helping his partner move quietly and peacefully on to death. These are special and private moments for the well partner, and most likely for the ill partner as well. In sharp contrast to the growing anxiety, at times frantic activity, and detachment, these periods are experienced as moments of calm. The well partner no longer feels alone, he experiences a re-kindling of the dialogue that has been so sharply diminished by the decline of his partner. "Stan was on a respirator, so he could not speak. We developed a system of eye blinks and squeezed hands and note writing. One day he wrote, 'I love Jack' on his note pad. I have saved and treasured it since."

The well partner guards these times with his ill partner and does his best to make sure he experiences them. "Mornings and early evenings were usually his best times. I made sure I was at the hospital then." Well partners are often concerned about their partners being alone. The fact is that both men are alone when separated and each needs to be with the other. "People were amazed that I slept with Walt up until he died. I did not get much sleep, but if I was in the other room, I did not rest for fear that I would not hear him if he needed something."

Calm and Peace can also be a time for settling unfinished business. A time for saying last "I love yous," or of explaining past behavior or feelings. If the rules laid down for negotiating the ill-ness deprive the well partner of this experience, he may choose to break them. "Mike started to come around and I ushered all of the family out of the room. He was so sick and could not move so I knew that I had him cornered. I bent over and told him in his ear just how much I loved him, how much I cared for him, and how much I was going to miss him. When I had finished saying what I had wanted to say, I asked if he wanted me to bring the family back. He opened his eyes wide and nodded. He was probably thinking, 'Please! Get them back and get out of my ear!' He may not have liked it but I was determined to say it."

Calm and Peace may also be shared by the ill partner's family. A nurse on a San Francisco AIDS unit related this account: "One of the patients was very close to death, and I heard before I left for the day that his mother was coming in from Colorado. I was uneasy, wondering how it would go. I am from the sticks of Colorado and I know how those people can be. She had never met his lover and probably did not know he was gay until he developed AIDS. Anyway I came on duty the next morning and found his partner in the bed holding him, and his mother next to the bed in a chair reading her Bible."

Chapter IX

Calm and Peace

He died here on the couch. I was surprised how peaceful it was. After he died, I just sat here with him for about an hour. I was glad that it happened here at home. No hospitals, no machines. Just the two of us and the cats. It was so peaceful, so quiet.

As the death of the partner approaches, *Calm and Peace* becomes a category of experience in its own right. It encompasses the death of the partner and often extends beyond memorial services. While the partner often has a considerable number of tasks to attend to, in contrast to the preceding and next area he feels a sense of calm, a lull in the storm. CALM AND PEACE may appear somewhat "thin" in comparison to the other areas of the experience. However, this is what gives this area its distinctive quality. While there may be a great deal of activity, the partner, perhaps for the first time in many months, feels peaceful. The activities of this category do not appear to be as significant for the partner as the peace he privately experiences.

Partners report the actual deaths of their partners to be quite peaceful with a quiet calm pervading the room. There is a feeling that a long, arduous journey has come to an end. "The last few hours were pretty awful. His breathing was so loud and labored. But then he started to slow down. When he died, it was so quick and peaceful. He just slipped off." "Tim's passing was very peaceful. His sister and I were laying down beside him, holding him, and quietly telling him it was okay to let go."

Partners often desire to be with their partner a few moments more and experience the peace. "After they turned off the machines, it was so quiet. After so much, it was peaceful again. The nurses were so nice. They said to take as long as I wanted. I just sat with him for a long time, thinking about all that we had been through. It was really hard to leave, as if by walking out the door I was closing a chapter of my life that I was just not ready to have end."

Some partners may decide not to linger with the body for a long period of time, wishing to remember the partner as he was, not as the disease had left him. "I went back for a few moments after the nurses were finished disconnecting all of the tubes, but I did not want to stay. He was so emaciated. I wanted to remember him as he was."

The length of CALM AND PEACE is highly variable. It may last a few hours, a few days, or several weeks. With the death of the partner there are funeral or memorial services to attend to. Several partners reported feeling a sense of quiet detachment for several days, often extending beyond any memorial services. "I was fine. There was so much to do. I kept busy. We were having people back to the house after the memorial service, so I spent several days waxing floors, even trimming the bushes out front. I probably looked like a wild man, but I felt pretty calm inside."

The memorial service is a quietly important event for the partner. The services were recalled with a sense of calm and very special, if not private meaning. "It turned out to be a beautiful service. The Gay Chorus sang, and several friends talked about him." "It was very moving, after going through so much, it was a peaceful ending." If, during his illness, the ill partner had made his requests for services explicit, the survivor views carrying his partners wishes out very seriously. "I made sure everything happened just the way he wanted it."

Some partners may feel that the memorial services are for other people, not for them. "The weekend after he died, we had kind of a weekend celebration of his life. We filled the apartment with flowers, because he loved flowers, and went to visit some of his favorite places. I was feeling pretty calm. Some of the people that joined in got pretty emotional. A couple of times I felt like I was taking care of everybody."

However, since memorial services involve a wide variety of people who may have their own agendas, they often have glitches. Partners may find conflicts that had been brewing with the parents carried over into the memorial service. This can represent an irritating intrusion into the calm and peace of the partner. "A man that Walt's father brought came up and introduced himself as a writer for a Christian magazine. He said he was writing a story on the pagan funeral services of homosexuals."

The surviving partner's family and their validation of his experience now becomes increasingly important. This need arises at different times in the mourning process for different men. For some, it begins with the service. The surviving partner may be disappointed. "I kept looking for someone from my family at the service. They all knew about it. But no one came." Other surviving partners will not be. "My parents were great. They came down to be with me when they found out Stan was dying. They were there through the service and all."

Often the surviving partner is surrounded (or surrounds himself) with family and friends. The person with whom the "special relationship" is formed often continues to be with the partner for several days or weeks. "Pam stayed on for a couple of weeks to help me get things settled with the estate and all." Hence, while he is alone now, he is not really alone. It is not unusual for men to return to their parent's homes for a while after the funeral. "I went back home with my parents after the service. I did not want to be alone in the apartment." "I went to visit my mother for a few days."

Often the first wish for the partner is to sleep. He becomes aware of how exhausted he is, and there is a desire to retreat into the sense of calm and peace that he is experiencing. "I wish I could keep on doing what I have been for the last week—sleeping late, laying around all day. For the first time in two years I do not feel a sense of enormous responsibility." Some men are able to do this by returning to their parent's home, or extending their time off from work and the demands of day to day life. Some men intuitively know what is coming and they actively extend CALM AND PEACE as long as possible. "I know as long as I am here and not back at the apartment and work that this is not reality. I am not ready to face it yet." "I was feeling better after a few weeks at my parents', but I started to get anxious as it came time for me to return back to the city."

Eventually, the person with whom the "special relationship"

was formed must return to his or her own life. Relatives and friends must also return to their usual routines. For the first time during the years of the relationship and the few days or weeks since his partner's death, the surviving partner finds himself alone. "I hated driving Jane to the airport. I was frightened and afraid to return home. I kept telling myself 'you are going to have to face this sooner or later.' On the way home I really felt alone."

Chapter X

Chaos

The hardest time was several weeks after he died. After so many months of taking care of him, then the funeral, then the estate, all of a sudden there was nothing. I realized just how big a part of my life he had become.

The duration and transitions in the previous areas of experience are largely determined by the disease course. The areas of experience that comprise the mourning process have more fluid boundaries and the transitions are often more discrete. There is a predictably unpredictable quality to the surviving partner's experience. The experience of CHAOS is easily reawakened during RETREAT and may be experienced during EARLY EXPLORATION. Similarly, experiences during EARLY EXPLORATION may send the partner back into the relative safety of RETREAT. Anniversaries or other events during BACK INTO THE WORLD may evoke experiences that are reminiscent of prior areas. However, they are short-lived and the affective qualities are considerably less intense. Essentially, in these areas of experience, the memories and the sense of there being a great missing piece in one's world, along with the associated affects, gradually come to occupy a less central position in the partner's life. While the surviving partner and the deceased partner are central figures, the person with whom the "special relationship" was formed, the surviving partner's family, the deceased partner's family, their friends, and for some men, the AIDS Quilt and other symbols of the loss, all play a part in facilitating or impeding the process. The presence or absence of HIV infection in the surviving partner imparts a powerful dimension to this process of finding new meaning in life.

CHAOS is a time of great emotional upheaval. The entry into this area is the partner's first experience of aloneness. It often takes him by surprise and the intensity of the experience is alarming. It is the first gut-wrenching realization that his partner is indeed dead and that he is alone. Then the surviving partner settles into an intense longing for his partner. His experience of himself and the world may be mildly to at times dramatically altered. Time may be distorted. The partner's sense of his self-worth may be greatly diminished. A profound sense of unpredictability and the absence of meaning in life evolves. The world comes to be experienced as an unpredictable and unsafe place.

The properties of CHAOS are: *The First Hit,* the first experience of aloneness and intense missing of the partner; *The Missing Piece,* an intense, at times all pervading, longing for the partner; *Altered States,* when the world no longer seems real, time is distorted, and the partner feels horribly insecure. CHAOS tends to last several days, or weeks. *The First Hit* is but the first of many *Hits* that will occur throughout RETREAT and EARLY EXPLORATION. Each *Hit* plunges the partner back into CHAOS. Depending on the nature of the *Hit,* the subsequent experiences of CHAOS are usually less intense and shorter in duration than the first. *The Missing Piece* and *Altered States* will extend into RETREAT, periodically resurfacing in the wake of a *Hit* in EXPLORATION.

THE FIRST HIT

I had a horrible time on my first layover after I returned to work. It was my first time being alone. Up until then, Patty or my brother had been with me. Whenever I was on a layover, I would always call home when I got to the hotel. I called and left a complete message for Walt. Then I realized that he was dead. I have never felt so alone in my life.

The First Hit is the first experience of aloneness, the first realization that the partner is indeed dead. It is often a terrifying experience, one that leaves the partner quite shaken. Up until this time, the quiet calm of CALM AND PEACE may have prevailed, perhaps with bouts of crying or sadness. *The First Hit* shatters the calm, and the partner is plunged into an experience that he has been ill-prepared for. "I had no idea it was going to feel this bad."

For many men, *The First Hit* comes when the special person returns to his or her life, when less central but sustaining people who may have stayed with him for a few days or weeks after the funeral return to their lives, or when the partner comes home from the place he has retreated to in an attempt to sustain CALM AND PEACE. The shared experience of loss found with the "special person" is a powerful sustaining force for the surviving partner. The loss or interruption of that relationship paves the way for *The First Hit*. "While his sister was here—he was her favorite, and she was his favorite—I had a companion. She liked me, and I liked her very much. I would say, including his family, she and I were the ones who missed him the most. But after a few weeks, she left to go back to Germany. After she left, there was no one to pal around with, no one who understood. It was like we were sharing something, sharing the grief and the loss. The hardest time was after she left." "Up until that time, I had never been alone. Patty stayed for a few days, and then my brother was with me."

Men who retreated either to their parents' homes or the homes of significant friends often had a foreboding of what might lie ahead when they returned to their home, and the daily routines that they once shared with their partners. "As long as I am here, it does not seem real. I am really afraid that I am going to lose it when I get back home. I have to go back to work, but I dread it. I am just not ready for it to be real." "When I was at my parents', things were kind of on hold. I missed him, but I felt safe somehow." What they find is that their anticipation of "losing it" becomes reality. "After being away from the apartment for so long, I started getting agitated. It built all day until I looked at his picture, then I fell apart."

Another central factor in the timing of *The First Hit* is the partner often going about a task or routine assuming his partner is there. In the course of a check-in call home, or turning to ask a question, he realizes that the partner is gone. "I was sitting and watching the news. A story came on that I knew he would be interested in and I called out for him. When I realized he was not there, it felt like someone knocked the wind out of me." "It was like someone kicked me in the stomach."

THE MISSING PIECE

I feel like so much has been ripped out of me, ripped out leaving huge holes.

Prior to *The First Hit*, the partner may have experienced periods of missing his partner. However, the first experience of deep aloneness opens the way for the profound, aching, at times agonizing experience of *The Missing Piece*. "I never thought I could miss anyone or hurt so much." There is very much the sense that a part of one's self is gone, leaving huge gaps, a hollowness that cannot be filled. "I miss you so much I cannot stand it. Without you I feel empty." Over the years of the relationship, the two men's lives had gradually become intertwined. Suddenly there is the profound sense that something incredibly important and sacred has disappeared, that half, if not more, of the surviving partner is now gone. That the time they shared together was much, much too brief. "We had only been together four years, but he had become a very important part of my day to day life." "He was such a good person."

At times the missing piece can take on overwhelming proportions. "Everything I do seems to remind me of him." The longing to have the partner back can be overwhelming. "I miss everything about you. I keep beating my head against this brick/stone wall that separates us over and over again." Though the missing mounts, and the longing continues, the partner does not return. "It sounds crazy, but there were times when I really wanted to get sick and die myself so I could be with him."

ALTERED STATES

The world no longer feels real to me. I feel incomplete. I feel cast adrift, cast adrift in an endless ocean of helplessness.

With the experience of *The First Hit*, subsequent *Hits,* and the *Missing Piece* comes the experience of *Altered States*. The surviving partner's experience of the world and of himself is dramatically altered. A world that once felt reasonably predictable now seems foreign and unfamiliar. The partner who once functioned as a "model of efficiency" during automatic pilot, now finds himself feeling enfeebled, incompetent and painfully unsure of himself. There is a profound sense of being irrevocably changed for the worse.

The intense experience of *The First Hit* leaves the partner fearing subsequent *Hits*. As he returns to work and old routines, he may find himself fearing a *Hit*. "I really was shaky those first few days at work. When I least expected it, I would find myself missing Stan, start to cry and have to shut my office door." The experience of time may be greatly altered. "It really was weird. Some minutes seemed like hours, some hours like minutes. I really thought I was losing my mind." The partner may struggle to make sense of all that he is experiencing. However, at this point in time, no sense can be made of the chaos he feels. "I cannot put any sense into this. There is no sense to any of it."

The condolences of friends and colleagues may be welcome, but carry with them the fear of "losing it." "People at work were great, but every time one of them said they were sorry, I took a deep breath, thanked them, and went on my way. I do not know how many times I almost burst into tears when someone said that." In the midst of CHAOS, the partner may find himself continuing to inform friends and colleagues of his partner's death. "It was awful at times. I would be feeling so bad, and the phone would ring. Someone would be asking how Walt was doing. I would take a deep breath and tell them that he died several weeks ago."

The partner may find himself feeling incompetent in his familiar routines, but especially so in tasks that the deceased partner usually performed. "Walt was the financial wiz. I sat down with some bills that came in since the funeral and promptly got overwhelmed." "I am afraid to touch the plants. Stan always took care of them. I am afraid I will kill them and then have nothing left of Stan." Though the now deceased partner may have depended on him greatly during the last few weeks and months of his life, the surviving partner comes to realize just how mutual the dependence was. "I felt so incompetent. A few weeks after Mike died, some friends were going to join me up at the cabin for the weekend. They called and asked me how to get there and I realized that I could not give them directions. All the years we went up there, Mike always drove. I freaked out. I realized that I did not even know how to get to my own cabin.''

Chapter XI

Retreat

The first six months after he died, life was like a Picasso paint-ing. Nothing felt real and everything seemed distorted. I was like a zombie. Trying to get through the pressures of work, dealing with his estate, thinking of him constantly, while peri-odically concerns about my own mortality would surface.

RETREAT is characterized by a withdrawal from a world that no longer feels safe, predictable, or meaningful. The partner with-draws into an intense, at times all consuming dialogue with his deceased partner. Photographs and special possessions that may have been acquired together or have special memories take on a great deal of importance. The dialogue often takes the form of imagined conversations with the deceased partner. The surviving partner reconstructs the relationship, the illness and the death of his partner. Often in the course of the reconstruction, the surviving partner finds many failures on his part. Any experience of having wished his partner dead comes back to haunt him with a vengeance. The missing which first arose in CHAOS continues at a high pace. Often the pain associated with the "missing" becomes a way of holding onto the dead partner. The more intense the pain is, the more the surviving partner may feel connected to the lost partner.

A longing for validation of the loss and accompanying pain and disorganization arises. At some point, partners invariably turn, or wish to turn, to their families. But often there is not the total accep-tance that partners yearn for. They may have to explain the signifi-cance of the loss. For some, their plight may be politely ignored or rudely discounted. Worse, some families may fear their son will expose them to the HIV virus. However, the person with whom the "special relationship" developed often remains an important source of validation and support. If the person lives far away, the relationship may continue in the form of letters, phone calls, and periodic visits. For many partners, the AIDS Quilt becomes an important source of validation of the experience, the relationship, and their loss. People who do not immediately validate the loss risk facing the wrath of the surviving partner. Having to explain the centrality of the loss, depth of their pain and disorganization, often feels like too much to ask — what survivors need, and often demand, is uncomplicated acceptance.

All the while there is a subtle process of moving on. The partner's thoughts at times turn to the future and future plans. At times, the plans may be quite grand. Often they are a bit much too soon. Invariably, the assumption that the partner is HIV-positive continues. Partners who know they are negative may doubt the validity of their results. Men who do not know their antibody status continue to assume they are positive, as well as that they are the next in line to develop AIDS.

For many men, RETREAT will prove to be the most painful and agonizing area of experience. The combination of shattered self-esteem, feeling acute vulnerability to being thrust back into CHAOS, the intense missing of the partner, and profound sense of an absence of meaning in life radically alters the partner's experience of himself and the world. While many men do have a sense at some level that they will indeed move on, that they will begin to feel better, this hope is often overshadowed, if not shattered, by the acute despair that they experience repeatedly throughout RETREAT. "It was like falling into a black hole, one that I often felt there was no way out of."

The properties of RETREAT are: *The Missing Piece,* the continued intense missing and longing for the partner; *Altered States,* the continued dramatic alteration in the experience of self and the world; *The Dialogue,* and at times all-consuming series of "conversations" with the dead partner, a process of reconstructing the relationship, the illness, and death of the partner along with rituals that serve to bridge the gap between the surviving and deceased partner; *The Guilts,* a series of at times painfully guilt-ridden ruminations over perceived failures on the well partner's part that may have caused the deceased partner grief during his illness; *Helpers/Spoil-*

ers, family, friends, and others who, by their actions and responses
to the surviving partner and his plight, either facilitate or impede the
mourning process; *Hits* experiences that plunge the partner back
into CHAOS; *Next In Line,* the conviction rather than the assumption that the surviving partner will be the next one to contract the
disease and follow the partner in death; and *Holding On/Moving
On,* a process that underlies the entire experience. It is the partner's
awareness that, as intense as the experience feels and as stuck as he
feels in it, he is indeed in a process. He finds himself wanting to
hold on to his partner, but also feels compelled to move on with his
own life.

THE MISSING PIECE

*I never thought I would feel this way. Just the daily, lonely,
missing Walt. It is a hurt every day and every moment. When
you are busy, you do not think about it, but when you slow
down . . . nighttime is a terrible time.*

The Missing Piece continues into RETREAT. In this area it becomes a daily, aching, at times agitating presence. A profound
sense of pain often accompanies the missing. For many men, the
persistence and sharp edges of the missing will be the most difficult
aspect of this area of experience. "Missing him is the hardest part
to get over." For many men, this is their first experience of the loss
of such a central figure in their lives. They are often surprised by
the depth of the longing and the hurt. "I never knew that it was
possible to miss someone like this. I love him so much, and miss
him so much."
    Partners find themselves missing a great deal of what they shared
with their partner. "I want to talk with him again, be with him
again." For many men, the loss of "body contact" is significant.
Many long to be held, but the person they want to be held by is not
present. "My body misses feeling you next to me at night." "For
four years, we slept together every night except when one of us was
away on business. The bed feels so big and empty now. I think that
is what makes the nights the hardest time."
    Men often find themselves missing the unpleasant times as well.

"Even the things that used to aggravate me. It is kind of silly, wishing to have the aggravation back. I would give anything to be aggravated by him." "When Mark snored, you would have thought a freight train was roaring through the bedroom. I had this technique where I would hit him with a pillow just lightly enough that he would stop but not wake up. It used to drive me crazy. Now the silence drives me crazy."

The dead partner often becomes highly idealized. In the wake of so much chaos, disorganization, and missing, the surviving partner continues to feel greatly diminished. In sharp contrast, the deceased partner may come to be viewed as a source of inspiration and the best thing that ever happened to the now very much alone surviving partner. "He really was a sweetheart." "He was a very basic, decent human being." "He really was a very brilliant man." If the partner knows he is HIV-positive, the deceased partner may be seen as a role model for negotiating the disease. "He was such a trouper. If I get sick also, I only hope that I can hang in there the way he did." In the wake of his own turmoil, the partner may evoke the image of his deceased partner. "Help me, baby. I am trying to be as brave in facing all of this, as you were in facing the disease."

ALTERED STATES

I guess the best way to describe it was that I felt fragile, that I could fall apart or break at any moment.

During RETREAT, surviving partners find their self-confidence greatly diminished. They often feel painfully unsure of themselves, and fear another *Hit* and a plunge into CHAOS. Work routines that they often performed without a second thought may now seem daunting. With the death of the partner, they often have to take on responsibility for the life — the home, the business, the investments-that the two men had built together. The partners continue to feel horribly insecure, especially in the tasks that their deceased partner had managed.

Partners are able to delay their return to work to different degrees, but invariably, they must return. For some, work is a welcome respite, a chance to get their minds off missing their partner.

However, they often find themselves feeling shaky and insecure. "My first trip after Walt's death was a disaster. Passengers can be very demanding and difficult, especially when they are intoxicated. Well, I had a whole cabin of them. I kept telling myself, 'You can do it'. But this one man got me so pissed off I wanted to say, 'Damn it, my lover died three weeks ago and I do not need this.'" If the partner's fellow employees do not know of the loss, his sense of isolation may be enhanced. "On one hand I loved the times when I could get absorbed into my work, but if I was having a bad day, not being able to talk about it at work felt very burdensome." "My boss kept giving me more and more responsibility. I knew if I was straight and my wife had just died he wouldn't. But there was no way I could tell him."

The home the two men once shared may at times feel like a burden. "The apartment is really too big for one person. I cannot really keep it up, but I am just not ready to move yet." Hobbies that the two men shared, or that the deceased partner was the motivating force behind, must now be taken over by the surviving partner. "Over the years, we built up this enormous collection of plants. Stan always took care of them. He could make anything grow. Even though I had a lot of plants before we moved in together, I really am afraid that I will kill them." If the now dead partner was the decision maker for the relationship, the surviving partner may feel overwhelmed by the decisions he must now make on his own. "Mike was a very dominant person. He tended to make all of the decisions for us. I used to resent it sometimes, but now I am afraid that I will make the wrong moves, that I won't be able to do it without Mike."

Often the sense of *Altered States* cuts into basic perception. "I walk down the street and it just does not feel the same. It is the same street we have lived on for years, but I just do not feel a part of it the way I used to." The partner may miss the joy he felt in life and wonder if it will ever return. "I used to always find something to laugh about, even in the hardest times. Now I wonder if there will ever be anything to laugh about." The joy in special places the two men shared together is often gone as well. "I went down to the beach that the two of us loved so much. It was not the same, something basic was gone." The world feels quite bleak. Reminders of special holidays for the couple are not welcomed. "I went shopping today, and they had Christmas decorations up already. I want nothing to do with Christmas this year. I never was into it until I met Adam. I finally learned to enjoy the holidays with him. We went all out. We collected ornaments on our trips. I am not planning on even getting them out this year. It would not be the same."

THE DIALOGUE

It was strange. I would constantly go over his illness, the whole thing, day by day, or think about how we met and the things we did. It became a daily ritual. I would get so wrapped up in it, I would look up and three hours had gone by.

Prior to the death of the ill partner, the dialogue was between two men. Now the dialogue is between the surviving partner and the memories of his ill partner. During RETREAT, the dialogue can become intense. Men find themselves carrying on elaborate conversations with their deceased partners, reconstructing the illness and reconstructing the entire relationship. When absorbed in the dialogue, several hours may go by. While some men may be disconcerted by the lapse of time, rarely are they truly alarmed. The intense dialogue is a relief from the conscious, painful missing of their partner. During RETREAT, partners often experience *The Dialogue* as the most meaningful thing in their lives. Rituals emerge, such as counting the days since the partner's death, weekly visits to graves, daily remembrances in prayers or a "good night" before falling asleep, and may continue for quite some time.

For many men, the home they shared becomes a sacred place, full of memories and reminders. "Sometimes I feel like I have turned the house into a shrine to Will's memory." The experience of CHAOS leaves partners feeling quite shaky. The world no longer feels like a safe and predictable place. There is a decline of interest in career pursuits and a lack of enthusiasm for activities that feel like an intrusion on the dialogue. But in the home he shared with his partner, and in the intense dialogue, the partner finds a sense of comfort and meaning that he feels is lacking in a world that no longer makes sense. "Sometimes I feel like a babbling old fool in my house. I will go around and pick up old photographs and talk to them, express my thoughts, things I never had a chance to say to Will." The dialogue also serves to buffer the intense missing that began in CHAOS. "The house is full of memories. At first, everything reminded me of him. I would walk through the house and remember when we bought a chair, or found a painting, or argued over which TV to buy." "Life is quite gruesome and lonely without him, but I can still reflect on our time together."

Partners spend a considerable amount of time reconstructing the illness, decline, and death of their partner. "The illness and his death are constant re-runs in my mind." "Two years is a very long time to take care of someone who is sick. Now, of course, it feels very brief." Critical points in the process, the first pieces of evidence, the diagnosis, the first realization of approaching death, the periods of renewed dialogue, and the death itself are all remembered. The partner then tries to fill in the gaps, in an effort to reconstruct the entire experience. "I remember the first night sweat." "I remember holding him and crying while he slept, thinking that he was going to die." Periods of reconnection are fondly remembered. "He had periods the last few days when he was much more alert." In reconstructing the partner's death, surviving partners begin to realize the enormity of the experience they have been through. As they look back, they often find things they did not notice during the illness. "There was so much going on, I realized that I was processing only a little of what was actually happening." While living through it with their partners, they may have felt buffered. But now the experience in some ways becomes more vivid. "At the time, it was hard to realize just how gruesome things really were."

The approach of an anniversary of a critical event — the diagnosis, a medical crisis, the last trip to the hospital, the death of the partner — tends to bring with it a heightening of efforts at reconstruction. "The first anniversary of Mike's death is coming up in a few weeks. I am spending more and more of my time trying to remember every detail of those last few days. I am not sure why, but it feels very important to remember as much as possible and to be able to play it all back on the day he died." Seasonal changes, holidays, or other anniversaries may all serve to trigger memories and a reconstruction. "Even several years later, during late fall, when it starts getting dark early, cold and rainy, I remember that this was the time when Stan really started to get sick." "He died several days after Christmas. He was such a kid at heart I think he wanted to squeeze out one more Christmas morning." "My sister was married the weekend after he was diagnosed. So now, her anniversary stirs up all that went along with the diagnosis."

Unanswered questions from the experience also make up the dialogue. "I keep wondering how long he knew he was sick. The doctor seemed shocked when I was so surprised by his diagnosis." If the couple did not do a great deal of talking about what they were individually experiencing, the surviving partner may wonder just what it was like for his partner. "I really wonder what was going through his mind. He would talk to his support manager, but not to me." "He never complained. I am sure he must have been miserable, but he is not the kind of guy who would let anyone know just how bad he was feeling."

Another aspect of *The Dialogue* is the reconstructing of the relationship. How they met, favorite times together, and things learned from the deceased partner are recalled. "I think back to those early days when we were first getting together." "We met on a blind date. It was a disaster. Half way through I was praying for it to be over – that I never wanted to see this jerk again – but things started to turn around after he confessed that he was anxious and trying hard to impress me." Over the course of the relationship the couple experienced a great deal and shared special times. "We had some incredible vacations to Canada, Michigan, Florida. His parents had a great cabin way up in the woods of Wisconsin. It was his favorite place." When two people join their lives, they often learn new things from each other. "He introduced me to the Puerto Rican world. It was a culture that I knew little about before I met him."

THE GUILTS

Since the time I learned he had AIDS onwards, it's been one form of guilt or another. Now, I look back at the things I wish I had not done, had not said and had not felt. If I could do it all over again, I would. There are so many things I would have done differently.

During the course of *The Dialogue*, the well partner finds many faults with the way he handled the partner's illness, and often the relationship as well, before AIDS entered their lives. Surviving partners often collect a great deal of evidence to confirm that they indeed let their partners down. If the survivor's antibody status is positive or unknown, *The Guilts* often include wondering whether he passed the virus to his partner. *The Guilts* often amount to a painful self-flagellation, despite the enormous amount of caretaking performed during the partner's illness.

In reconstructing the relationship, the partner often finds fault with himself. Old conflicts or longstanding problems between the two men are now defined by the partner as being all his fault. "I am so damned sorry for all the hurt I caused him, I never meant to hurt him." Issues that at one time were felt as having enormous stakes now seem trivial. "I wish I had not been so reluctant to settle down. If I had just gone with it instead of fighting it, we would have had two more years, and maybe we would not have gotten the damn virus." In sharp contrast to the idealized dead partner, the surviving partner sees himself as the villain and the culprit. With uncanny ability, issues that were clearly between the two men are now assumed by the partner. "Mike was very independent and insisted on his freedom. I wish I had not been so independent myself — I guess I wish I tried harder to keep him at home. If I had tried, he may not have gotten sick."

Invariably, the issue of transmission arises. "I keep wondering if it was me that gave it to him." "If it could ever be proven that I gave the disease to him, I could never forgive myself." Survivors may welcome evidence that the partner could have contracted the virus outside the relationship. "We sometimes took separate vacations. He went to San Francisco once with some friends of his. At a dinner party, someone accidently mentioned the trip to the baths." If the surviving partner is negative, he may feel guilty that he was somehow spared, and have mixed feelings about his own responses to testing negative. "What a strange world that he died and that indications are that I am negative." "I have to admit that I am relieved to be negative. He died a gruesome death, but somehow it feels disloyal to be relieved. I really beat myself up over that one."

In reconstructing the illness, the surviving partner often finds many faults with himself. "I am so sorry for the times I lost patience with him." "I really wish I had pushed the food issue harder. I knew he was not eating right, and he would get mad if he thought I was pushing, but sometimes I think he may have lived longer had he kept his weight up." A commonly perceived fault is the failure to talk about what was happening during the illness. "I am sorry I never tried harder to get him to talk about it. I guess I was trying to pretend that it was not real." Measures that the partner took to help sustain himself may be viewed as indications of selfishness. "The last few weeks I slept in the next bedroom. I could hear him if he needed anything, but I felt I could not sleep with all of that equipment. I probably could have, but I chose not to. I regret not having been at his side those last few nights."

Perhaps the most painful perceived failures are the partner's recollection of the times he withdrew from his ill partner and became preoccupied with his own welfare. "I keep finding myself thinking about the times I would wonder what was going to become of me, or of making plans for when it was all over, and I am horrified that I could have been worried about myself when he was lying there so ill." Most painful yet, are the recollection of times, if they occurred, when he wished for an end, the death of his partner. "As much as I hate to admit it, there were times when I was so exhausted I wanted it to be over." "One time, I was trying to do something for him and he screamed at me. I found myself thinking, 'I have had enough of this. Why don't you hurry up and die?'" Even when the wish was out of compassion, it returns to haunt. "The last few hours were really awful, his breathing was so loud and labored, I kept thinking, God, please let him die. But with his last breath, I wanted him back."

In a very real sense, the partner has failed. He has failed at his *Game Plan*, the plan that he so carefully constructed to keep his partner alive until a cure was found. The partner is dead. "I counted on being able to keep him healthy until they found a cure for this disease." "I find myself thinking that if I had done a few things differently, he would be alive today." The plan that the well partner had such hope for and often put so much energy and sacrifice into has come crashing down. The partner, in experiencing the failure of the plan, experiences himself as a failure. At times he may come to feel that he, and only he, is responsible for the state of affairs that he now finds himself in.

HELPERS/SPOILERS

Friends have been great. I feel like the poor widow. They are always calling, asking how I am doing and trying to get me out of the house.

Invariably, the partner experiences the responses of some people to his situation as more helpful than others. Depending on the response, some people will be experienced as extremely helpful and fondly thought of. Others will be experienced as very unhelpful and risk becoming the targets of considerable anger. *Helpers* are individuals who, by their words and actions, validate the depth of the partner's loss and his status as a grieving spouse. Those who either cannot tolerate the partner's sadness and retreat from the relationship, or do not acknowledge the importance of the relationship, are the *Spoilers*. The ultimate *Helper* is often the "special person." The similarity, the shared sense of loss, enables a deep and important validation. The ultimate *Spoiler* is the family that brings suit challenging the will, the insurance company that challenges a claim, or the friend who disappears. *Helpers/Spoilers* is actually a continuum. The depth of the partner's pain and sense of loss is enormous. Some people will be able to respond to his emotional state, others will respond in line with their own agendas. In the face of so much pain and disorganization, the partner's capacity to tolerate ambivalent or less than affirming responses is greatly diminished.

Friends who were pitching in to help take care of the ill partner often continue to "be there" for the surviving partner. If a strong "team spirit" evolved, often the team members find themselves getting together for several weeks after the partner's death. "The four of us really formed a team. Somehow we all kept congregating at the house for several weeks. Sometimes it felt like a bit much, there really were times when I wanted to be alone. But gradually, people stopped coming over as much and I missed all of the contact." Checking in on the well partner or taking him out of the home is often greatly appreciated. "It was nice. People would call, ask how I was doing. I never ate out so much in my life." "It felt good when the same people who were there for us were there for me." While the validation of his loss is important for the partner, the shared sense of loss with others is equally important. "We are all getting together Friday night to combine our pictures into one big book of memorabilia." Just as the sense of not being all alone in taking care of his partner helped sustain the partner during THE LONG HAUL, the shared sense of grief will help to sustain the partner during his experience of mourning.

A very meaningful experience for the surviving partner occurs when a friend or the special person relates a conversation with the deceased partner that affirms the relationship. "One of his friends told me that John had always wanted a relationship, that many times he told him how grateful he was for meeting me." "His sister told me that Mike had written to her after he was sick and said that he was worried about me, that I had built my whole life around his. He was worried that I would be resentful after he was gone. Well, I know I did that, and I do not regret it a bit." "Betty was his friend long before he met me. She told me how she heard about the progression of things between us from the start and she knew just how important I was to him."

However, the nature of the loss for friends is often quite different than for the partner. Their grief is less intense and they tend to return to their own lives faster than the partner. He may find himself feeling out of sync with people whom once he felt as sharing in his grief. "Gradually, people stopped calling as frequently and it was harder to get the old gang together." The partner finds himself very much preoccupied with his loss long after his friends and the friends of his partner. "It is hard sometimes, because what I really want to be talking about is how much I miss him, not their last vacation, new car, and certainly not their new boyfriend."

People often have a hard time tolerating another person's sustained sadness and depression. Partners are often acutely aware if they are making others uncomfortable. "I can tell when people are getting tired of hearing about it. If I told them what I was really feeling, I am afraid I would get carted off to a hospital." Sometimes partners find themselves getting angry at longstanding and trusted friends. "I got pissed at Ron the other night when he kind of hinted that maybe it was time I started getting over it." Friends who disappear leave the partner feeling disillusioned and enraged. "I found out who John and my friends really were. There are several people who I thought were real friends. Now I do not care if I ever see them again."

While the partner is deeply moved by the validation of his loss, the validation of his "making a new start" is important as well. Friends who acknowledge the many "firsts" that surviving partners face are often greatly appreciated. "When I got back from my first layover, there was a room full of people waiting for me. I was hoping to just crash, but it was really nice of them to be there."

Contact with the "special person" is often not as frequent due to geographic location. However, the contact may be quite intense, and anticipated with considerable excitement. "Paula is coming down this weekend. I cannot wait to see her." The shared sense of loss that is found with the special person is extremely important and validating. "Mike's friends loved him, but they miss him as a friend. I loved him, but I miss him as a spouse. Mike's sister loved him and she misses him as a brother. We both loved him in very special ways and it feels more familiar, for both of us." It is the special person that the partner often turns to during the first holidays after his partner's death and perhaps for subsequent ones as well. "I am going up to see Tim's sister for Thanksgiving. It will be the first one without him in five years. She and I held him while he died and I have not seen her since a few days after the funeral." "I called Mike's sister on Christmas Day and we talked and cried for a good hour."

Professionals that were experienced as being very helpful by the couple and the surviving partner during the illness are fondly remembered. Some partners find themselves maintaining contacts with these people. "Every now and then, I will go over to the hospital and stop and see the nurses in the infusion room or the nurses on the floor. They really were wonderful to Mike and I." It is not unusual for both partners to be followed by the same physician. If a positive alliance developed with the ill partner's physician, then the physician continues to be an idealized figure for the surviving partner. "When Mike died, Dr. S. came over to see me. That really meant a lot to me. She is such a compassionate person." However, some men, though they think highly of the physician, and though he or she is the survivor's personal physician as well, may initially want to stay away from the doctor's office. "I probably should go see Dr. K. It has been awhile since I have had a check up, but the idea of going into his office and remembering all the times I took Stan there just feels too hard right now."

The Role of Parents

> *I think that my parents finally got that Will and I were more than just "friends." I think they finally understood that I loved him the way they love each other.*

Invariably, the desire for validation is experienced in the context of the partner's parents and siblings. This will be a more or less complicated task depending on the people involved and the degree to which the relationship was acknowledged, validated, or known prior to the illness and death. Some men may have presented the relationship as a "friendship," while others actively pursued "married" status within their families. Others may not have informed their parents of their partner's diagnosis until well into the disease process. Some families will prove to be *Helpers*, others *Spoilers*. Most men will experience their families as a combination of each. In part this is due to the survivor's limited capacity to tolerate ambivalent acceptance or acknowledgment. In the depth of his pain and missing of the partner, the capacity to tolerate anything but total acceptance is limited. Some men will pursue the issue, explaining the relationship and the loss until the parents "get it." Others will be so disappointed on the first try that they give up, often feeling resentful and hurt. Unfortunately, some will experience a conspiracy of silence, a polite refusal to acknowledge the loss. And tragically, some men will find their families afraid of infection, which only enhances the sense of isolation and disappointment.

Invariably, any longstanding issues between the partner and his family regarding his gayness become intertwined with his need for validation of the loss. *Helpers,* by their response, cut into the sense of isolation and aloneness that accompanies the loss, while *Spoilers* accentuate the partner's sense of isolation. Often gay men have felt all alone with their gayness in the context of their families. Past experiences of less than total acceptance and memories of painful isolation because of being and feeling different come to the surface, and are often mixed in with his need, if not demand for a validation of the loss, and status of grieving spouse.

Surviving partners find the experience of their family validating the depth of the loss to be extremely meaningful. "When my nephew asked where Stan was and I told him that he had died, he burst into tears. Sometimes I felt that of my whole family, he was the only one who 'got it' right from the start — the only one who understood without my having to explain." The less complicated sense of loss that a child experiences may inspire other members of the family to respond. "He kept talking about the Monopoly game we all played. So, later that night, we all sat down and played a game to remember Stan by." While the condolences of friends are greatly appreciated, the unsolicited condolences of family are especially meaningful. "My cousin Pete stopped by while I was at my parents' and said how sorry he was. Aunt Kate and Aunt Bea sent a note."

Perhaps the highest form of validation is that of a parent sharing the son's grief as another adult. "I was home visiting my parents. I had stayed up late and was watching a rerun of one of Will's favorite TV programs. I started to really cry. I don't know whether I woke my mother up or what, but all of a sudden she was there. She sat down and told me about what it was like for her to lose my oldest brother and sister, that she thinks about them every day, and that she never really got over it. It was a real nice experience — her sharing that with me." Active participation by the family in the grief and mourning is deeply meaningful. "My parents and Stan's sister all gathered up at the cabin. We had a memorial service and buried some of his ashes by a marker that his father had placed at his favorite spot."

Often the family does not "get it," and the partner may find himself feeling irritated and/or deeply disappointed at what he experiences as polite acknowledgment, but not a total validation. Some partners, over time, will actively pursue their parents until they understand. "My dad was kind of saying that it was time to get on with things. I could not stand it any longer. Before I realized what I had said, I blurted out, 'How would you feel if Mom dropped dead? Do you think you would be over it by now?' To my surprise, he looked stunned and said that he was sorry." Some men assumed that they were accepted as a couple all along. If parental response is not in keeping with the assumption, they are often left feeling disappointed. "I really did not think that I would have to explain."

Some men will be left feeling deeply disappointed in, abandoned by, and alienated from their families. If the family failed to respond at the time of death, partners may feel acutely cut off from their families during RETREAT, which only enhances the loneliness and isolation. "They all knew about it, but I think they were embarrassed by the relationship. I kept looking for someone from my family to show up at the funeral, but no one came." "I got condolences from all over the U.S., but nothing from my family." Though they may long for their families, the hurt may be so deep that it feels too difficult to attempt to re-connect. "I have not seen or spoken to them since the day he died. Christmas is coming, and I would like to be there, but I don't know what to say to them. If one of my brothers' wives had died, my mother would have been there on the spot, helping out, anything she could do." With the death of the partner, some men feel that the cards are finally on the table, that the parents show their true colors regarding their son's gayness and the relationship. "All along I thought they accepted me. I guess I was mistaken." While there is often considerable anger at parents who respond in this manner, the partner may feel that there is something wrong with him. "I consider myself a good person, a loving person, but that is not the way they are treating me anymore."

Other men may not want to push for validation beyond the manner in which the relationship was explicitly known. "I always presented the relationship to my mother as a friendship. She knew we lived together, but it was never taken beyond that. She called me the day of the funeral to see how I was doing. That really felt nice." "I was dreading going home. In the past my parents and I could not talk about my being gay without it erupting into a fight. They knew Tim had died of AIDS and that we had lived together. It turned out OK. They had a few questions. We were able to talk about what happened and how I was feeling without it getting messy. I felt okay."

Perhaps the ultimate spoiling is family concern about AIDS contagion. "I went home and told them everything. They knew about Don and I, and that he had died of AIDS. I told them what it was like to see him go downhill. I also told them that I was positive. After that, they were edgy. I saw my mother handling my plates and silverware with extra care. It is pretty awful to feel contagious in the house you grew up in." Changes in the responses of sibs and their spouses are also noticed and may be felt deeply. "I thought my sister and brother-in-law were with it. From time to time, my niece and nephew had talked about wanting to come visit me in Chicago. My sister and brother-in-law always were receptive. Well, the kids are old enough now, and asked to come visit. My sister said she thought it was a good idea. Something happened. My brother-in-law never showed up while I was at home. I am sure he nixed the idea. I get so outraged that he would think that Uncle Dan would somehow give his kids AIDS. I am also pissed that my sister was not confident enough to tell him off."

Ties that developed or were solidified with the deceased partner's family often continue long after the death. "His mom, dad, and sister all said they want me to think of myself as part of the family." One cannot overestimate the sustenance derived from feeling a part of a family at this time. Often, the survivor may feel more akin to his dead partner's family due to the shared sense of loss. If relationships have solidified, they often feel that they do not have to explain. If the survivor's own family is unresponsive, then he may feel more tied to his partner's family. "His mom told me that she considers me an adopted son. To be honest, she has been more of a mother to me during this ordeal than my own has."

Other Spoilers

> *The mortgage insurance company has really been messing me around. They keep saying they are reviewing the case. Walt left the house to me, and the policy was there long before he got sick. It is mine. I deserve it and I want it.*

Spoilers come in many shapes and forms. Often the actions of institutions are the ultimate invalidators. Insurance companies that delay or attempt to challenge claims are a great irritant, "I got so upset every time I talked to them I finally turned it over to my lawyer,'' ''Every time I talked to them it was another run around — to them he was just another number — or another debit.'' The anger generated by these actions is often very disconcerting to the partner who is already in a vulnerable state of mind. ''I had to psyche myself up to call them and then allow a couple of hours to calm down afterward.''

The deceased partner's parents may challenge a will that leaves the bulk of their son's estate to his partner, creating a protracted battle that will greatly interfere with the partner's need to tend to his vulnerable state or later, pick up his life and carry on. ''Not two months after he died they were accusing me of stealing from him and demanding a complete accounting for the money spent during the time he was sick.'' Some parents will treat the partner as if he were trespassing on their property. ''I could not believe it. Right after the funeral, they told me they wanted to get into the apartment. I told them when I was ready for them to be in the apartment. His will was very specific, and if they think they are going to just come in and start carting things off, they have another think coming.''

The deceased partner's parents may assume that they have a right to their son's belongings. ''Right at the funeral dinner she said, 'Now when you are ready to sort through things just let us know,' then she called every week afterwards asking when we were going to go through things.'' Partners often feel very depersonalized and enraged by these demanding requests. ''It was as if it was his house, not mine. I wanted to say, 'I am still alive, you know.''' One could argue that just as the surviving partner needs and treasures his partner's belongings at this time, other family members may have similar needs. However, the request is rarely phrased in polite tones. ''If she would just have said 'I miss him so much, I remember how happy he was when he got that stuffed rabbit for his 6th birthday' — but no, it was as if she deserved it, and who was I to stand in her way.'' Partners often find themselves wondering if the partners' parents would treat a heterosexual in-law in this manner. ''I really wonder, do straight people go through this, or is there more respect?''

Often people who claim the deceased partner promised them things seem to come out of the woodwork. ''I was really disappointed in them, his brothers and nephews kept saying that he had promised them things I know he didn't. We discussed it. But there they were with the most sincere looks on their faces saying he had promised them this or that. What are you supposed to do?" "I wanted to say, 'you fucking vulture, he did not and you know it.'" Partners may feel betrayed when someone who was so helpful during the illness is now lying in order to have mementos. "She really was a great help, but then she had a list of things that he had supposedly promised her. Well, the reason there was no will in the first place was that he refused to acknowledge that he was dying. So I know he never promised her anything."

Parents who were supportive at the funeral may suddenly "turn on" the surviving partner. "At the funeral they were so nice, thanking me for all I had done, for all the care I had given him, but then four months later they called and said they wanted all of his belongings—his clothes, his furniture, even the sheets on his bed. I told them I burned the sheets—you can only wash urine and feces out of sheets so many times." If there is no will, then the partner may indeed be in trouble. "They called and said they would be up with a truck in two weeks. I panicked. There was no will. I called Howard Brown and talked to an attorney. He said I did not have a leg to stand on, but there was that line about possession being a key point of law and suggested that I take everything and get the hell out. So with the emergency help of a lot of friends I moved everything out a day before they were supposed to arrive." A forced move at any stage is disconcerting and traumatizing for a surviving partner. A move at this stage, when many men are so involved with memorializing their partners is very traumatic and demoralizing. When men most need to have a sense of order, and calm, when the world already feels traumatic, they suddenly find themselves in unfamiliar territory. "Four months after he died, most of the apartment was packed up in a storage locker, and I was living temporarily with the family of a former student."

The Role of the AIDS Quilt

We were very rushed. The Quilt was coming to town just a few weeks after he died. Janice, an old friend of Adam's and mine, helped me put it together. I sewed it on the machine Adam's mother gave us.

The AIDS Quilt has proven to be a very powerful source of validation for many people, especially so for some partners. The partner's experience of the Quilt in RETREAT will often be very different from his experience of it during EXPLORATION. "It was so intense. It was not all that long after he had died. I was not all that aware of what was going on around me. You had to walk through panels from other cities to get to the Chicago panels but I was only marginally aware of them. I just wanted to find and stay there by his panel." The partner may be deeply moved by the expressions of other people's respect and acknowledgement. "Someone that he did not even know had made a panel for him. I thought that was a pretty wonderful thing to do." "It was really great when friends of his came over to see me while I was there. Sandy, a longtime friend of his, came over and we lost it together."

NEXT IN LINE

But there is a bigger part of me that says "What is the point?" To be honest, I think I will be dead in a year.

The assumption of HIV infection that began in the earliest areas of the experience continues. The assumption tends to be present to some degree regardless of test results. Men who know they are antibody negative may, on some level doubt the results, doubt the integrity of the physician, or wonder if they have just not developed antibodies that could be detected. "The test turned out negative — according to what the doctor told me. I am not convinced. He may have kept it from me so I would not worry about it." "I am not positive . . . yet." Partners who struck a "devil's deal" fear that it has come time to pay up. "I kept saying, 'do not let me get sick, not now, I have to take care of him.' I always thought the symptoms would start after he died. Now, I am just sitting and waiting for it to happen." Men who know they are positive assume, in a more certain way, that they will follow the same fate. "I am positive also. I guess that means I will follow the same road."

Men who do not know their antibody status continue to assume they are positive, but during RETREAT, testing the assumption is not a strong desire. Perhaps more importantly, they feel too fragile to risk the trauma of what they assume is a confirmation of their fate. "I wonder about it. I probably will check into it, but later. There is just too much going on right now." "Things are all mixed up as it is. I am not going to risk putting myself over the edge." At this point, partners often do not experience a great deal of disruptive anxiety by the possibility of being positive or a desire to know their actual status. The assumption of being next in line is a quiet one, and at this point not railed against. Seropositivity also represents a tie to the deceased partner. In the midst of so much missing, pain and disorganization, joining the partner may not feel like such a bad possibility. "When I am at my gloomiest, being with him seems better than going on and feeling what I am feeling now." In addition, the surviving partner is more preoccupied with the loss of his mate, missing him, reconstructing the relationship, and holding on to memories. Preoccupation with antibody status represents a preoccupation with one's own self. At this point in the experience, the surviving partner does not feel nearly as important as what he has lost.

HITS

It is just something that happens, and I really do not know when it is going to happen. I do not know why, but, for me, it seems to be TV. I was watching "St. Elsewhere"—the episode where Brett the PWA died. It was so realistic, so similar to Wayne's death. It was like being faced with it all over again.

Hits are experiences that send the partner back into one or more of the intense properties of CHAOS. Experiences that trigger an intense sadness, intense missing, or intense disorganization are very disruptive for the partner. He is often left feeling that he is at the mercy of *Hits*, not knowing when or where they will come. The *Hits* impart a strong sense of unpredictability to the partner's experience of RETREAT. Often, they serve to reinforce the sense of vulnerability and of the world no longer being a safe and orderly place. "I do not know what is worse: the way I feel when it happens, or not knowing when it is going to happen." "Just as you think you have adjusted to it—Bam!" The partner may have felt stable, that he was getting back on his feet for several weeks and then, when he least expects it, he feels plunged back into CHAOS.

Hits remind the partner in a very intense and powerful way of the loss and absence of his partner. "We were watching *Kate and Allie* on New Year's Eve. During the end of the show Allie said, 'I have no one to kiss.' She realized that she was alone and it hit me that I won't ever be able to kiss him again." Hits can be triggered by a television show, coming across possessions of the deceased partner, or thinking the partner is present. "I had been having a couple of good days. I was going through some drawers at home and I came across some old things of Adam's. I just lost it." "The alarm went off one morning and I rolled over to give him a hug. No one was there. The rest of the day I felt that I was walking on eggshells, that I could fall apart at any moment."

Sexual encounters or threatened sexual encounters often provoke intense *Hits*. Some men, in their loneliness and body hunger may seek out a sexual encounter. It is often a mistake they will never forget. "I thought I was going to lose it for sure." "I was so lonely I went out and met this guy. Well, I no sooner got him home than I thought I was going to go through the ceiling. He must have thought I was crazy."

The surviving partner faces many "firsts": The first nights and weeks alone, the first holidays alone, the first major life decisions in several years alone, the first anniversary of their meeting alone, and the first anniversary of the partner's diagnosis or illness alone. All of these firsts can trigger hits and the intense feelings that follow.

Unsolicited offers of a relationship or sexual encounter often leave the partner feeling raped. "I could not believe it. Within the last two weeks, people that I considered old friends told me that they had always been attracted to me, and thought I was a wonderful person. They actually asked, if now that Adam was gone, would I be interested in a relationship with them!" A profound *Hit* may be experienced when a partner has developed a relationship with someone out of his loneliness and the other person wants to push the relationship in another direction. "I was devastated. He was a fun person. I enjoyed having someone to go out with, I do not think I was leading him on, but when I realized what was happening I freaked out."

HOLDING ON/MOVING ON

This pain and sadness is mine. It belongs to me. So, I am coming to sort of treasure it in some strange way. Right now it is still my link with him. In time, my link will be able to be there by itself and not need the pain.

Though partners may be periodically overwhelmed by the intense feelings that accompany RETREAT, they are aware, on some level, that they are engaged in a process that, by its very nature, is forward moving. In the long run it is a linear process, but partners may be somewhat disconcerted by its back and forth nature. It is one of *Holding On* to the memories of the partner, to their time together, and to the link that the sadness and missing often comes to represent. It is also a process of *Moving On*, beginning to say goodbye to the partner and the relationship, and redefining life without the partner. "You go a couple of steps forward and a couple of steps back."

Holding On and *Moving On* are different processes that often proceed at different paces. At times, partners may be very confused. In some aspects of their lives, they have made considerable progress in redefining and restructuring, yet times will arise when they are preoccupied with the pain and loss of their partner. Partners often feel relieved when they have made steps towards *Moving On* but also find comfort in *Holding On*. "I changed the answering machine the other day, everyone was complaining because it was Walt's voice. I changed it originally right after he died, but then I thought it was like turning off a switch. It was kind of comforting to hear his voice." In sensing that there is a forward movement, there is often a degree of relief. No matter how much comfort men may come to take in a seeming connection to their partner through the pain of missing, it is still pain. "Some day, I will let it in that he is gone. I am just not ready to yet. It hurts to miss him so, but it would hurt more to feel that I have nothing."

During RETREAT, *Moving On* is often a quiet voice, one that is easily overridden by the missing and vulnerability that men experience. It is always there in some shape or form. However, the partner's ability to believe it rises and falls. "As awful as I feel, as much that I am faced with that I do not want to be faced with, I do sense at times that this is an adventure, that there is a way out."

During RETREAT, many men will contemplate making major career changes, returning to school, or redecorating the apartment "their way." Often the plans are quite elaborate and though they are within the survivor's cognitive capabilities, they may prove to be too much too soon given his diminished confidence and resiliency. "I have so much time on my hands now. I am seriously thinking about going to a language school and learning Japanese. It would be great for my job. It would put me in a different rating and I could qualify for some pretty interesting assignments." "A friend keeps bugging me to go into a doctoral program. It is something I need to do. I think I used the relationship as an excuse to not get on with my education." Invariably, the partner finds that he is not ready during RETREAT to make such changes. He finds the available energy and confidence lacking. The plans may arise after several weeks of feeling better and more confident. Then a *Hit* is experienced, the partner is plunged back into CHAOS, and in the wake of his shaken self-esteem postpones his plans. "It was a good idea and I still plan on doing it, but not now. I do not know if I am just not ready yet or if I scared myself."

Contrary to what many people outside the partner's experience may assume, validation of the loss, and its accompanying feelings of pain and sadness, facilitate *Moving On* not *Holding On*. The "special person" often becomes a prime facilitator of the process. "Something got freed up after that phone call with his sister where we cried together." "I was having a real bad day, really missing him, I called up Patty, she was having a bad day too. I really felt better after that. I felt like a new person when I woke up the following morning." *Spoilers* often impede the process and facilitate *Holding On,* leaving the partner enraged and feeling alone. "His life insurance company said they were reviewing the case and, 'who was I in relation to the deceased?' I was his lover, damn it." "I feel so disappointed and cut off from my family. They just do not or will not understand what I feel like."

Chapter XII

Exploration

The world does not feel quite as bleak as it did. I still miss him a lot, but it is beginning to feel different. I am almost afraid to say it, but there are times when I feel excited again.

EXPLORATION is a transformational time. The partner begins to find himself trying out life on his own. *The Dialogue* and *Missing* decline and the world begins to be experienced as once again having possibilities. Early in EXPLORATION the partner continues to feel quite shaky and is easily plunged back into RETREAT or, in the wake of a *Hit*, CHAOS. Partners continue to define themselves as widowers, but also begin to examine their lives in terms of changes that they want to make for themselves. Living arrangements that the two men had together may not be feasible for one man to financially support. The partner may move or begin to give away his partner's clothes or belongings. The surviving partner also begins to think in a more concerted way about changes in career or other aspects of his life.

The thought of dating periodically surfaces. Some men will be able to form new relationships. Relationships formed during this period have the flavor of the partner negotiating two relationships, as he continues to mourn his deceased partner and the attachment develops with his boyfriend or potential new partner. Other men will not be able to tolerate a dating relationship or boyfriend, but will find activities such as country western dancing which involve a great deal of body contact in a structured environment to be very sustaining. Often men will volunteer for AIDS support services. The relationship with the special person and other *Helpers* continues to be very important. Some men will establish relationships with new people, who may also take on helper status. If the deceased partner's family have become *Spoilers* via lawsuits or other forms of hassling, then their activities become a source of irritation and preoccupation.

As the preoccupation with the lost partner declines, the surviving partner begins to become increasingly preoccupied with his own health status. In RETREAT, the assumption of seropositivity was a quiet one. In EXPLORATION it may take on obsessional qualities. Previously, the thought of joining the partner in death may not have felt so bad. In EXPLORATION the survivor may rail against it. He discovers that he no longer wants to die. He wants to live. Men who have not been tested often choose to test their assumption at this point. The results of the test will prove to have an enormous impact on the partner's ability to make new attachments and to continue on his journey of reconnecting to the world of the living.

The properties of EXPLORATION are: *Decline of the Dialogue*, the gradual waning of the intensity of thinking about the lost partner and the relationship; *Decline of Missing*, the gradual decrease in intensity of missing of the lost partner; *A Ray of Hope*, the partner beginning to feel excited, more self-confident and hopeful for the future; *Helpers/Spoilers*, people who validate or negate the partner's experience; *Next in Line*, the growing intensity and preoccupation with contracting AIDS; *The Fork in the Road*, the experience of partners who knew all along they were negative, or tested negative during their mourning process; and *The Tie That Binds*, the experience of the partner whose seropositivity is confirmed by testing.

DECLINE OF THE DIALOGUE

After a while, I started getting angry at myself. I would find myself still sitting in the same place at three in the afternoon, going over things in my head. I do not think it is good for me. It takes up too much time, and I am not getting anything accomplished around the house.

In RETREAT, *The Dialogue* is a welcome respite from the missing. It is a chance to once again feel a semblance of the familiar sense of shared experience with the partner, as well as an important component of the process of integrating, of making sense of the experience. However, in EXPLORATION it may start to feel intrusive, and the partner may find himself actively resisting becoming absorbed in his memories. "It was taking up too much of my life. If I started to feel it coming on, I would find a project to concentrate on." "It began to feel like pouring salt into an open wound." Partners may find themselves finding parallels between the dialogue and their relationships. "Jose was a very dominant person, he could be downright pushy, but I think I really let him dominate me. It was like I was allowing him to continue to dominate me from the grave." In RETREAT, often a component of *The Dialogue* was an attempt to answer unanswered questions left over from the experience, to deal with any unfinished business between the two men. Gradually, the partner may find that questions that at one time demanded answers lose some of their importance. "I came to realize, accept maybe, that there are just going to be a lot of things that I will never know for certain."

As in RETREAT, the approach of an anniversary may trigger an increase in *The Dialogue*. Often, it is not as intense as earlier, and men may actively "take charge" of the experience. "The anniversary of his death is coming around again. I am not thinking about him and the few weeks before he died as intensely as last year, nor do I let myself get carried away with it. I still am going to take the day off from work, though. It was a very significant event for me, and I think it is important to stop and be alone with my thoughts." For other men, the dialogue declines gradually and they do not realize that it has diminished. "I was surprised when I realized that the anniversary of his death is coming around again and I am not busy thinking about it." "For the longest time after Stan died, I would write him a letter in the journal I was keeping every night. Gradually, it became once a week, then once a month. I have not written him anything in months."

Gradually, surviving partners begin to feel that they have made sense of what happened to themselves and their partner. Initially, during CHAOS, partners find themselves feeling that they are not sure exactly what they have been through, except that it was hell. As they look back, they initially find a confusing jumble of painful memories and intense feelings. "I have come to realize that a lot of what I was doing was an attempt to sort it all out, to put everything that he and I went through into some kind of order." In putting the experience into order, men often find the *Guilts* subsiding. "I began to realize that there are other explanations for what happened other than failures on my part."

For some men, rituals that arose during *The Dialogue* of RETREAT continue and come to represent or encapsulate *The Dialogue*. "I go to the cemetery every week. I have confined my conversations with him to the graveside." Often, the rituals continue for several years. "I still go to the cemetery on his birthday, or our anniversary." Men have made enormous strides in redefining their lives, making many significant changes, and perhaps may be involved in a new relationship. But the rituals continue to have great importance, often extending well into BACK INTO THE WORLD. Men who establish new relationships may at times become confused, as they attempt to negotiate the new relationship and acknowledge the importance of the lost partner. "It was kind of confusing. It was Jack's birthday, and, as usual I went to the cemetery to put flowers on his niche and say hello. While I was doing that, David was back home cooking dinner."

DECLINE OF MISSING

There still are times when I miss him a lot. Actually, I probably think about him every day, but it is different now. It is not that painful anymore. The sharp edges seem to have smoothed out.

During EXPLORATION, the painful, aching missing of the partner declines and is gradually transformed into a more mellow experience. As with *The Dialogue,* some men may find themselves beginning to resist the missing. "I got this thing going where if I found myself missing him too much, I would think of some of the lousy things he did to me." The decline of *The Dialogue* and *Missing* may initially be somewhat anxiety-provoking for the partner, as he may fear that he is forgetting his partner. "I hope I do not forget him." For many men, the intensity of missing the partner results in their feeling more connected to him. "At first, I really was afraid that I was losing even more of him." Many men find that the new form that missing takes, one of bittersweet memories, is vastly more comfortable than the original experience. "I now find myself smiling when I think about him. It is not loaded with *angst* the way it used to be."

The idealization of the lost partner that was so prominent in the *Missing* of RETREAT begins to subside. Rather than being remembered as the greatest person who ever walked the earth, the partner becomes viewed in more realistic terms. "I had a tendency to put Mike on a pedestal, but I have also been able to say that he was an asshole at times. He was human. It feels better to be able to acknowledge both sides." In achieving a more balanced view of his partner, the surviving partner is able to gain a different perspective of himself. "I am beginning to realize the enormity of what I have been through. During these past few months, there were times that I felt absolutely crazy. I have come to think that it was all OK. I am human and I have human needs." "Losing your partner is bad enough, but the fact is that we, and I, went through hell."

Partners find themselves beginning to feel lonely rather than alone. "I used to feel all alone in the world. I have come to feel incomplete without a partner, but I am certainly not alone. I have a lot of friends who have been there all through Mike's death, and there for me since then." Some men may find themselves thinking about another relationship. "When he first died, the idea of another man in my life was distasteful, but lately I have been thinking that it would be nice to have a boyfriend." Early in EXPLORATION, men may intuitively sense that negotiating a relationship would be very difficult. "There is a part of me that would just love to jump right into another relationship, but I do not think that is healthy. He would only be a replacement."

A RAY OF HOPE

It has been a real growing couple of months. I am getting a little more comfortable with myself.

Gradually, the good days and bad weeks experienced during RETREAT turn into bad days and good weeks. The shattered self-esteem that dominated *Altered States* is transformed into the growing confidence and excitement found in *A Ray of Hope.* As the partner begins to explore the world and the relationships it has to offer, he begins to feel that perhaps there is a way out of the "black hole" that he fell into with the experience of CHAOS. As the partner experiences successes in negotiating relationships, successfully takes on tasks once performed by his partner, and finds enjoyment in new activities or renews his interest in old ones, he finds himself feeling stronger, more alive, and he senses that perhaps things can get better after all. Where before he may have felt incompetent, enfeebled, and acutely depressed, he now finds himself feeling excited. Evidence that he can succeed in new tasks, negotiate people, and have a good time is welcomed. For the first time in many months, he finds himself smiling. "One of the orchids bloomed the other day. I thought only Stan could get them to bloom."

Some men will find a "safe place" where they can be with other people, yet not feel threatened or overstimulated. For some, it will be volunteer work with AIDS organizations, which also serves to validate their experience as surviving partners and gives them a sense of mastery. Where they may not have been able to save their partners, they can help other people afflicted by the disease. They can also participate in a milieu that is comfortable and familiar. "A few months after Jon died, it felt real important for me to do something. I got involved in Chicago House after I heard about guys getting kicked out of their apartments and having nowhere to go. I had to feel like I was doing something, and it empowered me." In the course of their volunteer work they meet new people, people inclined to respect their experience. "I met some incredible people there and felt real comfortable. For awhile it was the only place that I did feel comfortable." For some men, being able to handle volunteer work will be an indicator that they are getting stronger. "I have started to volunteer at San Francisco General. The first patient they gave me was full of pneumocystis and on the verge of respiratory failure. That is what Mike died of. I was really worried walking into that room, but I was able to handle it."

Partners may also find a great deal of comfort and pleasure in new activities. "I have been taking country /western dance lessons. I keep thinking that the existence of that place, and the availability of it to me, has saved me in the past few months. The men that go there do not have a lot of overtly erotic things on their agendas. They go there to dance and have a good time. It is not an overtly cruisy bar. It's wonderful.'' Men find they can experience a good deal of body contact in the very structured and non-threatening environment that country/western dancing offers. ''I got so much out of it. I am down there a couple of nights a week.'' They may also find themselves becoming preoccupied with something other than their loss and the experience of the illness of their partner. ''I have become obsessed with country western music. It may sound weird, but it is a break from feeling so depressed and anxious and out of control.'' Men may also renew their interests in old activities. ''I started working out at the gym. That feels good too. I have made great strides in the last few months. Muscles that I developed years ago are coming back very quickly.''

As the partner negotiates social situations, he invariably encounters his shattered self-esteem that was so prominent during the *Altered States* of RETREAT. ''I am told that I am a reasonably attractive man, so why should I have all of these insecurities? It's hard sometimes, but I keep trying, and people are responding favorably to me, so that is reassuring.'' ''I kept thinking that I would meet somebody and when I told them that I was an AIDS widow, they would freak.'' To feel successful in venturing out on one's own, to negotiate a party, or a bar, perhaps on a first date, is a welcome sign for the partner that he is ''getting better'' and perhaps there is hope in a world without his partner after all. ''I went to Hawaii with a group of people. Hanging around with them felt fine for a while, but after a few days I was feeling claustrophobic. It was a big step, but I went out on my own. I ran into some people I knew from another city, and I ended up having a great time. I stayed out till three in the morning.'' ''When we were in D.C., the friend I was staying with wanted to take me out. I was very apprehensive. I have not been to a bar as a single person in five years. He took me to a western dance bar. I loved it. The guys were really nice. No one hit on me, except to dance, and I learned the two-step and the three-step.'' Another major event for the partner is the ''first date.'' ''I was really nervous. I have not been out on a date in 13 years. By the time the weekend rolled around, I was a wreck. I was not sure what to do or how to act, but it went fine." "That first date was a mile-stone for me. I had a great time. He had a great time. I began to feel that maybe I was not so weird after all."

The excitement builds as the partner finds evidence that he can be around people again, he can feel good about himself, and he can feel confident. "I was really on the edge, perhaps over the edge, but I have a grip on things now. My feet still feel that they are dangling sometimes, but I am slowly gaining enough strength to work myself onto a level surface." Activities that he and his partner used to do together, which at first may have been quite painful for the surviving partner, begin to be experienced differently. "I used to dread running Saturday errands alone. We always used to do that together but last week I was out running around, I had one of my favorite tapes playing and I found myself singing along and enjoying the spring weather." Confidence continues to grow as the partner feels himself taking charge of ever more aspects of his life. Where he previously may have felt inept in areas that his partner managed, he begins to feel that perhaps he did learn a few things from his partner and can now take them on himself. "I am taking a much more active stance in managing Will's estate. I want to know what is going on. It sounds cold, but Will was a great businessman and when it came to business he was as cold as ice." "John was an investment banker, so he always made the financial decisions. I took some classes on investments so I would know what I am doing when it comes to handling his estate."

HITS

I do not know what happened. I was feeling so much better, then something happened. I feel just as bad as I did at first. Is this ever going to end?

Partners are often sorely disappointed when their *Ray of Hope* is shattered by a *Hit*. A *Hit* that occurs during EXPLORATION will often trigger a brief experience of CHAOS and a more protracted experience of RETREAT. Often the *Hits* of EXPLORATION result from experiences with other men that evoke the memories of the lost partner. "I had met this guy. He was a lot of fun. We had gone out for dinner a few times. I did not think of it as a date or anything. But then in the course of a conversation, he said he wanted to have sex with me. I was floored. I felt raped." While the partner is feeling stronger and more confident, he is often still quite shaky, especially in the area of relationships. If someone comes on too strong, he may find himself feeling overwhelmed. In the wake of the hit, the shattered self-esteem, and the sense of missing, he may retreat home where he again feels safe. "After that, I just stayed home for awhile. It felt safe there. The world felt dangerous again."

Though partners may have been feeling considerably better, the approach of holidays or anniversaries or significant places can also trigger a *Hit*. "I was doing better, but as Christmas approached I started getting agitated. I made sure I was with friends on Christmas Eve, but I wanted to be alone on Christmas Day. It was pretty horrible." "I looked at the calendar and saw that it was the same day he was diagnosed." Partners may have purposely avoided places that they knew would be painful reminders, but as they begin to feel stronger, their vigilance may decline. "I always took another route home than the one that led past the hospital. I was in a hurry and not thinking and there it was, looming at me. I remembered the exact window of the room he died in, four windows from the end of the 12th floor. I lost it. It all came back as if it were yesterday."

However, the retreat will be short-lived. The partner invariably finds himself moving back into EXPLORATION. "The anniversary of his death came and went. Nothing momentous happened. I took the day off and went for a long walk." Men who find themselves overstimulated as they attempt to negotiate relationships may initially swear off dating, but often find themselves "back out there again." "Wasn't it last month that I had sworn off dating forever?"

HELPERS/SPOILERS

My mom is great at sewing. When I was home last, I showed her the design I had come up with for the AIDS quilt. She offered to help. We were really getting into it, and my dad started feeling left out and moping around. We needed four stars and just could not get them right. My dad is a draftsman,

*so I asked him to help us out. He sat down at his drafting table
and came up with a pattern that was perfect. It was really
wonderful having them all pitch in.*

The partner's need for validation of his experience continues into
EXPLORATION, though the quality is much different. It is not so
much the validation of the personal and often exquisite pain of RE-
TREAT, but the validation of the loss as a major event in his life. If
partners are not rushed by deadlines, it is during EXPLORATION
that they create a panel for the AIDS quilt. Partners tend to take
utmost care in planning and creating panels. "Adam used to design
his own Christmas cards. I took the design from one of his favor-
ites, then superimposed his signature on it. It was quite a task. I had
to borrow an opaque projector, project his signature on the wall,
make a pattern, then sew it on the quilt. When I heard the word
quilt, I thought they literally meant quilt. So I spent all of this time
quilting the top panel!"

The partner's experience of the AIDS Quilt in EXPLORATION
is considerably different than in RETREAT. He is more aware of,
and takes comfort in, the sense of shared loss of others. "This time,
I was much more aware of the other panels. I took time to look at
them as I worked my way towards the area where his was. There
really were some beautiful panels. I was also more aware of all of
the sadness and grief around me. I felt more a part of the larger quilt
and total experience than just Adam's panel." While aware of the
larger experience, the personal meaning of the panel is also important. "I was relieved that it was near a walkway. I wanted to sit
down by it and touch, talk to it. I was really taken by knowing that
it had gone all over the country, and that I had caught up with it
again."

Some men will find their encounter with the AIDS Quilt to be
just as deeply validating and subsequently freeing as an encounter
with the "special person." "It was a turning point for me. I am still
trying to sort it all out. I still feel in a daze. I know something very
important happened in D.C., but it has not quite sunk in yet."

If parental response during RETREAT was less than adequate,
some men will give up and look for validation elsewhere. Others
will doggedly pursue their parents until they "get it." "One day, I
really got angry and told them that I was really pissed off at the way

they had not been responding. He was my lover, my spouse, just like they are to each other. They got it. Things have been much smoother between us since then. Men who do not give up but continue to share their experience with their parents often find themselves on better ground than they have ever been before. One cannot talk about the loss of a partner to AIDS without talking about their experience as a gay man. The topic of homosexuality may have been difficult for both parents and their sons for many years. Some men may find a very open line of communication developing, and their long sense of isolation within their families beginning to disappear. "We have had some really great talks. I cannot believe the things we have talked about. I feel closer to them than I ever have as an adult."

Well into EXPLORATION, the approach of holidays may trigger the need to reconnect with the "special person." In many cases, the pain of friends of the partner and couple over the loss is well behind them. But for the partner, the holidays may evoke the profound sense of loss. Often he finds that the "special person" and/or the parents of his partner are feeling the same way. "I felt so awful on Christmas Day. I called his sister, and we cried for an hour. It felt so good I called his mother, and we cried for another hour."

The actions of *Spoilers* may continue to haunt the partner. The memories of families that were difficult during THE LONG HAUL often plague the partner. "When I think of some of the things she said, I still get furious." If the family contests the will, then legal procedures may be drawn out for a number of years. The partner may feel repeatedly pulled back into an experience that he is trying to put behind him. "It made me furious in the beginning, but I really am starting to get enraged with it all. This has gone on for three years. I am trying to move on with my life, but this lawsuit will not let me. I cannot give in because that would invalidate what we had, but I do want it to be over."

As in RETREAT, the partner still needs validation for his efforts at exploring the world and the relationships it has to offer. "I was on vacation in Hawaii with my brother. I got furious with him. When we were on the beach, if anybody said hello, he would get all agitated. And if I talked back to somebody, he would make me feel like a tramp or something. This one guy would come over to talk every day. One day he stopped. I know my brother must have told him that I was an AIDS widow. I was not looking for romance, just a friend or something.''

HOLDING ON/MOVING ON

I am torn between whether to put the picture of Jose on my dresser away, or out of the room, or what. It just stirs up too many memories. I am trying to get on with my life, but it somehow seems disloyal.

During EXPLORATION, *Moving On* gathers momentum. There is increased need and capacity to further define life without the partner. However, this process may also trigger guilt over moving away from the partner and the relationship, as well as missing. Partners may find themselves in a quandary over what possessions to hold on to. The fear of forgetting the partner arises, but what they gradually discover is that they cannot help but *Hold On* to the memories of him. ''I realized that no matter what I do, I will never forget him. He and the time we spent together will always be a part of me, no matter what happens.'' Many men will find themselves contemplating moves of their residences and wanting to disperse some of their partner's possessions. ''I really had to get out of the apartment. It used to feel comforting to be there, now it feels stifling. Plus, it is just too big for one person.'' As the partner contemplates the move, he encounters many of his partner's possessions. ''At first, it was painful going through his possessions. I would come across things that stirred up all kinds of memories. But gradually I got into thinking about who in his family would appreciate what.''

In moving, the partner encounters memories and the meanings various aspects of their home had for his deceased partner. ''In getting the house ready to put on the market, the agent suggested I take down the wallpaper in the kitchen and repaint the walls. It was really hard to do. He papered the kitchen himself and was so proud of the job he did.''

Men who decide to stay in their home are faced with what mementos to keep, or the possibility of redecorating. ''It really is crazy. I want to put some of his pictures away, but I am obsessing about which ones, how many are too many or not enough.'' ''I am getting used to the idea that the place is mine now. A lot of the furniture is looking worn. Sometimes I get excited about changing it, then I think about the nights we cuddled and watched TV on that couch. Other times, I wonder what his friends will say.''

Often a boyfriend will come along. If the partner can feel that his deceased partner would approve, the process is considerably easier. "I really think that is what he would have wanted. I certainly would want him to have someone in his life if I died.''

There will be times, however, even in the midst of so much forward movement, when the need to validate the loss arises. As in RETREAT, validation of the loss facilitates *Moving On*. "I met this guy, and there is something happening between us. I know it would not have been possible without what went on between Mike's sister and I on Christmas Day. It was the first time I really let myself cry.'' Partners may be confused at the way validation of the loss facilitates the process. In one day they may be engaged in two very different activities. "I did not think about it at the time, but I am amazed when I look back. That morning, I was at the AIDS Quilt, looking for Adam's panel and taking in the enormity of it all. That night, my friend took me out. There I was, dancing and having a great time.''

For some men and relationships, the AIDS quilt may not feel appropriate. "I thought about making a panel for him, but John was a very private person, so I decided against it. It was the kind of project that he would have believed in and given money to, but he probably would have been horribly embarrassed to have his name on public display.'' For these men, visiting the gravesite may become a meaningful experience, one that at times enables them to "move on.'' "I was feeling extremely blue on Christmas Day, so I went to his graveside. After my visit, I was quite content and enjoyed my day out with friends.''

NEXT IN LINE

I am beginning to be a hypochondriac. I am afraid to get tested. My active sexuality has come to an end. I have no desire to get close to someone out of fear of not knowing. I do not want to get tested, to find out what the situation is. As bad

*as it is, at this point I would rather be unsure than to know for
certain, but it is having a very big impact on my life.*

In RETREAT, the assumption that one is seropositive and will
follow the same fate often has the quality of a quiet acceptance. In
EXPLORATION, the partner begins to feel alive again. The possibility that he himself may become ill intrudes into the excitement
that he feels. "I really did not think about it that much while he was
sick. I was more concerned with taking care of him. But after he
died, I started getting more and more preoccupied with it. I expected it in the long run, but the more distance I got on his death,
the more I did not want it to happen." The partner has often experienced several "tastes" of what the world offers, either through new
relationships, evolving plans for a change in career, or for picking
up and carrying on with plans that he and his partner had made
together that are still meaningful for him as a single man. Now the
assumption of seropositivity and the possibility of illness and death
are resisted. Being seropositive or assuming that one is, begins to
feel like "a monkey on my back."

Preoccupation with contracting AIDS as their partner did is often
seen in men in all categories—those who know they are negative,
those who know they are positive, and those who do not know of
their antibody status. "Even though I may be considered a surviving partner, I consider myself to be in the category of the 'worried
well.'" Men who may have had difficulty believing their earlier
test results, now find themselves struggling to believe that they are
indeed HIV-negative. "I keep trying to convince myself I had a
close call with AIDS, and only a close call." "It is hard to believe,
that when you have been with someone for four years, and had sex
with someone for four years, that you would not have been exposed
to the virus, but the test says that I haven't." Men may have almost
convinced themselves, only to encounter a report in the media that
sends them back to wondering if they really are "out of danger."
"There was always this worry in the back of my mind that I did
have it. It was to the point of not trusting my doctor's saying that I
was negative. I had begun to settle down when I heard about a
report that said it could be 12 to 14 months after exposure that a

positive test would show up. That sent me right back to worrying again." Some men who tested negative earlier while their partner was alive will get tested again "to make sure." Others will find their preoccupation gradually diminishing the more comfortable they feel being out in the world again. "I went through a period being really worried that I was next, but it is not so central anymore. I think it has something to do with going out on my first date and just being with people again."

When the partner has previously tested positive, they experience the increase in AIDS anxiety with added certainty. "I just cannot get it out of my head. I remember what happened to Stan, think about my being positive, and find myself just waiting for it to happen." "It is making me nuts. I find myself looking for thrush and KS lesions as part of my morning routine." Some men who know they are seropositive but do not know their T-cell counts may decide to have this test performed in order to have an indication of their health status. Often for these men, the test result is viewed with as intense anxiety as the antibody test. "My doc wanted me to do it for quite some time. I always said no, I am not ready for that. Well, finally I went down and took it. Thank God, it was okay, for now . . .''

Men who do not know their antibody status begin to contemplate taking the test. "When Mike was sick, and after he died, I expected an AIDS diagnosis, and I was not afraid of it. I kept going to Dr. S., expecting her to find enlarged lymph nodes, and was almost disappointed when she did not. For a period, I almost wanted to get it. I don't anymore." Taking the HIV test is very anxiety-provoking for most gay men, but especially so for a surviving partner. "At first, I was adamantly against it. I was so hurt by the fact that John had died, and shocked, never having seen death before, or what the disease can do to people. It was so traumatic, seeing my lover dead in a hospital bed." "As much as I worried about it, I did not need any more indications that it could also happen to me."

The surviving partner has already been sorely disappointed; his *Game Plan* failed and his partner died. He is beginning to feel that *Ray of Hope* again. The results of the test are anticipated as indicating whether he will follow in his partner's footsteps or continue to experience the excitement and hope he feels as he re-engages with the world and senses new possibilities for himself. "I took the test, but did not go back for the results. The center told me they would keep it on file, and that I could come in and find out when I am ready. I am just not ready yet. It is information that once you know, you cannot take it back."

The ability to face test results appears to be related to the ability to begin to define one's self as a person in one's own right and not so much as an AIDS widower destined to follow the same path as one's partner. "At first I did not want to know for sure. Now I desperately want to know." "It took me two years before I got tested. I watched Jim die of the disease, and though I assumed I was positive, finding out would just have been devastating. But then, I was getting involved with this guy, and feeling a lot better about myself and I wanted to find out." As partners feel more sure of themselves, they are able to weigh evidence, not so much in terms of the tie to their lost partner, but in terms of their actual experience. "I really do not think that I am going to be positive. I did not have all that much sex back when the virus was infiltrating the community, and Mike and I were never into having a lot of sex during the years before he got sick."

Some men will decide not to get tested, but carry on with their lives as best they can. "I am terrified to find out. I need that edge that I might be negative gives me. My health is fine, my doctor is more concerned about my blood pressure. High blood pressure I can deal with, being positive, no way, not in the light of what happened to Jon." For these men, while they will have the edge they need, they will also have the uncertainty that often shades into the assumption of seropositivity and the "monkey on my back" or "the cloud over my head" that it represents.

If the partner does decide to be tested, he does so with considerable apprehension. "A friend of mine came with me. Even he was sweating." The results of the test will have considerable impact. It is as if partners intuitively know that if they are negative, they will be able to continue on in their process of moving back into the world in full force. If they are seropositive, their experience will be quite different.

THE FORK IN THE ROAD

I finally went down and got my test results. I was negative. I am still processing that. For the last five years, I have been assuming that I was going to get this disease. Especially since Mike got sick, I was positive that I was going to get it. Now I know I am going to live, not that I am going to die — at least not of AIDS.

When the results are negative, partners experience tremendous relief. They have been released from the very real possibility of following their partner in contracting the disease. For the first time in several years, the future is anticipated as one of unfolding possibilities, not one of uncertainty or of certain death.

Partners often feel that for the first time in several years, perhaps for the first time in their lives, they have been given an important gift. "I feel like I am incredibly lucky." They had hoped for a negative result and weighed their chances. Many feel that they have won their bet, beaten the odds. "There was a chance I was negative, else I would not have taken the test."

When partners receive their results, their first thoughts often return to their deceased partner. The issue of transmission feels settled once and for all. "When I found out, one of my first thoughts was, 'So I did not give it to Mike . . . and he did not give it to me.'" The results often trigger a return of *The Dialogue,* as the partner takes the new information that he was negative during his partner's illness and integrates it into the experience. Often, he wonders if he would have been there for his partner in the same way had he known he was negative. "I wonder, if I had known that I was negative during Mike's illness, if I would have been as cavalier, sharing sandwiches, open-mouth kissing him. I do not want to think that I may have been afraid of him."

Negative results represent a loss and a release. A tie to the partner has been undone, leaving the partner free to continue to find new meaning in life. However, it is an additional loss. One more piece of the connection to the partner is gone. "I always thought I was going to be joining Mike in the near future. Now I am probably going to have a longer life without him." "In a way, it is like I lost another part of what we had. To be honest, it is the only part of the relationship that I really do not mind losing, though I do find myself feeling guilty about it sometimes." Evidence for the power of the tie that seropositivity or assumed seropositivity represents is seen in a variety of ways. "While he was sick, I developed the same rash on my foot as he had. After he died it was always there, I would put the same medications on my rash as were prescribed for him, but it never went away. Two weeks after I found out that I was negative, it disappeared."

The partner finds his sense of the future changing dramatically. "Two weeks ago I did not think that I had any time in my future, now I have all of this time." "I guess I am going to have to carry his ashes around for a long time. We were going to have our ashes mixed and dispersed together." Partners who have been released often feel a sense of responsibility to their partner, and to themselves, to take life and themselves more seriously, to go on with plans for career changes, to finish degrees, to continue caring for others who contract the disease. "I always thought I needed the money we saved throughout our lives to die with. Now I can use it to live with." "Before, his estate felt like an insurance policy. Now it feels like a gift. I figured out that it is more than enough to get me through school." Partners find their *Ray of Hope* growing exponentially. In their excitement, they may initially fear that they will forget their partner, but what they find is that the memories of their partner take on a different, less complicated quality, now that the potential of contracting the same disease has disappeared.

In addition to the dramatic changes in his relationship to his deceased partner, the surviving partner may also find that his seronegative status complicates his relationships with his friends, especially if many of them are seropositive and he lives in a community that has been hit hard by the epidemic. "I learned pretty quickly that not everyone was going to be able to relate to just how happy I was. Right after I got the results, I saw a friend on the street and I told him the results. He just said, 'Oh.'" As with men who learned they were seronegative during the partner's illness, the seronegative surviving partner often feels that he has to squelch, or at least to be careful, whom he shares his joy with. "I called Dr. S., she said she was really happy. I called Mike's sister, she was glad also. I called my support group manager and she was really happy. She wants me to come in and tell the group. I really am having a hard time with that one. There are a lot of guys in the group that are positive.''

Partners who test positive may find themselves initially feeling isolated. Friends who know they are seropositive may retreat as they try to integrate their friend's new status. "Chuck lost his partner last year. He isn't really sick, but he isn't really well, either. We have spent a lot of time together these past few months, but it has not been the same since I got the results. I am afraid that he is thinking that, 'He is going to live, and I am going to die.'" The partner may find himself set apart as he attempts to integrate his new status, the implications for the relationship to the deceased partner, the implications for the future, and the excitement he finds growing inside him. "All of my long-term friends are positive. They have been having a hard time dealing with me. They think that I cannot relate to them in the same way as before." Partners may find that finding places to share their grief is easier than finding places to share their joy. "I am a lot more comfortable talking to my women friends about it than to my gay friends." "There should be a support group for people who test negative.'

THE TIE THAT BINDS

It really was a double whammy. In the face of losing my lover I found myself having to grapple with the uncertainty of my future. Though it was a confirmation of what I had assumed, when you know, you know. I very quickly went from feeling worried, but also hopeful, to feeling black, infected, diseased.

When the surviving partner tests positive, the implications are equally profound. Rather than the excitement of the man who tests negative, the surviving partner who tests positive experiences despair. He has not been released from the assumption that he will follow his partner. The future is viewed as a waiting game. He had often had the *Ray of Hope* that came from feeling reconnected to the world. Now, once again he is disappointed. Having lost his lover after hoping he would survive, he now feels that any hope he had of escaping AIDS himself has been dashed as well. "I was really beginning to feel better about losing Jerry. I had met a guy, and we were enjoying each other's company so I decided that maybe there was hope for me after all. When I turned up positive, it was the blackest day of my life." While he faces the same problems as other men who have tested positive—despair, loss of a sense of future, experience of themselves diseased and isolated—there is an added edge for the surviving partner. All through the experience, he has lived with the assumption that he was positive and would develop AIDS. This stems as much from the bond between the two men as it does from modes of transmission. The surviving partner now tends to feel all the more assured that his fate is sealed.

The asymptomatic partner who was able to have himself tested has gained a sense of distance from the despair he initially felt upon the death of his partner and in the months that followed. "I finally felt I was ready to handle finding out." He is able to begin to view himself as a person in his own right. With the positive test result, he returns in a very intense way to viewing himself in relation to his dead partner. *The Dialogue* is radically different for these men. Rather than integrate their being negative in reconstructing the experience, they now call upon their partner for guidance, as a model for facing the disease. "I found myself wondering if I would be as strong as he was. I remember thinking he was pretty strong, very courageous at times. I still think that. Actually, I think he was more so all of the time." "I found myself asking him to help me to be as strong as he was, to show me the way." Partners also find their thoughts turning to their status as single men. "I was there to take care of Stan. I saw how helpless he was when he was so sick. I find myself wondering who will take care of me."

Often, the effect of the positive result is to stop any forward movement. "In having lost my lover and faced with the possibility of my getting sick, for me it spelled, 'Hold on to the status quo, do not make any new commitments, stay right where you are.'" The partner who tests positive may become more concerned with maintaining his health than with reconnecting to the world. Maintenance becomes more important than *Moving On*.

Men who know they are positive and go through the period of increased AIDS anxiety often find it gradually subsiding. "About eight months after he died, I went through a period of being very preoccupied with getting sick myself. I was sure that I was going to die also, but it has mellowed considerably. I really feel like I am going to live." While they find it subsiding, the possibility of getting sick rarely completely disappears. "It is there, lurking in the background. Whenever I get the least bit sick it jumps up again. You would think that I would be used to it by now, but when it hits, it hits."

When the surviving partner who knows he is positive becomes symptomatic, the effect is often similar: stop everything and stay put. "I knew I was positive since shortly after Dan became sick. After he had been dead for a year, I felt ready to go ahead with going to culinary school. We had planned on doing that just before he got sick. A couple of days before I was ready to leave I decided to have my T-cells checked. They were 168. I decided I had better stay put. I was not sure how I would handle it physically and psychologically; the move, being back in school, a new career. I really was looking forward to it, but I decided to stay put. My friends are here. I did not want to get sick out there where I really did not know anybody." When lab results are onerous, the surviving partner feels that he has begun the same course as his lost partner. "I was terrified. I kept thinking about Stan and what he went through. It felt like what I had feared for so long was beginning." "I cannot begin to describe the terror I felt."

Surviving partners who become symptomatic may find themselves withdrawing. "I really did not want to be around people. It was like I was folding into myself." They may also encounter a great deal of difficulty in feeling hopeful, in believing that treatment regimens will indeed be effective. "I have had one game plan fail already. Why should this one be any different?" Perhaps the most difficult task for the symptomatic surviving partner is to view himself as a person in his own right, not a reflection of his dead partner. "At first, it was difficult to not think that what happened to John was going to happen to me, but I have come to see that physiologically we are two very different people. I am having some problems now, but they are not nearly as severe as what he encountered."

Chapter XIII

Back into the World

I am so excited. So many things have happened. I have so much to tell you about! I am working days, taking classes in the evening, and I have a new boyfriend!

BACK INTO THE WORLD is an ongoing, evolving category. It is also the area where the differences between HIV-positive and HIV-negative men that began to emerge in EXPLORATION become more clearly defined. Some of the differences are subtle, some are profound. While the quotes from interviews with these men indicate the differences to a degree, the affects of the men are the most dissimilar. One does not sense the same quality of excitement in seropositive men or those that assume positivity that one does in seronegative surviving partners. While the seropositive surviving partner at times may find himself getting excited, often this is in response to good news about his health. Hence, it is a contingent excitement, not the excitement that comes with viewing the future once again as a series of unfolding possibilities.

The experiences of the seropositive partner overlap into the general experiences of men who are seropositive. One cannot overestimate the psychological impact of testing positive for the HIV virus. Often, men who test positive go to considerable effort to regain a sense of connection to the world and to retain a sense of future, let alone hope for the future. Many find that being involved with social/support groups for men who have tested positive is extremely valuable for this process. The seropositive or symptomatic surviving partner has witnessed first-hand the effects of the virus. The same virus that killed his partner is inside him. For these men the challenge is to define themselves in their own right, to maintain

175

their hope in the face of the fear, and often the conviction, that they will follow in their partners' footsteps.

The properties of BACK INTO THE WORLD are: *Excitement*, the partner's excitement at once again feeling whole and of sensing the future as a series of unfolding possibilities; *Ordering*, the emergence of a perspective on the illness and loss of the partner; *New Relationships*, the partner finding new love attachments, or deciding to pass on relationships for the time being; *New Directions*, the partner following new career paths and interests; and *Holding Pattern*, a property unique to seropositive individuals and those who assume seropositivity, in which the emphasis becomes one of maintaining one's health, taking life one day at a time.

EXCITEMENT

It really is surprising, exciting, to feel this way after so many months of feeling horrible, of being in that darkness of mourning and grief. It is great to feel excited again.

After so many months of feeling acutely depressed, sad, depleted, diminished, and enfeebled, the partner finds himself feeling confident, capable, and most importantly, excited. The excitement of *Ray of Hope* in RETREAT may have felt tenuous, and it was. In BACK INTO THE WORLD, the excitement feels, and is, more solid and reliable.

The partner finds his shattered self-esteem being replaced by confidence. "I felt so bad about myself, so self-conscious, so unsure of myself. That is all gone now. I really feel that I can accomplish anything I put my mind to." Along with the excitement, a sense of strength evolves. "Not only am I happy, I feel stronger now than I ever have before." With great delight they contrast their current sense of self with their experience during the months following their partners' deaths. "If anyone would have told me a year ago that I would be feeling and doing what I am today, I would have told them they were crazy." Before, he may have felt that "half of me is gone," now he feel like "a whole person again."

Partners experience the excitement as they take off in new career directions and continue to experience successes. No longer painfully unsure of themselves, these surviving partners go at their pursuits with gusto. "I do not think that I have ever had as strong a sense of direction as I do now." "I can do it, I have been out of school for 20 years and I am 20 years older than most of the other students, but I also got higher grades than them." Not only does their sense of future return, but it often returns with a perspective that may have been missing before their partner got sick, and that certainly was absent during the months of mourning. "I feel like the future is one of endless possibilities."

In contrast to seronegative surviving partners, the seropositive or symptomatic, surviving partner does not experience the same quality or depth of excitement. "I thought I was pulling out of mourning Dan so much, but I am becoming aware of, like, a low-grade depression." They may sense that something is missing, that things are not quite right. They may feel very much back on track career-wise, but, again, something is missing. "I took on a new job, one that I am very capable of handling. The company wants me to oversee the opening of two more retail outlets. I should be excited, but I am not." "I have been given major new responsibilities at work. I have done an excellent job, but I do not get that excited. Something is missing."

Seropositive or symptomatic partners may periodically experience excitement. Often it is in relation to improved or stable lab counts. Hence, it is a contingent excitement, one that is not as stable, deep or reliable. "I got really good news from the Doc. My T-cell count is 700." "I am really relieved. My T-cells actually went up for a change." "I really feel great. After finding out my T-cells were so low, then the horrible bout with shingles and all of the pain, the new combination of pain meds my doc prescribed works like a charm, plus my T-cells went up 60 points. For the first time in four months, I am feeling great." Frustration or anger may result from feeling stuck. "I really get frustrated. I feel like I am sitting on a fence, looking at the other side, but every time I think it is safe to jump off, something else comes up, or I am reminded just how tenuous things continue to feel."

ORDERING

*Losing Mike to AIDS and the way I felt that year after he died
was the most traumatic thing that ever happened to me. But,
given how old my family tends to live, I have another 40 years
to look forward to. Mike occupied 14 years of my life. When I
look back at 80, I am going to realize that it really was a very
short time.*

In BACK INTO THE WORLD, one observes the partner *Ordering* the experience. The partner places the illness and death of his
partner into a larger life perspective. Before, caring for his ill partner and mourning his loss occupied the very center of his life. Now
he is able to feel that the experience is behind him, that it is a part of
his history, a very sad, painful part — often the most traumatic series
of events and experiences that ever happened to him — but nevertheless, only a chapter in his life, one that he can learn from and that
may enrich his life as he faces the future. The partner was faced
with many challenges, but he feels that he has overcome them,
often gaining a great deal of personal strength in the process.

Important contrasts in the *Ordering* of seronegative partners and
partners who are positive or assume they are positive can be observed. The differences in the experiences of HIV-negative and
HIV-positive partners that began to be observed during EXPLORA-
TION become increasingly clear and distinct as they move BACK
INTO THE WORLD. The seropositive surviving partner finds himself pulling out of the experience of mourning only to be confronted
with the challenges facing men who test positive or are manifesting
signs and symptoms of HIV infection. Rather than sense the world
as once again offering boundless opportunities, he faces an uncertain and frightening future. He may be convinced that the same
disease that killed his partner is in the process of killing him. The
loss of his partner, and perhaps several friends to the disease adds
weight to the conviction. For these men, there is not the sense of a
devastating chapter in their life being behind them and closed.
Rather the experience continues, and many fear that it will not be
over until they themselves succumb to the disease.

The seronegative partner, by contrast, finds himself feeling radically different than he has felt since before his partner became ill. He orders the experience of mourning, the experience of the partner's illness, and the relationship. In describing the experience of mourning the metaphor of darkness and light is often employed. "Things were so dark for me in the beginning, but I have made a lot of progress. It really does get better, a great deal better." "It felt like this summer was night. It finally started to get light out. I saw colors again and I felt a part of things once more." Partners point to key events in the process of mourning. "Testing negative was a real turning point for me. I was feeling confident again. It was like I was standing there, waiting to turn a corner. When I tested negative, I was free to go on." "D.C. was a real turning point for me. Being there with all of those people, all with their own grief, being with Adam's panel in the midst of a nine-acre quilt, it all just seemed to begin to fall into place. A few weeks later, I woke up one morning and said, 'Okay, enough of this. It is time to move on.' And I did."

A sense of satisfaction in how the partner's illness was handled may evolve. "You know, I really felt that we handled things right. We made the most of what support was available to each of us, and to us as a couple. Not that there were not some very rough times. It is a horrible disease that does horrible things to people. I know and am convinced that I played a central role in things going as well as they did." If the partner had been plagued by doubts about the way the disease was managed, the experience is more squarely placed between the two men. "I wish we could have talked more. Maybe it would have been easier on me or both of us. But he was stubborn as a mule sometimes. And, looking back he would always get more stubborn the more I got excited, insistent, or anxious about something."

The relationship and the particular meaning it had for the two men also achieves a perspective. Often, the surviving partner feels that as he moves on with his life he will not need the same characteristics in another partner should one come along. "At that time in my life, I desperately needed that feeling of being grounded that Mike provided. If I have learned one thing through all of this, it is that I can stand on my own two feet." "When Adam and I met, we were two people who desperately needed each other to feel complete. I do not feel that I need or want that kind of relationship with someone else. I feel very complete now.''

Partners often find themselves feeling radically different about who they are and what they have to offer. "In many ways, I feel stronger than I ever have. I feel like I have grown a great deal and am a much better, solid person." They may find a new sense of self-confidence evolving, one that they never felt before. "I have never felt this much sense of direction in my life." The deceased partner is far from forgotten. He has a place in the surviving partner's experience of himself. "I will always love him. He is a part of me, I learned a great deal from him. We had four years together and yes, they ended tragically. It is up to me to carry on and make the most of what I learned.''

In the *Ordering* of the seropositive or symptomatic partner, that sense of completeness and that the experience is behind them is lacking. The pain is more evident. These men still feel that they have learned a great deal, grown, and matured considerably, but they do not achieve the perspective of negative partners. Some of the idealization and pain so prevalent during the *Missing* of RE-TREAT is heard. "I am hurt by the past. I carry some scars about that traumatic experience, but three years later I am living much more in the present. My concerns have less to do with Jim. He left me a tremendous legacy." "It's not the pain anymore, it's more like a hurting, the mere fact that someone had to die, that kind of pain. The unfortunate circumstance of the whole thing. That someone had to suffer and die, but even more so, that it was Dave." "I still find myself asking, 'what would Jim have done?'"

These men feel that they also have grown and matured through the experience. "Along with the shock, a tremendous amount of wisdom came. I see the world differently, feel more mature. Out of the grief, a tremendous number of good things came out." However, they do not sense that they can carry their strength well into the future and use it to enrich their lives. They feel instead that they can use it to face the uncertainty that lies ahead. "Having been through it with Jim, in some ways I am less afraid of dying. I do not want to die, but I am less afraid of it.''

As they look to the future, a nagging question may arise: "Who will be there for me?" "I know what this disease is like. I know what it takes to care for someone. But who is going to take care of me? It is not the dying I am so much afraid of, it is the process. I do not want to die, I do not want to die alone, but I also do not want to put anyone through it, either." "I used to hope for a miracle for him. Now, I find myself hoping for a miracle, some sort of scientific breakthrough — for me."

NEW RELATIONSHIPS

I have a new boyfriend now. He is a wonderful person.

Surviving partners find a renewed interest and vastly enhanced capacity to negotiate new relationships. Some will find themselves becoming involved with one person again. Others will choose to "play the field" and focus on career pursuits. Still others will negotiate a new career or school program and a relationship. They may well be surprised by the energy they find available for such varied pursuits. Some men may have developed relationships during earlier areas of experience, but relationships that either last until the partner makes it BACK INTO THE WORLD, or those that develop during this time, have a much fuller and richer quality.

They may for a time find themselves frightened of sex. "I am afraid of sex. I saw what it did to Adam. I am negative and I want to stay that way." But if the right person comes along, they find themselves feeling very differently. "I was so scared of sex, so frightened by it, but it all melted away with him. It was so wonderful to find that I could feel again, to feel alive, to have someone touching my body."

Other men will enjoy the experience of dating, but not pursue another commitment for a while. "I have decided to pass on relationships. I am having fun dating, but getting on with my career is most important." As they find their confidence returning, they may find themselves being pursued, often to their delight. "I love it. I am going to go down to L.A. to visit this one guy next weekend. Then there is this other one who keeps calling from San Diego and wanting to come up here for a weekend."

In contrast to the relationships of the HIV-negative partner, the relationships of the seropositive partner are related in a very different manner. There is a tenuous, less joyful, more complicated tone about them. "I have a boyfriend. We have a very comfortable life. I am still having tremendous doubts about getting together with someone, about making a commitment, there are so many doubts about my own future. I am not sure that I have completely done away with the grief over Jim's death." "It has been difficult to establish a new relationship. I feel like I am living on borrowed time, that it just would not be fair to someone."

Other men may find that the interest simply is not there, that somehow new relationships just do not hold the same satisfaction that they had found with their partner. "I still feel, in a way, the satisfaction of my relationship. I have dated, probably fell in lust more than love. I wonder if I am carrying a torch or something, but I just have not felt the need to find a replacement or having someone there."

Often, surviving partners who are positive find themselves experiencing the same fear when it comes to relationships that is common among men in general who are HIV positive: the fear of abandonment. "Dave reacted much more positively than I did when I tested positive. I guess I was scared of losing him. He made it very clear that it did not matter to him, but the fear is still there." Men who test positive often encounter difficulty in negotiating relationships in the face of so much uncertainty. Again, the surviving partner has had first hand experience of the potential effects of HIV infection and the hardships, and at times anger at the ill partner that accompanies AIDS. "He says he will be there no matter what, but I have lived through it, I know what it is like." The fear of being abandoned while he is ill may compromise his capacity to trust that a new partner will indeed, as promised, be there for him, the way he was for his partner. The loss of his partner and the erosive psychological effects of being positive and in some cases symptomatic may further diminish the surviving partner's sense of self-esteem. For some men the future looks frightening; it may look even more complicated and frightening as they contemplate a new relationship. "I really do not think that I have a whole lot to offer someone. Bill and I were together for seven years before he got sick, what if I get sick in a few months?"

Some seropositive surviving partners may find that if the right person comes along, the excitement of the new relationship over-rides their fears. "He came along when I least expected it. I never thought anyone would be able to love me again, but it was one of those things, as soon as I met him I knew we were supposed to be together." If the new boyfriend or partner is also positive, it may feel less complicated. "I wonder if it would have worked if he were negative, with his being positive, it was one less thing to worry about. I cannot imagine trying to have a relationship with someone who was negative, I would constantly be worried about infecting him and I could not live with myself if I thought I had infected someone." The future for these men is still frightening, but the relationship may help buffer the fear for the future and maintain a focus on today. "Sure I live in dread of getting sick, but I haven't yet, and AZT helps me feel that maybe I have a future after all. So we are enjoying what we have now. We travel a lot and spend a lot of time at our house in the woods. I learned from Joe's illness that once you are sick there is no enjoyment, so we are enjoying ourselves now—for as long as we can."

NEW DIRECTIONS

I am really busy now. I went back to work in a hardware store. I really enjoy it. It's great to be out of the house and doing something again, though my feet are killing me.

Surviving partners often find themselves taking on new career pursuits, returning to school, or becoming re-invested in their original careers. Some men will find themselves going ahead with career directions that they had considered for quite some time. Others will find that in the course of caring for their partners new interests will have evolved. Again, there is that sense of gusto, and delight with both the challenge and successes they encounter.

Plans that had been considered but lay dormant during the relationship may come to fruition. "I went to an open house for a nursing program. I thought, 'What the hell, I have always wanted to do this.' So I signed up." Others will find that in the course of caring for their partners and learning about previously unfamiliar professions, a new interest will evolve. "I was very impressed with the nurses I encountered during Mike's illness, plus I found that I really enjoyed volunteering at San Francisco General." As in earlier areas of the larger experience, the partner may encounter a *Helper*. "The more I thought about it I wanted to go into nursing, but, at 42, I wondered if I would get accepted, if they would think that I was too old. I was at a luncheon for volunteers at the hospital and I was seated next to this woman. We got to talking, and I told her the whole story about Mike, and volunteering, and thinking about nursing school, but wondering if I was too old. Well, she turned out to be the Dean of one of the nursing programs in the city! She told me that I certainly was not too old, gave me her phone number, and told me that if I had any trouble getting in, to give her a call."

In the past, a several year plan may have felt overwhelming. Now partners find that they can easily commit to an education track that will take them several years to complete. "I have about 4 or 5 prerequisites to take before I can get into nursing school, then it will take me about three years to get my BSN." "It is a part-time evening program, it will take me three years to finish." A commitment to their communities and to others who have been impacted by AIDS is often evident. "I really want to go into nursing with AIDS patients. I feel a sense of responsibility." "I am co-leading a support group for significant others."

New Directions may be observed in seropositive partners, but they often lack the enthusiasm and long-range projections of the seronegative surviving partner. Those who assume they are positive but have not been tested may make long-range plans, but proceed with uncertainty. "It is a two-year doctoral program. It is a lot of work, but I think I can make it, assuming my health holds out." Some partners become very active in AIDS support organizations. "I am on the board of Test Positive Aware, I work at Chicago House and I am involved in the Names Project." While these men often give a great deal of time and energy, their perspective is different from that of the seronegative partner. The seronegative partner feels that he is offering himself to people whose experience he has shared but has now been released from. The surviving partner who is seropositive or symptomatic often finds a sense of belonging in these organizations.

Partners may find career plans blocked by medical problems, uncertainty regarding the future, or anxiety raised by switching insurance plans. As this quote from EXPLORATION indicates, new directions may be blocked by medical problems. "A couple of days before I was to leave for culinary school, I decided to have my T-cells checked. They were 168. I decided I had better stay put." "Sometimes I really would like to get out of the city. My company has offices in different parts of the country, some of them really nice places to live, but the thought of getting sick in a new city, where I do not know anyone and so far away from my family, is pretty scary."

Concerns over insurance coverage may also block *New Directions*. "I really would like to go into business for myself, but I really am afraid that I would be tested and unable to get insurance coverage. I know how expensive this disease can be." The *New Directions* some men will take will be the next property, *Holding Pattern*.

HOLDING PATTERN

> *I am reluctant to make any new commitments. I guess I feel most comfortable in a holding pattern.*

Holding Pattern is a summary and elaboration of the contrasts in the experiences of partners who are positive and/or symptomatic, described in the previous properties. Surviving partners face the same challenges as other men who are HIV positive and/or symptomatic: maintaining a sense of connection to others in the face of the isolation they often experience; maintaining their health; and perhaps most importantly, maintaining their hope in the wake of the deaths of their partners, and in the face of the progression of their own HIV infection, and perhaps the progression of illness in and deaths of friends as well.

A common experience among HIV-positive or symptomatic men is the loss of a sense of future. One cannot overestimate the impact of this loss on human psychological functioning. Some men, after becoming involved in support groups and/or psychotherapy, will find their sense of future returning. However, it is a contingent one, based on health indicators and lack of progression of the HIV infection to ARC or AIDS. For some men, letting go of despair over the lack of future and being able to live in the present is a valuable, adaptive achievement. "I am living in the present, not thinking a lot about the future. I am much more present-oriented than I ever was." An integral component in adapting to seropositivity is the feeling that one is doing something about the situation, taking an active role in maintaining one's health. "I am letting go of my long-term goals for now. I have taken a leave from work, and am focusing on my health." "I am on a macrobiotic diet, I go to the gym regularly, get plenty of rest and I am going to begin taking egg lecithin."

Being part of a support network is often very important for men who are seropositive. "When you are an HIV-impacted individual, you are going to need a lot of support." A common experience among test-positive men is isolation, feeling cut off, separated from the rest of the world. "One of my big problems was feeling isolated. I like feeling part of a group with similar hopes and fears." In the group experience, the sense of isolation may wane. "I really enjoy the group. It feels like we are all helping each other out." These men may not only find their sense of isolation waning, but find their hope returning as well. "It gives me a sense of community and identity. I see a lot of good role models, people who are in the same situation and are active, contributing members of society. It has a tremendous effect."

In the wake of so much uncertainty and the required efforts at maintenance, individual relationships may be experienced with considerable anxiety. While survivors often derive a great deal of pleasure and support from their new relationships, they find a nagging question remains: "Do I want to put him through what I went through with Jim?" If the person with whom the partner is involved is negative, then they may feel that it adds to the complication. Again, a group may provide a buffer for the survivor's fears and experiences. "I have talked to other HIV-positive individuals who are in a mixed dating situation. These issues seem to be pretty common." Some will find a man with the capacity to maintain a relationship in the face of the challenges confronting the seropositive surviving partner. "I really appreciate Don. He always has accepted me just as I am."

Ultimately, the symptomatic surviving partner must rely on hope to sustain him. "You always hold out until the end. Throughout the entire experience of the past three years, I have learned that hope is really one of the great virtues that we as human beings have. Always hope for the future. It will get you through the worst situations. Sometimes you make it, sometimes you don't. Hope keeps me going."

Chapter XIV

Mourning Theory Reconsidered

The reconstruction of the experience of men whose relationships were impacted by HIV infection and AIDS in the previous chapters can be viewed from many perspectives. Indeed, as Glaser and Strauss (1967) stated: ". . . since the categories are discovered by examination of the data, laymen involved in the area to which the theory applies will usually be able to understand it, while sociologists [in the case of clinical ethnography, clinicians] who work in other areas will recognize and understand theory linked with the data of a given area" (p. 3-4). This reconstruction represents an historical account of these men and their experience of AIDS. For men currently trying to organize and understand their experience of AIDS, it offers the potential of a healing encounter. For clinicians, the data offer an illustration of clinical theory with considerable implications. The data demand a review of our existing theory, and a push forward to fill in the theoretical gaps that currently exist. Recent advances in the clinical theory of the self and the integration of linguistic and communication models into psychoanalytic theory make this endeavor possible. Consequently, new territory will be charted in an effort to elaborate a theory of mourning from a self psychology framework. Again, the data demand that attempts be made to give a theoretical accounting for the differences in the mourning experiences of seropositive and seronegative men.

To do this, I will discuss the development of psychoanalytic mourning theory, the problems with the theory in general and for the understanding of gay men in particular, offer a more elaborated self psychological model, illustrate the theory with the study results and theoretically account for the observed differences in the mourning process of seronegative and seropositive men.

THE MOURNING PROCESS

The basic formulation regarding the nature of the mourning process that has guided our theoretical and clinical understanding for more than 70 years can be found in Freud's (1912-13) work *Totem and Taboo*: ". . . Mourning has a quite specific task to perform: its function is to detach the survivor's memories and hopes from the dead. When this has been achieved the pain grows less, and with it the remorse and self-reproach." The two interrelated and enduring elements are: (1) mourning concerns two central figures, the mourner and the deceased, more specifically, the memories, hopes and affects — essentially the meaning of the particular relationship and its loss, (2) mourning is a process that, in an undistorted form, consists of a reorganization of the ego of the mourner. Essentially the loss of a central person and the accompanying psychological manifestations of loss gradually move the person from a central, painful and often overwhelming aspect of the survivor's experience to a less central, affectively charged position. When this reorganization has been achieved, the survivor is able to again feel a part of the world of the living and have the psychological resources to actively participate in new love attachments.

With the publication of "Mourning and Melancholia" (1917), Freud laid out a theory of relationships, their loss and subsequent role in the structuralization of the mind. The process consists of a libidinal cathexis to another person. With the loss of the person, the libidinal energy must be withdrawn. The ego initially protests and resists as this represents the abandonment of a libidinal position. In successful mourning the object is eventually preserved in the form of an identification and libidinal energy is available for new attachments. In pathological mourning or melancholia, the object is not decathected due to unresolvable ambivalence; rather the libido is withdrawn into the ego and the ambivalence towards the lost object becomes an aspect of the ego's structure.

Pollock (1961), in the framework of analytic ego-psychology, describes the process as a gradual realignment of the self representation and the object representation — representations being internalized intrapsychic counterpoints to the individual's experience of the world. Object representations consist of the images and experiences with individuals whom the person has formed attachments, while self representations consist of images and experience of the person himself. Over the course of the lifecycle, reality calls for modifications in self and object representations. In the case of mourning, the process consists of integrating the reality of the loss.

The object representation is decathected, giving rise to the pain associated with the loss of an attachment. A component of the process is the mourner experiencing a gradually shifting series of identifications with the deceased. Gradually, the self representation is modified and "reshaped," partially in the image of the dead individual. Two potential pathologicial outcomes to the process are: (1) an excessive identification with the lost individual, in which the object representation becomes incorporated into the self representation; or (2) an inability to tolerate the process of mourning, in which the object representation remains intact and the fantasy evolves that the person never died. Crucial to this process is the ability to work through ambivalent feelings toward the deceased. As the ambivalence toward the deceased is resolved, the object representation is transformed into a set of memories, cathexis is withdrawn and the individual is available for new attachments. Pollock also points out that the work of mourning is never fully completed, that often on anniversaries the mourner will consciously or unconsciously recall the deceased.

The emphasis on the ability to work through ambivalent feelings toward the deceased indicates the extent to which traditional analytic theory is based on drives and their organization or psychic structure as being the primary determinants of behavior, consequently key determinants in the ability of the individual to mourn. The ability to resolve ambivalence is contingent on the resolution of the oedipal phase and the consequent laying down of the repression barrier. A reflection of this problem is seen in the debate among psychoanalysts concerning what ages and levels of intrapsychic structure a child must theoretically obtain in order to be able to mourn. (See Shane and Shane 1990 and Palombo 1981 for more thorough reviews of this literature.) This is the aspect of traditional analytic theories that makes them problematic in understanding the mourning process of gay men. In the traditional analytic framework, homosexual men and women have not reached the oedipal level of drive organization (Lewes 1988). Consequently, children and homosexuals are considered to be infantile in terms of psychic structure, hence theoretically unable to mourn.

The theoretical consequences of an unmourned loss in an individual incapable of mourning are considerable: "Without the capacity to adequately mourn an overwhelming loss, the child's development is significantly impeded. It is postulated that because the child cannot mourn—that is, give up (decathect) the attachment to an investment in the representation of the lost person—or cannot preserve the relationship in the form of an identification, the search goes on forever for the parent whose death is unconsciously denied and the person remains, in an important sense, the child at that phase or age when the loss was sustained. Thus, the fantasy that the parent still lives and can be found again precludes the possibility for true replacement, not just in childhood, but throughout life" (Shane & Shane 1990, p.116).

CLINICAL THEORY AND HOMOSEXUALITY

Before moving on to a discussion of mourning in a self psychological paradigm, a brief detour into a theoretical discussion of homosexuality is in order.

Clinicians who strive to practice from a depth psychology model with gay men or lesbian women face a central theoretical problem. Until fairly recently, all of our depth, or analytic, psychological models were rooted in libidinal drive theory. Over the last twenty years, self psychological theory has assumed increasing influence on analytic theory and clinical practice. Clinical understanding and intervention with homosexual men and women within a self psychology framework provides a better model than libidinal and ego-analytic theories, which rely heavily on the cornerstone of oedipus and the heterosexual functioning that successful resolution represents. Freud (see Lewes 1988 for a thorough account) struggled for years to reconcile his clinical and personal experience with homosexual men and women, and the developmental aspects of his theory which placed them in a less psychologically capable position.

Isay (1989) has attempted to describe clinical intervention with gay men within a drive theory based theoretical framework. However, his selective inattention to key aspects of the theory, especially the resolution of the oedipal conflict and the formation of the superego, the laying down of the repression barrier and the difference between homosexuality and neurosis, essentially leave him operating from an atheoretical position.

The basic issue comes down to the role of sexuality in the development of the structure of the mind. Does the development of sexual or libidinal drives shape the mind (in the orthodox analytic view with significant implied deficits), or does the self's organization and coherence influence the experience of sexuality and the ability to form relationships that are mutually enhancing? Clearly the general direction that analytic theory is currently moving indicates that the latter provides a broader explanation of the phenomena than the former.

In clinical work with gay men, "the issue is not what caused the patients' homosexuality, it is the meaning that being homosexual has for the particular person" (Shelby 1989). In the course of development, homosexual children live in the context of a selfobject environment (both parental and the larger environment) that is culturally phobic if not outright hostile towards homosexuality and its sexual expression. Consequently, the developing self often experiences numerous selfobject failures and outright narcissistic assaults. However, It would be too simple to merely blame a homophobic society.

Clearly, the shared sense of sexuality or masculine competence is an important element in the mirroring and alter ego components of the father/son dialogue and often dramatically affects the idealizing sphere as well. Subsequently, the homosexual child does not experience these selfobject functions in an uncomplicated manner, and the self organization begins to include the experience of being different, incompetent, and at times attacked because of the differences.

A series of meanings becomes structured around these often painful experiences, and a distance or gap in experience often develops in the father/son dialogue that is difficult to mediate. These early experiences become the organizers for which messages from the larger homophobic environment are understood and become the basis for the self experience which Maylon (1982) has referred to as "internalized homophobia." In the course of the mourning process, these experiences and meanings are often reawakened. If the environmental response is nonsupportive or attacking, they may take on a central significance.

MOURNING AND SELF PSYCHOLOGY

In the self psychological model, the loss is viewed as the loss of a selfobject relationship which brings about an imbalance in self-esteem (Palombo 1981, p.82). In many cases, the imbalance in self-esteem is more acurately described as a massive disorganization of the self and shattering of self-esteem. Relationships will vary in the degree to which individuals rely on one another for specific selfobject experiences, hence each relationship will vary in terms of the meaning of the loss and consequently, the psychological impact on the mourner.

Shane and Shane (1990) extend formulations of mourning theory within a self psychology framework. Though they focus on children, they assert that it is not the degree of psychic structure that enables the child to mourn, rather the presence and ability of the surviving parent or other adult to tolerate, mirror, sustain, and share the range of the child's affects regarding the lost parent, essentially to provide "compensatory self-structure . . . to repair the weakened aspects of the self, but facilitate continued or renewed development" (p.119).

In the face of the massive loss of selfobject functions of the deceased parent, the surviving parent (when not overly compromised by his/her own grief) serves as a selfobject that facilitates the mourning process. When this supportive environment is available, the child is able ". . . to face the impact of the loss without feeling the risk of being overwhelmed, annihilated, or fragmented (p.118). ". . . The pain of the loss can be borne and the necessary capacity to think, talk, and reflect about it can be sustained if the child is helped to mourn" (p.119). The authors postulate that for many children, the surviving parent's inability to perform these functions results in a double loss for the child and accounts for the considerable pathology observed later in life. The loss of the parent is further complicated when the surviving parent is so compromised by his/

her own grief as to be unable to provide the sustaining selfobject environment to support the child's mourning process. Hence, in the face of an overwhelming loss, the child is once again abandoned.

It is reasonable to assert that adults as well as children require selfobject experiences to facilitate the self reorganization that mourning involves. While Shane and Shane (1990, p.19) indicate that the presence of a required "optimal selfobject environment, [is] more available to the adult," they do not elaborate on the nature of the role of the selfobject matrix in adult mourning. Indeed, the results of this study clearly demonstrate the central role selfobject encounters with individuals who exhibit their understanding and tolerance of the mourners' affects, concerns and general psychological state play in facilitating the reorganization of the self that mourning involves.

At this point in time an elaborated theory of mourning in a self psychological framework has not been posited. The basic elements exist in the literature: Kohut's (1978) assertion that "[there] is no mature love in which the love object is not also a selfobject, or, to put this depth psychological formulation into a a psychosocial context, there is no love relationship without mutual self-esteem enhancing, mirroring and idealization" (p.141); Palombo's 1981 statement that "the loss must also be viewed as the loss of a selfobject relationship which brings about an imbalance in self-esteem"; and Shane and Shane's 1990 indication that there exists a "required optimal selfobject environment" for the mourning process. The results of this study[1] and recent advances in clinical theory enable us to make a beginning in the formulation of a theory of mourning within a self psychological framework.

In recent years, many theorists have worked towards integrating linguistic and/or cognitive theories into psychoanalytic theory. Since the time of Freud, analytic theory has tended to develop in a context of its own, generally ignoring advances in cognitive and

---

1. One could argue that I am using analytic theory, but not analytic level data — that is, men in the study were interviewed periodically versus the considerably more intensive experience of psychoanalysis where one presumedly has greater access to unconscious processes. I am attempting to begin the process of reframing mourning within the framework of self psychology and other theoretical advances.

linguistic theories. (Krystal 1990). This reexamination of psychoanalysis in the context of other theories so basic to human experience — cognition, language and developmental research — has resulted in a necessary revision of the philosophical underpinnings of
clinical theory — how the mind develops, is organized and perhaps
most importantly, the nature of the therapeutic process itself (for
example, Stern 1985; Saari 1986; Basch 1988; Goldberg 1990; Palombo 1990).

Palombo (1990) presents an integration of numerous theorists
into a cohesive theory of the nature of meaning, the processes by
which it is organized into the structure we refer to as the self, and
the process we call psychotherapy. The central stance concerns the
innate aspect of being human — from birth onwards, humans strive
to organize or give meaning to their experience. "Meanings are
constituted of the sense a person makes of his/her lived experiences.
They are residues from these experiences which are retained by the
person . . . go beyond the facts of the experience itself; and are the
definitions a person uses to organize and integrate experiences."
Central to the organization of meanings is the role of others in the
environment. "Meanings evolve out of the early affective states
which in infancy occur in interaction with a caregiver who attempts
to both give significance to the affective states, to modify them, and
to share in them. Meanings then, whether personal or shared, are
embeded within a matrix of affectivity and cognition." The inter-
play between affect and the role of other individuals in the formation of meaning is a key component. "The integration of affect
serves to organize experience. Affects constitute a signaling system
which when joined with cognitive faculties and a caregiver's responses result in a residue of comprehension of the experience by
the child." This is the process by which the narrative — the individual's account of his own experience — is formed. In defining the
narrative, Palombo (1990) quotes Stern (1985) and his concept of
RIGs, or Representations of Internalization Generalized. RIGs form
the nucleus around which model scenes are formed. The model
scenes form part of a script, and scripts finally become the components of a larger narrative.

Language plays a central role. For Palombo (1990), "Language . . . is a medium through which meanings become encoded

and are capable of being recalled and of being communicated to others." Thus, language is the central tool by which we encode personal meaning and participate in the larger world. Palombo states that "language mediates experience" and in a similar vein, Goldberg 1990, p. III states "The use of language as a link to other people produces a different kind of orientation that says that the signifiers allow for a developmental process to take place, which process allows for the completion of a configuration, in this case a configuration called the self, one that was not completed during development."

For Palombo, the nature of the mind or the self is defined as a "hierarchy of meanings,"; "psychic structure may be defined as a set of symbols that remain stable over time." "Eventually the hierarchies of the meaning systems acquire a coherence that defines the personality. This coherence is experienced as a sense of cohesion . . . the sum of these coherent systems may be said to constitute a personal narrative." While there is a considerable degree of stability to the self's organization, elements are subject to change and reorganization. "Experiences and events may not retain their original meanings but are constantly re-interpreted."

While the basis of these theories is the development of meaning in the context of childhood development, they also form models that can be extended as part of a dynamic process throughout the life span. As human beings living in the context of the larger world, we are exposed to events and experiences that tax our psychic resources, reactivate old meanings, challenge us to form new meanings and engage in relationships that often serve a central role in the process.

Thus while psychic structure is reasonably stable over time, elements of our personal narratives are subject to change and revision. In defining the therapeutic process, Palombo (1990) quotes Saari (1986) as saying that it: "involves the organizing of old meanings into newly constructed consciousness. What is curative, is not so much the recovery of deeply rooted repressed material, but the reordering of structures that underlie personal meaning and the symbolic capacities of the individual so the new meanings can be differentiated, constructed or abstracted (p.27).

TOWARD AN ELABORATED THEORY OF MOURNING

Any attempt to redefine or elaborate the process of mourning must take into account and integrate recent clinical advances. Drawing on current clinical thinking I am proposing the following definition of mourning: It is a process that involves a reorganization of central aspects of the self, of major affect states, and consequently of the meaning of the loss into a narrative that can be integrated into the overall structure of the self. Mourning begins with a state of acute disorganization of the self, with a resultant lack of coherence and disequilibrium in self-esteem, brought about by the loss of a relationship in an individual's life. Central to the disorganization and self-esteem difficulties is the massive loss of selfobject functions that the survivor experienced within the context of the relationship, the loss of the shared experience or dialogue that occurs within a relationship, and any particular meaning that the loss entails (in the case of an AIDS-related death, the potential that the survivor may also die of the same disease).

Mourning as a process involves a gradual and often painful reorganization of the affects secondary to the loss and the integration of the meaning of the loss into the self. The degree of disorganization and intensity of the affects involved depends on the centrality of the relationship and the degree to which the individual relied on the deceased person to complete his own experience of self. Initially the self is in a deficient state — the person has lost the sense of coherence because it is impossible to integrate the meaning of this experience, and the affects associated with it. Consequently, the emphasis is on the missing of the lost individual, the desire for the experience of the lost individual, and behavioral expressions that offer the mourner a sense of their prior experience of the lost individual.

A crucial distinction must be made here. The mourner is not missing, yearning for, or searching for a "lost figure," "object," or representation thereof; rather what is absent is his particular, unique experience of that individual and the shared experience — the dialogue that an intimate relationship entails. Goldberg (1990), using cognitive and linguistic theories, presents a thorough and convincing argument for essentially dispensing with the concept and theory of representations. He argues that analytic theories of representations are not consistent with the findings of cognitive and linguistic science, that the mind is not structured or "mapped" by a series of object representations, but rather that there are no "objects" in our minds, only the subject-ourselves. For Goldberg (1990, p.110), "The Kohution analyst is not concerned so much with the hidden representation of the object as with the representation of the deficient self."

If mourning does not center on the preservation of the object in the form of identifications or realignment of self and object representations, then just what does the process entail? The process is one of the reorganization of affects and the construction of a new or modified narrrative: an account of the meaning of the death that can then be integrated into the self organization. The person who has become increasingly accustomed to an intimate, ongoing dialogue on the bedrock of shared experience with another must now integrate the experience of being alone. Secondary to this disorganized and vulnerable state, affects are intense and volatile, self-esteem is diminished and unstable, and consequently the environment feels very unsafe and unfamiliar. The work of mourning concerns the gradual reorganization of the affect states and integration into the experience of the self. As the affects become less intense, a narrative can be formed; hence, the mourner makes meaning out of his loss-language and the narrative gradually surplant shifting affect states. As this is achieved, the narrative can be integrated into the overall self organization. The loss and the experience of the loss become viewed as complicated and painful events in a larger life experience.

The central figures are not so much the mourner and the deceased, but the mourner and the selfobject environment. By responding to the mourner's affect states, and the meaning or centrality of the loss, the environment assists in the organization of affect, and consequently the construction and integration of the narrative (referred to as Ordering in Chapter 13). Stolorow et al. (1987) state, "Selfobject functions pertain fundamentally to the integration of affect into the evolving organization of self experience" (p.86). The problem with this definition is that other people cannot integrate our experience; we as individuals integrate our experience.

Hence, selfobject encounters serve to help modulate and regulate the intensity of affects, which enables the individual to integrate the meaning of his experience. Ultimately, the result of the mourner's encounters with the responsive selfobject environment is the transformation of the experience from one of massive selfobject failure, with its attendant fragmentation states and loss of coherence, into a very sad and painful event in one's life, but one that has been lived through, overcome, and has often stimulated renewed growth.

Affects are soothed and organized and the narrative formed through the mourner's private interactions with symbols of the loss and his shared experience with the deceased, which in a private way completes the configuration that represents the deficient self; and through the empathic response of the selfobject environment, which completes the configuration in a shared experience with living people. Public encounters serve to orient the self towards the world of the living and rekindle the hope that the self can become enriched through participating in ongoing shared experiences with the living, versus finding meaning and solace in attempts to recreate the shared experience with the deceased. Ultimately, these experiences often result in the formation of idealizing relationships with living people that can spur further growth, enabling the person to take on new career challenges, and/or form relationships that reflect a higher level of self organization.

ILLUSTRATION

The results of this study can be used to illustrate this theoretical reconceptualization of the mourning process. The categories encompass the gradual organization of the experience and the particular use of the environment at different points in the process. To illustrate the role of the selfobject environment, it is neccessary to begin in the area of experience that precedes the death, THE LONG HAUL. It is in this area that the relationship with the special person in particular, and other relationships supportive of the needs of the well and ill partner are formed. Many of these relationships will endure throughout the mourning process and play an integral role in the survivors' integration of his experience.

The Long Haul

An integral component of the couple's adaptation to living with AIDS appears to be the ability to engage a sustaining matrix of relationships. Friends, the physician, other professionals, family, and the members of support groups, who know of the diagnosis and take an active role in helping the partners negotiate the disease and the hardships it creates, all serve valuable and crucial roles for the couple. The individual and collective loss of coherence and consequent depression and anxiety following the diagnosis often begin to ease as the matrix is formed. The couple once again experience themselves not as being alone and isolated, but rather as attempting to negotiate a traumatic experience with the support, expertise and often camaraderie of other people. A central figure in the matrix is the person with whom the "special relationship" forms, usually a sibling, most often the sister of the ill partner. The relationship tends to solidify as the ill partner declines, and serves to buffer the well partner's growing sense of "aloneness."

The strength of this tie is related to the shared experience of the meaning of the impending loss and often mutual sadness over the decline of the components of the relationship. Several partners pointed out that they experienced themselves and the "special person" as deeply understanding the meaning of the anticipated (and later actual) loss of the relationship. Partners indicated that the special relationship had great sustaining power and enabled them to keep going, to keep caring for their partner in the face of the aloneness and the mounting tasks that caring for a gravely ill person entails.

The results indicate that an integral component of adaptation to the experience is the availability of one or more persons with whom the well partner shares the affects associated with the decline and future loss of the dialogue with the ill partner. In this shared understanding, the aloneness that accompanies the decline and alteration of the selfobject dimensions of the relationship is buffered and the self retains its coherence.

Elements of the three central selfobject needs are observed in the well partner's description of the special person: He or she is often idealized; the well partner experiences the special person as being empathically attuned to his sadness; and in the face of the decline of the ill partner, there is a sense of the two people forming a team with common goals. During the early areas of the experience, the well and ill partners experience themselves as being "in this together." As the ill partner declines, the well partner comes to experience himself and the special person as "being in this together." The special person will continue to play a central role in the experience by facilitating the mourning process of the surviving partner.

The basic assumptions underlying the concept of anticipatory grief and mourning are indicated not only in the definitions of the concept, but in the semantic structure of the concept as well. The concept is labeled and defined as grief in *anticipation* of a loss. Following the accepted definitions of mourning as a process and grief as the affective component of the process, Lebow (1976) defines anticipatory mourning as "the total set of cognitive, affective, cultural and social reactions to *expected* death felt by the client and family." Aldrich (1974) defines anticipatory grief as, "any grief occurring *prior* to a loss . . ."

The authors' model of human relationships appears rooted in an object relations theoretical framework. While they identify the stressors that accompany the situation of caring for a dying family member, they do not identify these events and circumstances as indicating or representing actual losses of components of the relationship. Rather, the central aspect is again the anticipation of the loss of the person with whom the relationship exists. If we view the selfobject functions and the shared experience of the dialogue as integral components of the relationship, then anticipatory grief and mourning also involve the responses to the decline and alteration of these dimensions. An integral component of the process appears to be an attempt to reconcile and tolerate the experience of loss of vital components of the relationship in the face of the continued physical presence of the partner and often tremendous demands that caring for a critically ill person requires.

The participants in the study reported an increasing sense of aloneness as their partner physically and often mentally declined. While the demands for caretaking on the well partner's part mounted, they experienced their partner as becoming increasingly withdrawn and unavailable. These men were highly aware of a painful sense of aloneness as they gave more and more to their partner, but experienced less and less in return. Periods of acute despair appeared to be in response to an expression of anger, or a sudden or protracted withdrawal on the ill partner's part. The well partner's growing sense of aloneness can be understood as stemming from the decline of shared experience in the relationship, while acute despair indicates the experience of a selfobject failure, which results in anger, rage, and/or depletion.

Clearly, there are elements that reflect actual anticipation of the loss of shared experience. Participants reported periodically emerging thoughts of the partner's eventual death and the possibility that the meaningful event or shared experience (holidays, vacations, times of renewed connection) they were having with their partner might be their last as a couple. Early in THE LONG HAUL, the dialogue, the well partner's hope of its restoration, and faith in his *Game Plan* help to counter this anticipation.

Aldrich (1974) and Lebow (1976) have described and the results illustrate how the mutual knowledge of the approaching death potentially interferes with the relationship as the individuals, in their denial and grief, withdraw from each other. Many men reported being very much aware of their mutual sadness, but also having a great deal of difficulty talking about it together, which resulted in a sense of distance at a time when they desperately needed to experience each other's emotional presence. Here again, members of the supportive matrix can help to buffer this experience either through sustaining relationships, or as is so often the case of support groups, sharing their similar experience. Ultimately, this serves to organize the affects secondary to these disruptions, often giving them new meaning other than personal faults of one or both of the partners.

The terminal illness of the partner places a great deal of strain on the selfs of the partners and the dialogue. The social stigma of AIDS tends to add to this burden, as do any difficulties in negotiating families. The stressful nature of the situation taxes the self and often causes regressive trends. The self under stress tends to seek out more archaic selfobject encounters. Indeed, one observes strong idealizing elements in many of the relationships that form the matrix. While this often greatly assists the self in maintaining its cohesion, disruptions in the relationship with the physician or other key members of the matrix (just as disruptions between the partners) can result in considerable narcissistic injury with its attendant affects of rage and depletion.

Fever Pitch

For the majority of the experience, evidence that the ill partner is indeed dying often is lacking. The well partner tends to be more focused on maintaining the dialogue and may not be fully aware of the extent of his partner's decline. The partner's realization of approaching death often emerges from his own perceptions, the information conveyed by physicians, and the reactions he observes in other people. This realization is at once alternately disorganizing and organizing. The name of this category stems not from the often considerable activity in this area but from the private experience of the partner. There is a sense of tension, of harried activity, of considerable affect being kept at bay. In sharp contrast, periods of renewed dialogue between the two men are calming, comforting and highly meaningful. At this point men may attempt to put a sense of closure to their dialogue. Longstanding conflicts may be laid aside, and apologies made for past behavior, slights or injuries. The perception of settling of old conflicts is very important for the well partner, especially if there were considerable difficulties during THE LONG HAUL. The experience of being "forgiven" will leave the well partner less plagued by guilt during the mourning process.

The special person is often present, and is experienced as a strong ally. As death approaches, other family members and friends often gather as well. Relationships that formed and began to solidify around the shared sense of loss may become even stronger. Difficulties with the ill partner's family may be temporarily placed aside, or individuals in their panic over the approaching death may renew conflicts as a displacement or diversion from their distress. While realizing that the partner is indeed dying threatens a loss of coherence, the dialogue with the ill partner, the many tasks, and the continued presence of the special person and other members of the supportive matrix serve to maintain the self's organization and focus.

Calm and Peace

The death of the ill partner often is anticipated as carrying with it a great deal of chaos, turmoil and despair. In sharp contrast, the experience is often quite peaceful. Rather than feel the experience as the partner being ripped away from them, partners tend to feel a sense of calm. As funeral or memorial plans are made, and observances attended, the partner is surrounded by a matrix of relationships that share the sense of loss. Thus, while he is alone, he does not feel alone, nor does he lack relationships that maintain his coherence.

Some men may be somewhat baffled by the intense affect expressed by others. They experience a sense of calm and purpose. They may experience periods of sadness, but they do not become significantly disorganized. In many ways, carrying out funerals or other observances in accordance with the partner's wishes is an extension of the dialogue. Observances of the death also represent a shared experience of grief and loss.

Chaos

Pollock (1961) states that the initial phase of mourning is one of numbness — the ego has not integrated the reality of the loss. If we define mourning as the loss and gradual restoration of the self's coherence following the loss of a central relationship that was an aspect of the coherence, then it is more appropriate to state that the process begins with the experience of CHAOS.

The experience in this area is essentially a fragmentation, which ensues when the individual first realizes that the partner is indeed dead and he is alone. Until this time, the surviving partner has not lost his coherence; he may have experienced bouts of crying or sadness, but not the degree of disorganization central to this area.

Two factors are integral to the advent of this experience. The first is the loss of the presence of the special person or other sustaining relationships. While surrounded by relationships that provided selfobject and shared affect experiences, the surviving partner did not feel alone. The second factor involves the survivor acting as if the shared experience with the deceased partner still existed in its familiar form. Over time, the dialogue between two people develops familiar patterns or configurations. Rather than the usual response or completion of the pattern by the now deceased partner, the survivor experiences its absence. He realizes in a very different way that his partner is indeed dead. He is flooded by disorganizing affect, and intense and painful missing of the partner. The self loses its coherence, causing the world to feel unfamilar. Self-esteem is disrupted and the partner feels inept, especially in concrete areas or activities that the deceased partner excelled in, a reflection of the loss of the ongoing selfobject experiences integral to the dialogue of the relationship.

Retreat

This area is characterized by a withdrawal from a world that no longer feels safe, meaningful or predictable. The self is in a deficient state and consequently is highly vulnerable to being over-whelmed by intense and volatile affect or overstimulated by the environment. Periodic disorganization similar to that seen in the previous area *Chaos* is experienced when the self is overtaxed, or when the partner is reminded of his past shared experience and its current absence. These experiences tend to occur when the partner is operating outside of the sphere of his supportive matrix or when there is an empathic failure in the matrix. This area is dominated by the self's efforts at soothing protection from overstimulation, beginning efforts at constructing the narrative, and a periodic reaching out to the environment for responses that reflect an understanding of the self's current diminished state and preoccupation.

The intense missing of the partner continues, especially when the survivor is not distracted by career or other tasks. Missing of the shared experiences of intimacy and body contact as well as the more abstract but fundamental regulation of the self's equilibrium. The survivor tends to feel diminished and simultaneously idealizes his deceased partner. In the context of the idealization, the survivor experiences a degree of comfort and protection that at this point in the process he may not be able to experience elsewhere. Self-esteem and confidence continue to be diminished, as well as varying states of depletion.

The dialogue that gradually developed between two people takes on a new form. Now it the private dialogue of one man. It is in this component that two of the three central organizers of the mourning process occur. The survivor spends considerable time reconstructing — consciously recalling events in the development of the relationship and his partner's illness and death. He attempts to answer unanswered questions and account for particular events that he did not understand at the time they occurred. This represents the beginning construction of the narrative. At this point, the narrative is a rather concrete, factual recall of events that tends to lack nuance.

The other aspect is the cherishing, intense value and meaning that photographs, the deceased partner's possessions, and shared possessions, often the home itself, come to have. Talking to photographs, wearing the partner's clothes, and holding onto possessions, represent efforts at experiencing a semblance of the shared experience of the partner. The experience of recollection of memories and interaction with objects is quite meaningful and soothing, a sharp contrast to the experience of the world, which often feels harsh, overstimulating, unsafe and demanding. As stated earlier these efforts do not reflect a series of identifications with the deceased, rather they are efforts to soothe the self. Recalling Goldberg, these efforts are attempts to complete the familar configuration with the lost partner. The current deficit state is a result of the loss of the components of the relationship, hence the self attempts to recreate familar, but now lacking configurations.

Guilty ruminations often plague the mourner and can be accompanied by a great deal of shame. The survivor often experiences periods of feeling that he is to blame for the loss of shared experience, and the regulatory experiences of selfobject functions in the dialogue. He tends to gather evidence of failures on his part. Failures to be attuned to the states of others in the past may have caused disruptions in the dialogues of relationships, and he tends to view his experience of becoming enraged, depleted or withdrawn as contributing to the demise of the dialogue with the partner. Attunement and failure of being attuned become confused with the failure of the Game Plan — the hope that if everything was done right, the partner would not succumb to the illness.

The third organizing element of the process concerns the selfobject environment. Friends who may have helped care for the ill partner now turn their attention to the surviving partner and play a central role in sustaining him and organizing his experience. Initially, the survivor often feels comfortable only around people who were intimately involved in his experience, whom he does not have to explain anything to and often have a great deal of silent respect for the centrality of the loss. When he has to negotiate people outside of this matrix, and outside of the home and his dialogue, he tends to feel vulnerable. However, the loss for friends is often quite different, and their process of mourning considerably less protracted. The special person often tends to mourn at a pace more in keeping with the surviving partner, hence their affective states will most likely be in tune with the survivors' for a longer period of time.

Visits and phone calls with the special person are very meaningful events. A consistent pattern was the survivor seeking out conversations or visits with the individual, or other members of his partner's family, especially on holidays or anniversaries when the missing of shared experience and consequent sense of aloneness are intense. Often the special person or other family member is also deeply missing and contemplating the loss as well. Invariably, these conversations evolved into a dialogue regarding their mutual loss and the mutual experience of a great deal of affect. Following these encounters, survivors related feeling revitalized, stronger, less tormented by their missing, more interested in holiday events, and relationships with others who did not share the loss so deeply.

Clearly these encounters included selfobject experiences as well as the sharing of mutual affect. A communication regarding the self's distress was responded to, and a configuration was completed with a living person. Consequently, affect was organized, the self revitalized, the partner reassured that he is not alone in his grief, and the self a bit more oriented toward relationships with living people versus consolation through attempts to recreate the dialogue with the deceased. The shared sense of loss is crucial. Often both individuals experience the other as a connection to the deceased. Hence the surviving partner is also assisting the special person and others who deeply share the loss in their process of mourning.

Invariably, partners desire to turn to the people who first com-

forted them in times of distress and helped to organize their experience – their parents. Parental ambivalence about their son's homosexuality, the centrality and validity of the relationship, and the
partner's own ambivalence about his parents knowledge of his sexuality and the true nature of the relationship all potentially complicate and diminish the soothing and organizing ability of these relationships. At this point in time, the partner has little tolerance for
responses that are not in tune with his need for comfort. They are
experienced as further narcissistic injury to an already diminished
self. Past experiences and injuries due to parental ambivalence can
resurface, and the situation can become complicated and volatile.

Responses that affirm the partner's distress are experienced as
comforting, soothing and organizing, and a reassurance that he is
part of his family. If these responses are not immediately forthcom-
ing, some men gave up and retreated, experiencing a great deal of
hurt that became mingled with any past experiences of isolation
from their family. Other men pursued a dialogue, explaining if not
demanding recognition of their current experience. If the family is
amenable, then a dialogue may open up that ultimatey addresses the
partner's current distress, as well as past injuries regarding his sexuality, which ultimately left him feeling isolated and distant from his
parents. The optimal response appears to be a parent who cannot
only respond in a comforting manner to the partner's affect, but
share their own affectual experiences of loss, grief and mourning.
The effect of these responses is as powerful as encounters with the
special person. The partner's affect is responded to and organized, a
mutual affect sharing occurs, and the partner not only feels a part of
the world of the living but a part of his family as well.

Families who refuse to acknowledge the partner's experience,
insurance companies who delay or attempt to withhold payment, or
families who hassle the survivor or challenge wills, often cause
considerable rage and disorganization. These actions represent further narcissistic injuries to an already vulnerable self. When the self
is in need of comforting and soothing, these represent woefully out
of tune intrusions that only serve to enhance already volatile affects
and subsequently disrupt the self's attempts at organizing the experience of loss. The rage represents not only an affront to the self's

needs, but also an affront to the centrality and validity of the relationship.

Public symbols may have comforting and organizing characteristics as well. The AIDS Quilt has come to serve as a powerful symbol of loss and grief and ultimately represents the efforts of thousands of individuals to comfort the self through creating memorials to deceased partners, friends and relatives. The partner's experience of the quilt and his partner's panel in this area will be more akin to the comfort he receives through his private dialogue. The focus is on his partner's panel and his loss; he is not so attuned to the communal expressions of grief as his own.

The infectious nature of AIDS presents a complicating factor in the partner's attempt to organize the affects associated with his loss. In this area, the partners tended to assume that they too were infected, regardless of test results. At this point, there is not a great deal of disorganizing affect associated with the possibility of infection. The self is diminished, the world of the living is experienced as unsafe, unpredictable and often devoid of meaning outside of the loss. In the intense missing of shared experience, much of the self's activity is directed towards regaining its coherence of that experience. Illness and death may offer this possibility, and the self does not resist. Biological factors aside, infection in the surviving partner represents a continuation of shared experience with the deceased — one that will profoundly affect the nature of the narrative and its capacity to be integrated in a benign and organizing manner.

While the person feels varying degrees of depletion, vulnerability and disorganization, he still senses that he is in the midst of a process that is forward moving. Periods of acute disorganization are contrasted with periods of soothing and feeling understood. The need to become absorbed in the personal meaning of the dialogue is contrasted with the need to feel understood by the environment. Days progress into weeks, the self continues to live and attempt to organize its experience. The empathic response of the selfobject environment serves to gradually restore coherence and to reorient the self toward the living and rekindle the hope that meaning and vitality can be experienced through participating in the world of the living.

Exploration

Exploration is a period of considerable transformation. The person is not as vulnerable; he feels more confident and alive. At this point in time, surviving partners still consider themselves to be widowers, but also engaged in a process of healing and redefinition. He is less concerned with protection and more oriented towards once again exploring the world and its possibilities. There is a greater interest in participating in the world of the living. While the self is oriented more towards participating in limited relationships with others, times will arrive when the environment may overstimulate, and anniversaries or holidays result in the need to acknowledge the loss, and consequently the need to soothe and organize affects.

The intense painful missing of the partner and the shared dialogue declines as does the need and desire to become absorbed in reconstruction of the events of the relationship and its loss. Missing of the partner and the relationship is not as painful, and becoming absorbed in memories often comes to feel intrusive. Questions that at one time demanded answers no longer feel so pressing and guilty ruminations subside. Rituals, such as weekly visits to gravesights, often take on more of the flavor of a routine, a quietly important activity rather than desperate attempts to regain shared experience.

In this area, the narrative becomes less factual, is not as intensely personalized and a greater range of nuance is evident. As the intensity of affects subside, the experience of the relationship and its loss is viewed in a larger perspective. Men experience themselves as actively putting some order or organization to their experience of loss. The initially intense idealization of the partner declines and the partner's experience of himself vis-à-vis the deceased partner shifts to a more confident and capable position. Partners come to experience themselves not only as widowers, who have sustained a major loss, but also as individuals actively engaged in a process of healing and reorganization. This represents the narrative evolving to a point where it can begin to be integrated. A greater degree of coherence evolves as the self experience includes an active effort toward healing, integration and organizing.

Men often find their sense of hope and excitement beginning to return as they experience successful encounters with others and the self begins to regain its confidence and vitality. Survivors begin to find themselves feeling lonely, rather than alone. Partners may seek out encounters with others that are challenging yet "safe," in that they do not threaten to overstimulate the stronger but still vulnerable self. Volunteering with AIDS organizations places the survivor in a position of challenging the self to reach out to others without overly personalizing the experience and keeps the partner in a social context where his status as a survivor will be respected. Social settings that offer more structured contact with others lessen the possibility that the self will be overstimulated by an erotized gesture, but also offer the experience of the self being responded to for its own qualities, not forwhat it has lost.

The partner, though stronger, is still vulnerable. He may be overwhelmed in the course of negotiating relationships via an erotized gesture, or when unexpectedly reminded of the loss of the dialogue. These events may result in a degree of disorganization and a brief return to soothing through activities that recreate the shared experience as seen in earlier areas. However, the degree of the disorganization and the time it takes to recover is often considerably less.

Anniversaries or holidays may trigger a return of missing and painful affect. Here again, survivors often seek out conversations with the special person. The configuration is identical to that observed in RETREAT. In the face of missing his partner and their shared experience, the partner seeks out a dialogue with the special person and/or relative of his partner. During the interchange, the mutual experience of loss and affects are shared, the self is revitalized, the painful affects that were so dominate lose their intensity, and the self is able to participate in dialogues that often center around celebrating life and the meanings of holidays, rather than participate in activities that acknowledge and soothe the experience of loss.

Partners in this area tend to seek out responses from the environment that are not so much attuned to the painful affects and disorganization of RETREAT, but are more attuned to the loss as a major event with considerable consequences, and the partner's own efforts at making a "new start." Dialogues with parents that opened up regarding the loss and the son's sexuality often continue, and include efforts at reworking old meanings in the context of the son's experience of feeling different and misunderstood. If parents are unresponsive, disappointment may continue. If these disappointments are not too devastating both in terms of current experience and the evocation of past failures, the partner often turns to his deceased partner's family or other relationships for these experiences.

In this area, efforts to memorialize the partner often arise. Partners may make a panel to add to the others of the AIDS Quilt. Again, the participation of family or friends who either acknowledge the validity of the activity or join in the creation as a way of sharing their own sense of loss is highly meaningful. The partner's experience of the AIDS Quilt is quite different in this area. The partner tends to feel a part of the larger, communal experience of grief. While his own private experience of his partner's panel is significant, he is much more aware of participating in a shared experience. He is a part of the many people who have lost relationships, and he takes comfort in feeling a part of the communal experience of grief.

Here again, the partner's private and public interaction with the AIDS Quilt and/or private experience during a visit to the gravesight help to organize affect and revitalize the self. The partner who earlier in the day was absorbed in the communal and private experience of grief during a visit to the AIDS Quilt is learning to dance in the evening and feeling a joyous sense of participation in the larger world. The partner who woke up on Christmas Day feeling depressed and isolated visits the gravesight of his partner, and later finds himself joining in holiday celebrations.

As he continues to feel more alive, the possibility of the surviving partner being infected with the same agent often becomes railed against. It is an intrusion into the rekindling hope and joy the self is experiencing. In RETREAT and CHAOS, this continuation of shared experience with the partner and the possibility of joining him was often quietly accepted. In this area, it comes to represent a thwarting of the hope of being able to participate in the world once more. In earlier areas, the survivor does not feel nearly as important as what he lost. As the self gradually reorganizes, he feels stronger and more alive, and the desire to share experiences with others supplants the desire to recreate the experience of the lost relationship.

Partners who at this point still do not know their antibody status approach testing with considerable apprehension. Some men will choose not to be tested, but continue their process of re-engagement with the world the best they can. Others will choose to settle the matter. The ability to face the anxiety and potential trauma of testing reflects the degree of cohesion the self has attained.

Testing negative represents a release and a loss. It is a release from a potentially deadly element of shared experience with the deceased partner. It is also a loss, in that one more element of the shared experience has disappeared. A return to reconstructing the experience in light of the new information is often observed. The partner now works at integrating into the narrative the fact that he was negative all along, his partner died of a disease that he has not contracted, and that he can go on in his process of integrating the loss and finding new meaning in life. The partner often seeks out individuals in the environment who can share in his joy and sense of relief and release. The shared response with individuals in the matrix furthers the process of integrating these affects and again revitalizes the self as a participant in ongoing human experience.

Before, the surviving partner's sense of future felt tentative, now the possibilities again begin to seem endless. The process of reorganizing and redefining oneself now proceeds with vigor. As this information is integrated into the dialogue, self-esteem and confidence tend to grow and solidify. Challenges via academic and/or career pursuits that once were only tantalizing possibilities may be actively sought out.

When the partner tests positive, or already knows he is positive, often the effect is equally profound. He must now attempt to integrate the meaning of his partner's death, which becomes entwined with the meaning of his own death. He does not feel released from the experience; rather the experience is ongoing, perceived as ending only with his own illness and death. The serpositive surviving partner often must struggle to define himself in light of his own experience rather than that of his partner. Rather than continuing to diminish, the idealization of the lost partner often reawakens and he is held up as an example of strength in the face of adversity, from which the survivor may draw strength of his own. Considerable intense affect is associated with this continuation of experience;

consequently, the narrative does not proceed to be integrated in a
benign form. Self-esteem continues to be shaky, and in the face of
the narcissistic injury of being positive, often declines. Rather than
continue to seek out and participate in new relationships, seropositive men often retreat. The future once again looks bleak, often
including elements of terror and further losses.

The relationships they do seek out often focus on helping them
adapt to the impact of seropositivity. Social/support groups for men
who have tested positive may feel the most meaningful. However,
the focus tends to be directed towards maintaining and enhancing
the self in the face of the uncertainty of being seropositive, not
towards efforts at enhancing and challenging the self in the context
of ongoing life experiences.

Back into the World

This area of experience is ongoing and evolving. The surviving
partner is primarily preoccupied with participation in the world.
Often the dominate affects are excitement and optimism. One observes few attempts at completion of the familiar dialogue with the
deceased partner save ritual visits to gravesights or quiet acknowledgment of anniversaries. A narrative has evolved and gains considerable integration into the self experience. The self is reorganized and revitalized, no longer in the deficient state that once
dominated the surviving partner's experience. The emphasis shifts
to responses from the environment that assist the survivor in new
career or other pursuits. New relationships may be pursued, and the
self's revitalized state often contributes to the possibility for their
success.

A sense of excitement may come to dominate as the survivor
views the disorganization and painful affect states as now being
behind him, a part of his past, not current existence. In this area, the
narrative has evolved and has been integrated to a degree that enables him to acknowledge and appreciate the past, look forward to
the future, and be vitally involved in the present. The loss of the
relationship and its painfully disorganizing impact is viewed as an
event in the course of a longer life, and, perhaps more importantly,

a traumatic event that has been overcome. After considerable suffering, the self has reorganized and continues to live, if not thrive.

Dialogues that opened up between men and their parents regarding the sexuality of their son often result in the reworking of old meanings. Consequently, affects regarding feeling painfully different, if not narcissistically assaulted, may have also reached a higher degree of integration, with men feeling a greater sense of belonging in their own families. The optimal responses of the environment may also have served to address any sense of isolation due to a homosexual orientation, as well as more basic past experiences of not being responded to in times of acute distress. Consequently, the narrative regarding the loss may be integrated, along with experiences that serve to re-organize past experiences of isolation, the result being a self that is considerably more comfortable, flexible and optimistic in its narratives or experience of self.

This self state represents an ability to engage in new relationships. Individuals who negotiate relationships once the narrative has been integrated may find themselves seeking out relationships with very different qualities than the dialogue they had with their previous partners. A self that has achieved a greater degree of integration and cohesion will naturally seek out encounters that reflect this level of organization. People are not attempting to find a "replacement" for their experience of their previous partner, but a dialogue that reflects the self's current needs, pursuits and interests.

For some men, the new career pursuits reflect certain elements of the experience of the partner's loss to AIDS. Several men in the study pursued academic tracks to enter the field of nursing, and two of them intended to work with AIDS patients. One man had periodically entertained the idea, the other participant's pursuit clearly evolved out of a new exposure to the profession and his idealization of the individuals he encountered during his partner's illness. While altruistic and identificatory elements are evident, the overriding dimensions concern the self's continued striving for new potential and challenging experiences.

The experiences of men who know they are seropositive tend to be quite different. Rather than experiencing a renewed sense of excitement, they are often aware of the lack of it. Life may come to feel very complicated, and the future percieved as tenuous. Consequently, new career plans may be approached with a degree of uncertainty and apprehension. Men who are being medically monitored may experience excitement, but it is a contingent excitement that accompanies medical reports that indicate their condition is stable, not declining. These men tend not to seek out new relationships that challenge the self, but rather seek those that provide a degree of comfort and predictability. Some men may withdraw and become quite isolated; others seek out a sense of belonging through participation in support groups for men who have tested positive. The self works at maintaining, not so much at a challenging re-engagement with the world.

A continued idealization of the deceased partner is often evident. Some men may continue their private dialogue with their partners for considerably longer lengths of time. The death of the partner and their own potential deaths become entwined. The infection of the surviving partner represents a continuation in shared experience with grave consequences. Considerable intense affect accompanies this experience and the subsequent difficulties to redefine the self. In the face of the tenuous sense of future, the uncertainty, and decline in resilience that often accompanies seropositivity, the self attempts to block or disavow the affect. A degree of comfort and safety can be found in the dialogue with the deceased partner. Intense affect may be experienced as threatening a dialogue that is providing a sense of comfort and coherence. The affect may be intensely experienced when these men become ill, or experience a decline in medical status.

While these men may experience an acute disorganization and loss of coherence, if one listens closely, one can hear that they are often being flooded with images of their deceased partner and the loss of that dialogue. The experience is often markedly similar to their first experience of the loss of cohesion following their partner's death. Consequently, the affect impedes the evolution of a narrative that can be integrated in such a manner that enables the self's process of redefinition and reorganization.

Men may become preoccupied with the fear of dying alone without the comfort they provided their partners. This feeling may only be enhanced by difficulties in negotiating new relationships. Men may find their damaged self-esteem emerging in the course of attempting to meet new people, and may become disorganized and retreat from such relationships. The issue is not the reality-based availability of men willing to form relationships with seropositive surviving partners; it is the diminished self state that views the self as isolated, infected, ill, and alone, with little hope of experiencing a sense of vital, sustaining connection.

The encounters with the selfobject environment that facilitate the mourning process via the organization of affect are in response to the readily recognizable and often shared — by virtue of our humanness — affects that accompany the experience of loss. The affects and experience of being infected with the same agent responsible for the death of a partner are not so readily understandable, are more complicated, and, as previously described, may not be readily available to the conscious experience of the surviving partner, let alone publicly shared. Thus the ability to form and integrate a narrative is hampered both by the gravity of the situation and the lack of potential selfobject encounters to organize the associated affects.

There appears to be range in the ability and quality of the relationships formed by seropositive/symptomatic surviving partners. Some men are simply not able to form new attachments to other men and instead rely on friend and family relationships. Others form relationships that as they describe them have a highly tenuous flavor. Here, the self of the other person plays an integral role. These men appear to be able to tolerate the sense of tenuous connection and the lack of unbridled optimism on the part of the surviving partner. Still other men are able to form new relationships that are vital and provide both members with a sense of excited belonging. It appears here that the selfobject dimension plays a crucial role, i.e., the organization the self experiences via mutual idealizing and mirroring dimensions may buffer self-esteem difficulties to the point that new sustaining and mutually enhancing relationships are possible.

SUMMARY

This chapter has presented a beginning reconceptualization of the process of mourning within a self psychological framework. Analytic theory has advanced considerably since the work of Pollock, hence it is also an attempt to bring our understanding of mourning into the context of current theoretical thinking. As linguistic, cognitive and developmental theories become integrated into analytic theory, a re-examination of the basic experiences of being human is in order.

Very early in the process of collecting data for this study, I began to observe phenomenon not accounted for in the analytic literature, i.e., the integral role other people played in helping the ill, well, and later surviving partner negotiate his experience. Analytic theories emphasized the nature of the intrapsychic task of mourning and the necessary level of drive organization to accomplish the task. These models ultimately negate the richness of human experience. They take the mourner out of his selfobject environment, and describe him/her as a solitary figure attempting to integrate the loss based on individual ability to accomplish such a task.

This reformulation of mourning theory addresses the integral, if not crucial, role the environment plays in the process. The central issue pertains to the role other people play in the structuralization of our minds. Clinical thinking is moving far away from the once sacred concept that our minds are structured with discrete analogues or representations of other people. Currently the view is that others serve to help us organize and integrate our experience of self, which profoundly influences our experience of others. Clearly, mourning involves some sort of psychic reorganization. In the context of current advances in clinical theory, it involves the reorganization of affect, and efforts at integrating the meaning of the loss.

Chapter XV

Clinical Intervention

THE CLINICIAN'S TASK

In a strictly biological sense, HIV infection occurs on a continuum: the point of infection, often lengthy period of non-apparent symptomatology (save perhaps laboratory indicators), emergence of symptoms, development of opportunistic infections, decline in physical and often mental status, and finally death. Parallel and integral to this process are the person's emotional responses to the risk of or actual HIV infection. Individuals must acknowledge the need to modify behavior in the face of the presence of the disease in their social milieu. Balancing the fear of knowing with the fear of not knowing, individuals often struggle with the decision to be tested for presence of HIV antibodies. In the wake of testing positive, people experience the emotional upheaval and often significant self reorganization that accompanies the knowledge.

Depending on the status of the infection once it is identified, people may essentially be symptom-free but face a several year period of knowing they are infected. This time period often taxes the person's resiliency. The loss of a sense of future, and the self experience of being infected and ill, tend to have an erosive effect on self-esteem. With the emergence of symptoms and/or the need to begin AZT or other pharmaceutical treatment, people often experience another period of emotional upheaval and yet another as they experience the first opportunistic infection and the official diagnosis of AIDS. The diagnosis of AIDS places the need for the person to integrate the changes in self experience secondary to terminal illness and often subsequent decline in physical functioning. Eventually, the person experiences the process of dying. However, the often extended time period infected individuals encounter does offer the possibility of further growth, as many people form numerous meaningful relationships in the service of managing the experience of being HIV positive and/or ill.

The continuum actually continues as surviving partners, friends and family members experience the processes of mourning the loss of a central person in their lives. Far too often, an integral part of carrying on with life for these people includes the experience of their own HIV infection. Martin (1988), in a 1985 sample of gay men, found that 27% had experienced the loss of a lover or close friend, one third of whom had experienced multiple losses. Five years later into the epidemic, it is reasonable to anticipate the percentages are even higher. Thus, we as clinicians working with HIV-related problems must understand the effects of loss, perhaps many losses, on the individual's experience of HIV infection. This chapter will address clinical intervention with people whose lives, experience of self, and consequently, efforts at integrating the meaning of their own infection, have been profoundly influenced by the loss of a relationship to AIDS.

In making a clear distinction between biological and emotional processes, I realize that I am walking into the perilous realm of Descartian mind-body dualism that has plagued clinical theory since the time of Freud. However, I make the distinction for a reason, i.e., to underscore our tasks as clinicians. As psychotherapists, we can do nothing to stop viral progression. We can do our best to help an uninfected client modify their behavior in the face of viral presence in the social milieu, but if a client is infected, our task becomes exercising our clinical skills to help the client secure appropriate medical treatment, follow through on recommendations, and integrate and manage the emotional responses that accompany the physical and psychological effects of infection.

This may seem like an obvious point, but in the intimacy of the client/therapist relationship, its distorting as well as holding power, it is an important reference for keeping the treatment on track. Both the client and the clinician have often witnessed far too many deaths to AIDS. Just as the well partner may have hoped that if he did everything just right, his partner would not die, this hope can and often does arise in the transference-countertransference continuum. As clinicians, we assist our patients by engaging them in a mutual dynamic effort—a dialogue that serves to soothe and organize affects, consequently, to sort out and help integrate the often myriad meanings of their experience of HIV infection. There is considerable difference between a dialogue that serves to help soothe and organize the self, and combatting a viral infection.

The mutual hope between therapist and client, that this person will not become ill, or that somehow, the right combination of therapies will be found, potentially interferes with the clinician's ability to help the client tolerate the uncertainty of HIV infection. Ultimately, the fact is that the infection is with him, will not go away, and he has no other choice but to attempt to integrate the meaning of its presence. When HIV infection is viewed on a continuum, then it is clear that the process of dying actually occupies a relatively small portion of the experience. However, for many men who are infected, and consequently the clinicians who work with them, the specter of death is present. We must all learn to tolerate this, and attempt to place the possibility of death in its proper perspective. Far too often we will have to help a client in their process of dying, of saying goodbye to their world. However, this chapter relates to helping patients remain vitally involved in their worlds, to keep living, and often growing, in the face of powerful psychological forces that may cause them to retreat, long before they become critically ill.

Granted, research (Spiegel 1989) has indicated that female breast cancer patients who became involved in support groups that addressed their emotional experience lived almost twice as long as their cohorts not involved in such endeavors. If assisting the person in their process of organizing and integrating the many affects and meanings involved in illness helps them not to fall into despair and be overtaken by the illness so readily, so be it. However, I feel we are on much firmer theoretical ground to state that we are helping the person integrate the meaning of traumatic, life threatening experience. The ultimate issue is the quality of life. Though time may be shortened, a great deal of living can be achieved when the person is not depleted and or struggling to retain a sense of coherence in the face of repeatedly overwhelming affect. For many infected individuals, the amount of time they have may be considerably greater than they are able to anticipate. For some, it will be far too short. Ultimately, the issue is the quality of life, not the length.

Another crucial aspect of working with HIV-related problems is that HIV infection does not exist in a vacuum. People impacted by HIV vary widely in terms of their cohesion, coherence and general life experience. Thus, the personal meaning of the infection will vary considerably from client to client. Ultimately the pre-existing state of self structure will, to varying degrees, affect the individual's experience of the infection, and consequently their ability and the nature of their efforts to remain engaged with their world. Often we are dealing with the interface between pre-existing self deficits or psychopathology and efforts at maintaining coherence in the face of the narcissistic injury that HIV represents. The results of this study provide a general frame of reference from which to view the particular experience of our patients. Clearly the experience of losing a partner to AIDS is long, complicated and traumatic. Consequently, there are numerous points where personal meaning can distort or amplify the experience of an individual, with the personal meaning coming to have a life of its own, potentially distorting the larger experience.

Humans do not exist in vacuums either. We have family, friend, love and collegial relationships. Just as the individual faces a series of emotional upheavals, to varying degrees the individuals in the matrix will also be affected. An integral factor in integrating the experience of HIV infection is often the ability to engage a supportive matrix of relationships. Individuals will vary in terms of their ability to engage or develop a matrix. Existing matrixes will vary in terms of their ability to respond to the individual's distress.

As clinicians, we become a part of the individual's supportive matrix. Our role is to facilitate integration through the soothing and organization of affect, the mutual understanding of the meaning of the problem and often attempts to identify the distortions personal meaning may bring to their experience of HIV. Often in extended treatment we become engaged in the process of reworking old meanings. The transference may seemingly take us far afield of the impact of HIV, but invariably it represents the patient's efforts to understand and organize a previous experience that has been activated in the course of their experience with HIV, and the therapist's willingness to help.

The framework from which the following cases are viewed is that HIV infection is experienced as a narcissistic injury that also carries with it the threat of the actual destruction of the self. Self-esteem is disrupted, if not shattered, and the individual's narratives are challenged as well. Human beings, for most of our lives, tend to operate on the assumption of life being an ongoing, if not infinite experience. With the knowledge of HIV infection, this assumption is often shattered, and the individual experiences himself as terminally ill, as a person who is dying. This tends to have considerable distorting power, in that we tend to perceive life either as infinite, or able to be lost at any time. The future becomes viewed as tenuous, if not terrifying. Affects often become intense and labile, the experiences of the self as incompetent or deficient are enhanced and the person may no longer experience himself as a vital participant in the world.

When HIV-infection occurs in the context of an ongoing relationship, the dialogue is disrupted. There is often a disruption in narcissistic equilibrium for both parties, resulting in a disruption of the dialogues' familiar selfobject areas of idealization, mirroring and twinship. Just as individuals have their own styles of managing affect, so do couples. Similarly, couples may find themselves having difficulty managing affect in the relationship. Conflicts may become more frequent and intense which further adds to the confusion, sadness and anger over the presence of HIV infection in one or both men.

The work of treatment involves providing a relationship to help organize and soothe affects and to sort out meanings that have been activated by the experience of HIV infection, ultimately to assist in the restoration of coherence. Selfobject transferences that emerge in the course of the client-therapist dialogue, will serve to modulate affect as the often radically altered experience of self is organized and to varying degrees, integrated. The personal narrative must now include the presence of HIV infection, and its implications. In working with couples, the therapist often serves to help modulate affect which enables issues and problems to be addressed in a productive manner. Just as individuals need to integrate the meaning of HIV infection, the couple faces a similar task.

The implication for infected individuals of course is being on a continuum that eventually leads to severe illness and death. As the following cases will illustrate, one of the central aspects of negotiating the experience is being able to place oneself on the continuum and proceed with life accordingly. The cases also illustrate several experiences that can distort the person's capacity to "read" the body's signals, to integrate medical information and utilize relationships at their disposal.

The following cases represent clinical intervention with couples who were experiencing difficulty managing the presence of HIV infection in one of the partners and men whose experience of HIV infection was profoundly influenced by the loss of central people in their lives. Not all of the individual cases represent the loss of partners. The loss of friends, and other individuals central to peoples' lives are all events that people in this stage of the epidemic are likely to experience. Hopefully, the cases also illustrate the complexity that clinical work with individuals impacted by HIV often entails.

CLINICAL WORK WITH COUPLES

Donald and Sam

Donald, 28, and Sam, 39, sought treatment due to the lack of sexual expression in their relationship of four years. Sam was well established in his career and enjoyed a prominent status in his profession. Donald had just begun to make his mark professionally, but was beginning to receive considerable attention. Sam tended to be warm and engaging but subtly aloof and controlling, while Donald often appeared bored, disinterested and at times passive-aggressively provocative. The presenting complaint was quickly surpassed by numerous other complaints and conflicts that left each man angry and frustrated with the lack of progression in the relationship. The fact that Sam had tested positive approximately a year earlier was raised periodically, but little fruitful discussion would come of it as the couple quickly diverted onto one of their numerous points of contention.

Gradually the transference elements and related myths emerged. Sam was the "together"one, who was to take care of Donald. Donald was the incompetent kid that needed and wanted to be taken care of. Sam tended to present the couple's problems as being all Donald's fault, while Donald portrayed himself as the victim of Sam's numerous neuroses. There was often a very elusive quality to the sessions. The issue of Sam being HIV positive surfaced periodically, but would quickly slip away, as the couple argued about a fault of the other partner. Sam's being positive began to have the feel of a family secret; there but not there, exerting its influence but somehow untouchable.

Several months into treatment a series of escalating arguments occurred. The arguments centered around Sam wanting Donald to respond to his distress, but Donald was being oblivious and unresponsive. A session was held in the wake of a particularly bitter fight in which Sam demanded Donald leave and find another place to live. During this session it became clear that Sam wanted Donald to respond to his growing distress over being HIV positive. Two of Sam's close friends had died and he found himself increasingly depressed, preoccupied with contracting AIDS and panicked at the possibility. As Sam tearfully related his distress and his experience of being terminally ill, Donald became more and more withdrawn, at times appearing distracted and bored. When questioned about this, Donald related that he was frightened by what Sam was saying.

With prompting on my part, Donald related his considerable fear of Sam becoming ill, questioned his ability to care for him having seen what a mutual friend had gone through with his partner, and his desire to protect his own negative antibody status. When I related their difficulty to the transference elements of their relationship, the two men began to see what had been happening. Sam desperately wanted Donald to comfort his fear and anxiety, yet he viewed Donald as incompetent and incapable of being a steady reliable figure. He too was frightened that should he become ill, Donald would be unable to tolerate the strain. Donald felt incapable of responding to Sam due to his strong dependency, his need to *be taken care of, and because he found the idea of Sam becoming ill so frightening. Sam's frequent attacks were further eroding his confidence and creating a growing level of anger and resentment that was preventing him from wanting to respond. Sam had been thinking about joining a support group for seropositive men, but had not followed through for various reasons. I pointed out that Sam wanted the support of his partner, not a group and had been locked in a conflict around his lack of support in the relationship. I also pointed out that there is only so much support a partner can give and recommended that he join one of several groups.*

The nature of the sessions changed dramatically after Sam joined a group. Sam presented fewer complaints about Donald and the intensity of affect on both men's parts declined dramatically. Eventually an important event occurred. Sam became distraught over the loss of yet another friend. Sam ended up crying with his head in Donald's lap, with Donald not withdrawing, but being supportive and consoling. Eventually the treatment began to address the presenting complaint – the lack of sexual activity in the relationship. This was related to both men's disappointment in each other, Sam's lack of interest in sex since testing positive – sex was now experienced as something dirty, and dangerous with his semen loaded with the AIDS virus – and Donald's fear of contracting the virus regardless of safer sex practices.

There are numerous theoretical frameworks for clinical intervention with couples. The approach consistent with this book is for the therapist to be attuned to the selfobject components of the relationship's dialogue – the areas of idealization, mirroring and twinship. This prospective conflict in couples tends to be about narcissistic injury resulting in the failure of one partner to perform a needed selfobject function (see MacMahon 1991 for a thorough review of couple work in a self psychology framework).

When one or both partners tests positive, it often greatly impacts on the dynamics of the relationship. Both consciously and unconsciously, the impact is experienced and reacted against. However, the expression of the impact occurs within an established dialogue and is experienced within the context of established dynamics. In the case of Sam and Donald, the development of the relationship had been stalled for some time prior to Sam testing positive. Neither man could experience the sense of partnership they wanted, given the problematic dynamic components of their dialogue. Clearly the HIV-related problem was entwined with the other aspects of the relationship and could not really be addressed or understood by any of us until it was brought into sharper focus in the context of an established treatment relationship.

In this case Donald had a strong need to idealize Sam through which he gained a sense of confidence, stability and direction. Sam's initial attraction to Donald was that he was incredibly attractive, and took great pleasure being in the company of such a handsome man. However, over time, Sam was increasingly frustrated by Donald's dependance on him, while Donald was increasingly confused and angry by Sam's numerous complaints. When the couple was tested, Sam was positive and Donald negative. Initially Sam was moderately distressed but seemed to recover quickly, though conflict increasingly dominated the relationship.

The increasing conflict was most likely related to Sam's need to idealize Donald in the wake of testing positive. Sam now needed to feel secure, stable, and to feel that he could rely on Donald, even though he viewed him as unreliable. With the deaths of several friends, Sam's increasing distress and Donald's withdrawal helped to bring the problem into focus. In other words, HIV infection resulted in a pronounced shift of selfobject needs in the relationship. Sam's transference experience of Donald, Donald's need to idealize Sam, Donald's withdrawal, and his fear of Sam's distress, as well as potential illness were preventing Sam from obtaining the experience of being soothed and comforted.

Often men in relationships who test positive will tend to look for, if not demand a great deal from their partners. Often, the emotional needs of people who test positve are realistically beyond what the partner is able to provide. People often fail to realize the degree to which being HIV-positive has diminished self-esteem, resiliency and their ability to modulate affect. Men realistically may need more archaic selfobject encounters to compensate for these self deficits. In the context of the relationship, they may become locked into a frustrating pattern of wanting, but not receiving support that the partner may have trouble providing due to their proximity to the situation and/or as in this case pre-existing self deficits. The combination of the positive partner joining a group and experiencing sustaining selfobject encounters, specifically in the context of HIV infection and the therapist helping both men express their concerns and fears, will often help to ease the tension in the relationship. This will ultimately to help both men sustain and support each other to the best of their ability.

Brian and Cal

Brian and Cal were both in their early thirties when they entered treatment. Brian is a lean, rather constricted, obsessive-compulsive man. He holds an MBA, is meticulous about money, housekeeping and any other task he takes on. Cal is a rather large guy, big-hearted, not well educated but very adept and respected in his line of work. He is very likeable, spontaneous, at times impulsive and very quick to identify with people he perceives as victims. Several months into the relationship which was initially characterized by an unusually high degree of limerance, the two men decided to be tested together. Cal was positive, Brian negative.

Several months after being tested, Brian called, requesting couples treatment due to the problems Cal was having with being positive. He went into great detail about how Cal was showing all the signs of someone having difficulty with being positive that he had read about in an article. Cal had refused to join a group, but had agreed to couples work.

During the initial session both men presented the history of their relationship, how deeply they felt for each other and their plans for a holy union. However, since Cal tested positive there had been numerous arguments. Cal was feeling increasingly depressed and out of control, was experiencing mood swings and periodic anxiety attacks. Brian related that he had no problems with Cal being positive, that he fully intended to remain in the relationship, but was very concerned about Cal's emotional state and wanted to know what could be done to help him.

At this point Cal began to cry. He related how Brian only made him feel worse. Since the testing, Brian had been reluctant to kiss him, sex had fallen off to nothing – Brian always seemed to have an excuse for not engaging in sexual activity – he found himself feeling like a leper and enraged with the man he had been so deeply in love with several months earlier. Sex was very important to Cal, he tended to enjoy passive anal intercourse and "wild and free" spirited sex. They had great sex before the testing, that was safe, but also spontaneous and exciting. As Cal was relating his sexual desires, I observed Brian cringe. With little prompting, Brian went into an elaborate, anxious and constricted monologue about safer sex, and how no one knew what was really safe, what should be done with Cal's semen?, should it go into a towel?, what if he had a rash, or a break in his skin? what then? After several minutes of Brian's anxious concerns, Cal became acutely upset, relating how badly he felt – the longer Brian talked, the worse he felt and that perhaps it would be easier to just terminate the relationship. Cal wanted to "forget" about his testing positive, to just shelve the problem and get on with life, get things back to normal; however, Brian's concerns kept it in the forefront of his mind.

Over the next few sessions I pushed each man to talk about their individual fears about Cal being positive. With a good deal of support and structure, Cal related his intense fears of becoming ill, how he felt damaged, diminished and dirty. He tended to experience himself as the least successful member of his family, always messing up, and that he had really messed up with this one. On top of everything else, now he was going to get AIDS. Brian was shocked, but very interested and empathetic as Cal related the extent of his distress. Brian continued to deny any difficulty on his part. With some very provocative maneuvering by myself, Brian was able to relate the extent of his concerns – his fear of losing Cal, his devastation that the only man he felt he had ever loved may become ill, his own intense fear of diseases and illness. Cal was shocked. He had increasingly viewed Brian as cold and rejecting, not devastated in his own right.

As the work progressed. Cal related how he had taken care of his father as he slowly died of brain cancer. He knew firsthand how hard it was to care for an acutely ill person. As is often the case, there were times when Cal was so exhausted, that he wished his father would hurry up and die. He had tended to view Brian as very steady and together, but now he wondered if Brian could really handle taking care of him should he become ill. Each experience of feeling rejected further eroded his confidence in Brian and accentuated his guilt over wishing his father would die. Brian was shocked by the degree of Cal's disillusionment. I pointed out that there is considerable difference between having sex with and caring for an ill person and that in all probability illness was farther away than either of them imagined. The issue at hand was managing the fear and anxiety they both were experiencing which was only enhanced by their being so out of tune with each other.

A common dynamic seen in couples when one partner is negative and the other positive is for the negative partner to minimize, if not disavow the extent of his distress and fears. The dynamic is similar to that of the Game Plan discussed in the study results, the negative partner often focuses on being steady, organized and concerned about his partners' well-being. Privately he is often acutely disappointed, sad and terrified in his own right. The potential problem becomes the positive partner experiencing the affect for both men. Hence on top of his own stress and secondary to being positive, the affective intensity is further enhanced, and disorganization protracted. Negative partners are often reluctant to relate the extent of their fears to their partner, however I will push them to do so. The fear is there and is impacting on the affect life of the relationship. Rather than feel rejected, positive partners are often relieved and feel more connected to their partners following the verbalization of mutual fears. Often the therapist will serve to modulate affect for the relationship so that fears and concerns can be expressed and heard, rather than reacted to.

Cal had a long history of using sex to modulate affect and self-esteem. In the wake of his disorganization, anxiety and fear over being positive, he was seeking out intense sexual encounters that provided him with considerable mirroring which in past times of stress had modulated his self-esteem. Ultimately, he was looking to sex to modulate his intense feelings of being damaged and diminished. When Brian became anxious and pulled back from sexual encounters, Cal was flooded with feeling damaged and rejected. As this was pointed out, and Cal helped to verbalize the extent to which he felt damaged, the intensity of his need for sex declined.

The combination of problems in the sexual arena, Brian's tendency to focus on Cal's problems and minimize his own fears resulted in the dialogue becoming increasingly disrupted. Both men were reacting as much to their disappointment over a relationship that they had such high hopes for as they were over the issue of seropositivity. Neither man was experiencing the other as they had been accustomed to in the early limerant stages of their relationship. As Cal's search for reassurance via sex was pointed out, and the extent of Brian's fears verbalized, the intensity of affect declined considerably.

The differing character structures of these two men would probably lead to difficulty in any relationship. However when the HIV-infection was identified, the intensity of the anxiety and differing defensive styles resulted in each partner being acutely out of tune with the other. One often observes couples having difficulty with sex following the identification of HIV-infection. The emotional experience of assuming a person is positive and having safer sex with them, is often very different than *knowing* someone is positive and having safer sex. Given Brian's obsessive-compulsive character structure, he was bound to have difficulty with sex in general. In the wake of knowing Cal was positive, his anxiety was expressed in terms of germs, messes and correct safer sex procedures.

As the intensity of affect declined and the two men began to feel more in tune with each other, our work focused on restoring their sexual dialogue. There are numerous possibilities for intense, satisfying, safer sex. Given the intense affect and disappointment that sex had come to represent, the couple needed considerable help in finding mutually comfortable ways of reengaging in a sexual dialogue. The work of treatment gradually came to focus on the two men's individual self-esteem issues and characterlogical differences which often put them at odds with each other.

Jim and Eric

Jim was in his late 40s and Eric in his late 20s when they were referred by the medical social worker who had worked with Jim for several months following his AIDS diagnosis. Jim presented himself in a very quiet, reserved, at times highly constricted "cut and dry"

*manner. Eric was very verbal, anxious, at times histrionic. Neither
man could present a definite problem but it was clear that there was
a great deal of tension in the relationship. There had been a series
of escalating fights to the point where Eric had threatened to leave
if things did not change.*

*The two men had lived together for less than a year. They had
met several years earlier and maintained a long distance relationship. During this time Jim was diagnosed with AIDS. The relationship continued and Eric eventually moved to be with Jim. Several
months after they moved in together, Jim had another bout of PCP.
He quickly recovered; however, conflict had been escalating between the two men since the illness.*

*Jim's medical condition was stable though somewhat tenuous. In
general he was functioning quite well, working full time and involved in several political and social groups. He maintained a
fighting stance, tended to minimize his condition and focus on his
numerous medical problems in a matter-of-fact manner. He stated
adamantly that he had no intention of dying from this disease. Jim's
former partner had died several years before, and he had taken
care of him and was quite familar with dealing with the problems
that came along with AIDS.*

*Eric related that he was not familiar with AIDS, he was learning
since being with Jim, but that Jim would never discuss anything. He
recalled the last bout of PCP. Following his discharge Jim was still
fairly ill — as much from the medication as anything. Eric became
increasingly distraught, frightened by the IV equipment, afraid that
something was wrong and called Jim's physician and social worker
repeatedly. At this point Jim angrily accused Eric of making a big
deal out of everything, pointing out that everyone knows the medication is a big if not bigger problem than PCP, and that it takes
several weeks to recover. Eric angrily responded that he did not
know, that Jim never tells him anything about the illness and he is
left worried and terrified. Jim responded that there is nothing to
worry about, so don't be.*

*As the work progressed it became clear that there was a strong
pattern of Jim minimizing his anxiety and resenting the intrusion of
Eric's fear. The more anxious Eric became, the more Jim would
alternately withdraw or attack with cutting, dismissing comments*

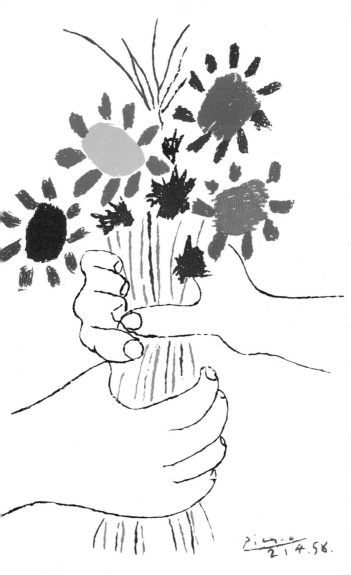

that left Eric hurt, enraged and even more anxious. Eric began to feel more ungrounded and insecure in the new city and relationship, consequently becoming more needy, anxious and disorganized. Jim was highly intolerant of all three states and became increasingly withdrawn and short-tempered with Eric.

The work often entailed modulating Eric's often intense anxiety so that Jim would feel comfortable enough to formulate his thoughts and verbalize his concerns. He was clearly overstimulated and disorganized by Eric's intensity. With the intensity modulated, Jim was able to express this dynamic as well as relate more of his own concerns and fears. Though he minimized his condition, Jim did feel that he was walking a tightrope and experienced Eric's anxiety as upsetting his balance which he thoroughly resented. Eric was becoming increasingly angered by Jim's cutting remarks, and felt his attempts to help were soundly dismissed. The more he tried, the more Jim pushed him away.

Gradually the intensity in the relationship diminished. Jim was able to verbalize more and Eric became less anxious and needy. The two men became involved in their relationship development, began looking for a new apartment, attended a support organization for people impacted by HIV, and attempted to start a self-help couples group. During this process the dynamic of Eric having good ideas, but presenting them in an overstimulating manner and Jim rejecting him and the ideas repeatedly occurred. Gradually the individual meaning of this pattern for each man was related and the intensity subsided. The treatment came to an end as the two men found a new apartment and went about making it their home.

The study results indicate just how much organizing power the Game Plan has for the well partner. The experience of having an important and integral role in the partner's illness provides a great deal of structure and ultimately helps to organize and modulate affect. Idealization of the ill partner is also an aspect of this process. With Jim and Eric, we see how Jim's difficulty in allowing Eric to participate in his illness by sharing this aspect of his life was leaving Eric isolated and panicked. By the time Eric moved in, Jim had several years of negotiating the illness as a single person. Though the illness was an integral aspect of their lives, both men most likely participated in a process of minimizing its influence in lieu of the hopeful excitement that goes along with a new and developing relationship. With the second bout of PCP, the men did not have prior experience in negotiating acute illness together. Jim's defensive stance of "it's no big deal, I know how to manage it" only served to heighten Eric's anxiety by isolating him from the illness, while Jim's cutting remarks impeded Eric's ability to idealize him.

As in the previous cases, we see two men with radically different temperaments and character styles. Jim tended to be constricted, somewhat withdrawn, very private with his experience and had a strong tendency to minimize affect; and Eric was highly demonstrative, talkative and tended to heighten his affective experience. With such differing temperaments both men were bound to be out of tune with each other. Though his defensive style was cutting and devaluing, Jim was highly overstimulated and disorganized by Eric's anxiety and style of communicating. Eric of course felt increasingly isolated, angered, and anxious which only caused him to try harder to get Jim to talk.

Initially during treatment, it was necessary to help modulate Eric's anxiety to take the pressure off Jim so that I could get a better sense of what was underlying Jim's defensive stance. As Eric's anxiety eased, and I was able to develop a rapport with Jim, I could then work with him to verbalize his concerns and anxiety rather than minimize his distress. At times this took some provocative maneuvering on my part, but it was an approach that Jim responded well to. Jim's being able to relate how he got overstimulated by Eric's anxiety was an important area for the couple. Jim could then empathize and understand Eric's experience rather than be attacked, criticized, and consequently enraged.

I often point out to couples such as Jim and Eric that, though their styles are very different and may put them at odds, perhaps they could help each other out a great deal. If one listens to couples, there often is the hope and belief that something can be gained from the other. When conflict comes to dominate a relationship, this hope may be dashed. In this case Jim needed to "loosen up," to be drawn out of his isolation. Eric needed to "tighten up," to be better organized and contained. When one partner is ill and the other is not, there is often still a pull for the development of the relationship to continue. The well partner will usually push for a new home or pet — activities that symbolize the evolution and growth of the relationship. The ill partner may resist, at times greatly so, but on some level can also be grateful, as this helps him to feel connected to and participating in the world. As the epidemic continues and management of AIDS continues to increase longevity, we are bound to see more relationships that form after the diagnosis of one of the partners. Better clinical understanding of the potential pitfalls of these relationships will help ensure their endurance.

CLINICAL WORK WITH INDIVIDUALS

Distortions in the Mourning Process

When he entered treatment, Mr. B. was forty-one years old. His partner of ten years had died approximately 1 1/2 years earlier. Mr. B. had known that he was seropositive for a number of years prior to his partner's death. His chief complaint upon entering treatment was "something is wrong, I am not excited about anything, I have this new job with great opportunities, I should be excited — but I am not." The clinical interview revealed several other problems: a significant level of depression, periodic acute anxiety, though his t-cells were in the 500 range and had been for several years, he was convinced he was dying, his self was organized around the assumption of impending death and he clearly perceived himself as being more ill than he actually was. He had developed a reputation in his seropositive support group as a rebel, actively challenging what he called the leaders' "recipes" for seropositive people to remain that way and not contract AIDS. He pointed out that his lover was a vegetarian, took massive quantities of vitamins, did not do drugs and went to the gym daily for many years before he became ill, and died anyway.

Mr. B's partner had died in California. After the death, he moved to a city were he had lived previously, in which several family members resided. He moved in with his sister, and took "time to heal." After several months, he took a job that was well beneath his capabilities to "get back into practice." After several months he took the more challenging position that he had when he entered treatment. He reported that both he and his partner's families had been very supportive and that he felt his need to mourn had been respected and validated by them. However, in the community he felt like a pariah. He experienced the reactions of several old acquaintances as becoming anxious and withdrawing when he related that he had returned to the city because his partner had died of AIDS. If he attempted to go out and meet new people he quickly become anxious and withdrew, fearing that he would eventually have to tell people about his partner and positive status. Consequently, he avoided contact with people outside of his family, or the relationships he had developed in his support and self help groups.

In general, he felt that no one understood or cared to understand, though he was not quite sure what he wanted people to understand. He felt that moving had been a mistake, and longed for California where he felt being a surviving partner and being positive was more readily accepted as the "norm" rather than the exception; perhaps there, people would not treat him differently. Though he assumed he was dying (he knew his lab counts via a research study) he was not being followed by a physician, and resisted my attempts to get him engaged in a medical assessment, stating that when the time came that he needed a physician he would find one. Though he had developed a number of friends in the seropositive support organization, he was beginning to alienate them. It was their complaints about his soap boxing, many interrupted dinner conversations with his "carrying on," and consequent urging to get help that led him to seek treatment.

As treatment progressed, Mr. B. related more of his private experience. He continued to carry on elaborate conversations with his deceased partner, and a strong element of idealization of the dead partner was evident. He initially was reluctant and felt very embarrassed to relate the extent of these conversations, fearing that he would be labeled as crazy. Severe self-esteem problems were evident: he felt diminished, unable to function as well as previously in job or social settings, panicked at the idea of purchasing new clothes, feeling that everything looked terrible on him, and profoundly anxious at the idea of looking in the mirror with sales people nearby. It became increasingly clear that he felt desperately out of control and that his anxiety over feeling out of control was as disabling as his clinical symptoms.

Mr. B. was a recovered alcoholic. He began attending AA meetings and stopped drinking in the years preceding his partner's illness. His father died of cancer when Mr. B. was in high school. He recalled being relieved at his father's death. The relationship had been complicated and conflictual. Mr. B. was rather short in stature and did not have his adolescent growth spurt until he was in college. In contrast, his father was well over six feet tall and imposing. In addition, he experienced his father as belittling the activities he found meaningful and excelled in. A potential career in figure skating was derailed because his father would not allow him to attend intensive training camps run by Mr. B.'s instructor whom the father openly viewed as a "fag." There were other memories of experiences with his father that left him feeling acutely devalued and humiliated, several in the presence of other men or peers. Mr. B. deeply distrusted and was fearful of his father, but was not exactly certain why. These feelings were not so much associated with his father's actions as they were with a basic experience of him. (Mr. B.'s sister was in treatment as well. Several months into the course of Mr. B.'s treatment, his sister recalled events that confirmed just how seriously disturbed the father was.) Mr. B. was plagued by his lack of height, and learned to actively engage people in conversation so he could feel accepted and surrounded by his taller and presumedly more adequate peers. He quickly discovered that alcohol left him feeling tall and so began his extensive social drinking. In many ways he experienced himself as an "underdog," a man who had to try harder than others, but still succeeded.

After several weekly meetings, he requested twice weekly sessions, which was agreed to. He quickly formed an idealizing transference; initially some erotized elements were evident, but not to the extent that it threatened to disrupt the treatment alliance. The erotized elements diminished over the next few weeks and were replaced by a more solid idealization of the therapist.

Very quickly, I pointed out that I thought a great deal of what he was experiencing was due to his being a seropositive surviving partner, that yes, he should be getting excited again and probably would if he was not carrying the same virus that killed his partner. I

*also validated and attempted to normalize the continued dialogue
or conversations with his partner. I was also interested in what he
talked about with his partner. I encouraged his relating of the story
of their relationship, and his partner's illness and death. Initially,
in a very real way, it felt as if there were three people in the consulting room: myself, Mr. B. and his partner.*

*Mr. B. proved to be a vivid dreamer and his dreams often beauti-
fully and succinctly summed up the current themes in his treatment.
Over the first two months of our work, he related three dreams:*

1. *Jay (his partner) and I were on an island in a river, Jay was
   sick and laying on a cot, the river was raging, it was storming,
   there was chaos all around us. I was worried about keeping
   him dry and was busy making sure he did not get wet. Though
   there was chaos all around us, I felt calm inside.*
2. *I was going somewhere on a train. All of sudden I was outside
   of the train. I felt fine until I thought that I should hold onto
   something, since the train was moving so fast. I panicked
   when I realized there was only a little rail to hold onto that I
   could barely get my fingers around.*
3. *I was getting on a plane to go to Florida. I sat down in the
   cramped and shabby tourist section. The stewardess approached and said there had been a mistake, that I was to sit
   in first class. She pointed to an escalator that was going up. I
   rode up and was in a first class section, that had plush seats
   and huge windows. I became anxious and thought, "I do not
   belong here, I am going back to tourist were I belong."*

The dreams were dealt with in the manner proposed by Fosshage
(1987): "Dream images are poignantly meaningful representations
that serve as thematic or organizational nodal points. The primary
clinical task, in contrast to the translation of dream images, is to
amplify and elucidate the meanings of the chosen images." These
dreams paralleled our early attempts at understanding and organizing Mr. B.'s current experience. Mr. B.'s experience of himself in
the context of the relationship with his partner sharply contrasted
with his current state of depression, confusion and anxiety. The first

dream[1] was understood to summarize the common experience of men caring for their ill partners: though their world may feel that it is falling apart around them as the partner becomes increasingly ill, the well partner does not loose his coherence. He has an important job to do—caring for his ill partner. The sense of duty and the sustaining power of the relationship help the partner to feel grounded and to not be as vulnerable or buffeted by the chaos that he feels in the wake of a disruption in the relationship, or with the death of his partner. Thus, in the face of chaos, the world still makes sense and has meaning. The second dream was understood as representing his loss of coherence—the panic that he came to experience as he realized the world was still moving on, perhaps even to his own illness, and how little grounded he felt, let alone secure that there would be relationships that could sustain him the way he sustained his partner. The third dream was understood as relating to his own damaged and diminished self-esteem that ultimately was preventing him from engaging in relationships that could help him feel grounded and secure, consequently enhancing his feeling of not belonging.

Over the next five months of treatment, Mr. B.'s depression lifted considerably and his anxiety diminished. The dialogue with his partner diminished over the first several months of treatment and he became more interested in other people. He became increasingly comfortable with himself, and was less abrasive in his support group. He pursued other interests, took another more challenging job, and hosted a holiday party. This was especially significant in that he and his partner were avid entertainers, and each event was very much an effort in team work. Soon after the party, Mr. B. began to bring in his experience of attempting to negotiate new people outside of the milieu of his seropositive support and twelve-step groups. At first, if anyone approached him, he would become overwhelmed and panic. He was flooded with his experience of damaged self and torn between his desire to want to be understood given his experience with his partner, and current status, but also

---

1. This series of dreams can also be understood as reflecting the deepening transference. The explanations are not mutually exclusive.

fearing that he would be rejected if this information was known. Gradually, his anxiety in these situations subsided, he was able to carry on conversations with people, and eventually began dating a man.

Discussion

This case illustrates several important aspects of intervention with surviving partners who are seropositive. I am going to focus on the handling of the continued idealization of the deceased partner, the active introduction of knowledge regarding the distorting effects of seropositivity on the mourning process, and the interface between meanings derived from past experiences and the current experience of mourning.

The continued idealization of the deceased partner must be handled appropriately and empathically else one risks traumatizing, if not enraging, the client. A common countertransference experience is the therapist feeling somewhat uncomfortable as the extent of the ongoing dialogue and continued presence of the deceased partner in the survivor's ongoing experience becomes evident. The idealization and continued dialogue can not be "interpreted" away, rather it must be allowed to gradually subside. Recalling the formulations in the previous chapter, the dialogue is serving an important function: the survivor derives a degree of comfort and coherence and it often represents the most substantial sense of connection for these men. It has become a part of the ongoing self experience. While it may be a factor in difficulties forming new relationships, it is only one aspect of a larger constellation.

In a very real way, the relationship with the therapist offers the opportunity for the survivor to negotiate and develop his first new intimate relationship after the death of his partner. The clinician must do his or her best to ensure that it is a successful one: successful in that the client will not be overwhelmed by anxiety relating to damaged self-esteem, and successful in that it offers the hope of making meaning out of the confusing array of affects and private activities that, while important to the mourner, may distress others.

Survivors have been through a traumatic experience, often a series of traumatic experiences. The deficient self state leads to the experience of the world and unfamiliar people as potentially over-stimulating if not damaging, and hence a great deal of effort is often employed to protect the self from further trauma. A negative transference is often apparent or in the background. The therapist may have to actively but gently help the client settle in to treatment; to experience the therapist as attempting to understand, rather than make demands that the self cannot tolerate or accommodate. This probably accounts for why surviving partners and spouses tend not to seek out treatment early in the mourning process. Though they may be experiencing considerable disorganization, pain and anxiety, beginning treatment represents engaging in a new relationship which the mourner may experience as potentially overstimulating.

As the clinician is able to be empathically in tune with the surviving partner's experience of mourning, and is able to sustain and soothe anxiety rather than enhance it, the transference will deepen and solidify. As this happens one will also observe the idealization of the deceased partner gradually wane. By showing interest in and being empathically attuned to the affects related to the relationship, its history, the illness and death of the partner – ultimately its meanings, the clinician is assuring the client that he is not attempting to "take the relationship away," but rather attempting to understand its importance. Recalling the conception of the work of mourning in the previous chapter, the clinician is participating in the process of the mourner's attempts to complete the configuration lost with the death of the partner. As the survivor becomes more attached to and comfortable with the clinician, one often observes him becoming more comfortable outside of the therapeutic relationship and beginning to feel lonely, rather than alone. The clinician's response to attempts to complete the lost configuration and subsequently organize affects to the point where meaning can evolve serves to orient the partner away from the world he has lost, to the world of the living.

As in this case, erotized elements may emerge in the transference. If these are not distressing to the client and/or so intense that they threaten to disrupt the treatment then no interpretation is in order and the erotized elements will also wane as the transference deepens. If the client is showing signs of distress, then discussion from the framework that the erotization is a sign of his feeling un-

derstood, comfortable and excited about the possibility that perhaps
he is capable of forming new attachments may be called for.

Another aspect of work with these men is the therapist pointing
out the distorting influence of seropositivity. While this may potentially be an intellectual intrusion into the dialogue between the client and the therapist, it offers an important structure with which to
help the client organize his experience. The client is already feeling
depressed, anxious isolated, and perhaps most painful of all, feeling
weird and different — apart from the rest of the world. The client
often explains his ongoing experience to himself in these terms.
Suggesting to the client that part of what he is experiencing is due
not to his personal "pathology," but rather to the distorting effects
of something beyond his control, helps to organize the experience
into something considerably more benign, cuts into the negative
experience of self that has often come to dominate the self organization, and offers him the opportunity to relate his fears about his own
health and life, and their connections to the loss of his partner.

This also provides the opportunity for the client to experience
with the clinician any angry affect surrounding his experience. Several men have related considerable anger — feeling cheated, and that
the situation is "unfair." I tend to respond that yes, they have been
cheated, AIDS has taken a great deal away from them and they have
every right to be angry over their situation. This can be especially
helpful in that often these and other seropositive men have adopted
a "walking on eggshells" stance — fearing that the experience of
any angry affect (save perhaps a projected anger towards institutions or unhelpful individuals) may disrupt their equilibrium. The
threatened loss of coherence is experienced as the potential for the
world to come crashing down — essentially that they will become
ill.

For Mr. B., numerous and complicated meanings from the past
had come to dominate his current experience. He had spent considerable energy throughout his life attempting to compensate for long-
standing and complicated feelings of incompetence and inferiority,
with a vigilance being kept in anticipation of hostile assault. Once
again, he found himself thrust back into his experience of latency
and adolescence and the profound feeling that there was something
terribly wrong with him. This time he could not view himself as the

underdog — there was no seeming way out of his experience, other than his own demise. Mr. B.'s pronounced panic at feeling "out of control" did serve him in that it was an important factor that brought him into treatment. It also proved to be a complicating factor in the process as well.

If the themes and experiences he brought to a particular session could not be neatly wrapped up or put into a coherent language-based cognitive mode he would frequently panic. In part this was due to his experience of twelve-step groups where everything could seemingly be neatly labeled and organized into a "this is what you are doing wrong, this is what you need to do" formula. The transference aspect was related to feeling incompetent in the clinician-client relationship, that he had not been able to "get it," to grasp and organize unfamiliar data. Hence, he found himself experiencing himself as vulnerable and panicked. His hope of being understood was overridden by the fear of being traumatized.

One could argue that this was related to the unmourned death of the father. For Mr. B., the death was experienced as a relief, a seemingly neat solution to the complicated relationship. One could argue that it was not so much the failure to mourn the relationship, but the inability to view himself as a competent adult vis à vis his father. We often see patients who have difficulty experiencing themselves as competent in relation to their parents. Mr. B. probably would not have been able to accomplish this without intensive psychotherapy, regardless if the father still lived. The information that emerged that confirmed the extent of the father's pathology only served to further complicate, but also explain, a complicated and painful experience in the context of a central relationship of childhood.

Emergence of Symptoms and the Ability to Hope

The emergence of symptoms for surviving partners is often a terrifying event. For many years they have lived in fear of their own illness. The emergence of symptoms and/or need to begin taking AZT is often experienced as the beginning of the end. The clinical question is what is the terror related to? In work with these men it has become clear to me that the terror they experience has much to do with the illness and loss of their partner. They experience a fragmentation with the emergence of symptoms, often profoundly withdraw and attempt to manage their terror. However, the terror seems related to the experience of relationships and sustaining connections being ripped away from them.

If one listens closely, it is as if they are experiencing a similar state as when they first realized their partner was dead, and they were alone. The intensity of the reaction is due to just this state; in the self organization, they are unable to recall the presence and past experiences of benign and helpful people. It is often helpful if the alliance is solid enough to point out to the client that AIDS did rip the relationship with the partner away; however, he has a number of relationships at his disposal that will be there for him.

At the point when he became symptomatic, Mr. G. had been in twice weekly treatment with me for three years. The treatment relationship began with him and his partner due to difficulties they were having managing the partner's illness with AIDS. His partner developed pneumonia and died after several sessions. However, Mr. G. continued in a treatment that addressed his experience of mourning, the complication of his own infection and eventually considerable pre-existing self pathology.

In a very rapid succession, Mr. G.'s T-cells dropped considerably. Just as he had achieved a degree of equilibrium secondary to the disruption caused by the decline in lab values, he developed a severe and extremely painful case of shingles. He canceled several sessions, often just before they were to begin, saying he was not feeling up to leaving his home. After the third cancellation, I gently insisted that he come in. He had spent the last ten days holed up in his apartment, groggy on pain medication and attempting to keep at bay the terror he felt. He related that he feared if he sat across from me, he would experience the terror full force. (Though his physician had explained that the shingles were not necessarily HIV-related, he experienced them as the "beginning of the end.")

In the course of the session, he indeed did experience considerable intense affect, however, with considerable relief. He related that he felt intense terror, he kept being flooded by images of his partner on his death bed, he alternately felt acutely alone, isolated, terrified and enraged. In the session he repeatedly experienced these states and affects. He experienced himself as now in the process of dying, the events that he had feared for so long were now happening, he too was dying just as his partner, and it had come too soon, much too soon. At the end of the hour with some surprise he reported, "you are still here, and I am still here, there were times when I felt you slipping away, but we are both still around."

After this experience, Mr. G. attended sessions regularly, but a pronounced withdrawal was evident for several weeks. Granted, in part this was related to the narcissistic withdrawal often experienced by people during illness, but the other crucial aspect was his preoccupation with the death of his partner and his own death. He was avoiding contact with his family—relationships that had solidified considerably since his partner's death—as he experienced their concern as overstimulating and triggering his anxiety. I tended to doggedly pursue him during this period. Gradually, the terror, withdrawal and preoccupation with his partner eased as we were more firmly able to establish his symbolic connection of his symptoms to the ripping away of his relationship with his partner, and he was once again able to take considerable comfort in the number of relationships that he indeed had at his disposal. Eventually, he related the experience of the several weeks following the emergence of shingles to that of his partner calling to him as Captain Ahab beckoned from Moby Dick, with myself on the other hand calling him back. There was also a transference connection. His wish was that, in the context of the idealizing transference with me which he experienced as very sustaining, if he did everything right, he would not get sick. The emergence of symptoms thus also represented a transference disappointment. This same sequence was experienced several months later in a much milder and less protracted form when Mr. G.'s T-cells declined to the point where his physician recommended he begin taking AZT.

This case offers a number of potential insights into the experience of surviving partners as they face their own illness. In making initial explorations for the study, numerous professionals related their experiences with surviving partners who became ill. They all tended to be struck by the degree of withdrawal, often rapid decline, and

lack of enthusiasm for their own treatment. Several of the symptomatic survivors I encountered in the course of the study tended to
have to varying degrees, an "as if" quality about them. They were
only partly here, as if they were going about the motions of living.
Several were actively, saying and doing all the "right things" in
regards to their own treatment and outlook for the future, but were
actually far away. Essentially, their private dialogue was very different from their public dialogue.

Mr. G.'s experience offers a potential glimpse at the dynamics
that contribute to this sometimes, dramatic turning inward, if not
gradual shutting down, of the self and its involvement with the
world of the living. Recalling the formulations of the previous
chapter, the intense and often complicated affect secondary to infection of the surviving partner makes it extremely difficult to form
a narrative where the surviving partner's potential illness and death
are experienced as separate from the illness and death of his partner,
hence illness and death represent an ongoing shared experience. In
the wake of the trauma of illness, the self organizes along these
lines, and the survivor views his current experience as an extension
of that with his partner. If the survivor is already significantly ill
when his partner dies, or symptoms emerge early in the mourning
experience, this process may be difficult to buffer or reverse.

This shades into the nature of the capacity to hope and hope itself. Hope ultimately represents the past experience of available and
sustaining people and the subsequent integration of these experiences into the self organization — that at a time of trauma, overstimulation, or anxiety, a relationship has calmed or soothed and helped
to restore coherence. Hence it is ultimately related to the idealized
parental imago, the self structure that develops out of the idealizing
selfobject relationships with the child's parents. In patients that
have severe deficits in this area, ultimately due to selfobject failure
or severe disapointments, one often sees an inability to hope, let
alone trust that people can be useful in helping them manage anxiety or trauma. The seropositive surviving partner has already experienced several severe, often acutely traumatizing disappointments.
He often has hoped that he would be seronegative, he hoped that he
could sustain his partner until a cure is found, and he hoped that he
would not become ill himself. The emergence of symptoms ulti-

mately represents another disappointed hope. Repeated disappointments, the assault on the self that AIDS represents, and the overall erosive effect of a protracted immersion in the experience of HIV-related problems taxes even the most resilient self.

When the client is not severely traumatized, and is able to make use of the distinction, it is often useful to point out the difference between hope and contingent hope or wishes. The hope of being negative, of sustaining their partner until a cure is found and of not becoming symptomatic themselves are ultimately more related to wishes or contingent hope. By this I mean results that are often contingent on doing things right, of being a "good person." It is often helpful to point out to the client that while their wish to remain symptom-free has been dashed, and their wish to not lose their partner to death was also dashed, and the relationship was ripped away, their hope comes from the experience of others being there for them — the therapist is still available, as are other sustaining connections. However, in the face of the terror of becoming ill, patients may not readily be able to call upon them. The therapist's task becomes to handle the client in such a way that he can feel calmed and reassured and once again begin to call upon his past experiences, and the available people at his disposal.

Throughout Mr. G.'s experience of mourning he maintained at times a high degree of withdrawal from the larger social networks potentially available to him. His experience of mourning and being in therapy resulted in considerable reworking of his experience in his family. Just as a dialogue regarding long-standing self experience of being weird and different opened up in the dialogue of the treatment relationship, a dialogue evolved with his family, and he began to experience himself as an actively involved member of his family of origin. A model scene from childhood (Stern 1985) involved his mother's failure to help him negotiate the world outside of his family. He recalled that at around five years of age he was invited to go to a birthday party. His mother met him on the steps of the school, to walk him to the event. He became anxious, protested that he did not want to go to the party and focused on wanting to know what the present was that his mother had purchased and wrapped. His mother replied that she would tell him if he did a dance. He became increasingly upset, finally performing a brief, agonized dance. His mother informed him what the present was and he was not forced to go to the party. (One could argue that the more helpful approach would have been to recognize the child's distress, and offer to accompany him to the party and "help out the other child's mother." If the child settled comfortably into the peer activities, then the mother could leave him to participate. However, his mother was a second generation immigrant, and a degree of suspicion and distrust was evident for the community outside of the strong cultural ties of the family and the immigrant community. This may have contributed to the mother's difficulty in helping her child bridge to the larger world.)

Mr. G. had made several attempts to attend the meetings of a large seropositive support organization. However, he frequently became anxious and overstimulated, especially if anyone attempted to strike up a conversation. Frequently, he would make plans to attend but then fall asleep and miss the meetings. He was at once chagrined by this behavior and relieved. In the transference he would ask me for help and dare me to do anything about it. Recalling the model scene, approximately one year after the experience described previously, I suggested that he might want to join the group for seropositive men that I was forming. He was anxious but interested; I took a neutral stance. He eventually decided not to join, but would periodically ask about the group. Several months later an opening was available in the group and I related this to him. He again was anxious but interested. This time I casually remarked that, "I just might insist that you join." Mr. G. laughed, and the next week announced that he wanted to give the group a try.

During the first several sessions he experienced considerable anxiety about revealing that he was a surviving partner, and interpreted several group members' responses as attacking and overstimulating, but was also surprised that there was another surviving partner in the group. For several weeks, his individual session (which followed the group several days later) was spent in helping him to organize his experience of the group, and the acute vulnerability he felt. Very quickly his anxiety diminished and he became an active member.

Five years after the death of his partner and 20 months after the experience initially described in this discussion, Mr. G. is enthusiastically engaged in his family of origin, the large support/social organization for men who test positive, is an active member in the group led by myself and has begun to attend social events of a group of gay men and women who share his vocational interests. In a recent group session in which the members were talking about their experience of isolation, he remarked, "looking back, being so isolated was like being dead." One can only wonder where this man would be today, had he not been engaged in treatment and continued to strive to manage the intense affects and pull towards isolation that he experienced when he became symptomatic.

The Loss of a Therapist

Just as the loss of a partner can have profound effects on the surviving partner's experience of HIV-infection, so can the loss of a client's therapist. This particular man had experienced several traumatic losses in the course of his life. With the unexpected death of his therapist from AIDS, affects and meanings from his series of losses came to dominate his experience. Once again he was left feeling alone in the face of a great hardship. His treatment initially consisted of a process of accounting for the meaning of each of the losses.

Mr. S., a 33-year-old man, contacted the therapist after he had reached an impasse in his treatment with a clinician he had been seeing for several months. He was acutely agitated, disorganized and depressed. He was having extreme difficulty accomplishing tasks that his job required. On the weekends he tended to drink and use cocaine heavily, often returning home alone late at night and engaging in a masochistic piercing of his nipples. He felt acutely lost, without a sense of direction, and terrified. He was afraid of people and withdrawing from several important relationships. While he was experiencing a great deal of depression and anxiety, these feelings appeared "fused" and were not readily distinct. Initially he could barely tolerate being in the same room with me. Every 10 to 15 minutes, the flow of conversation would suddenly stop as he felt acutely anxious, exposed and vulnerable.

He related the following events. His therapist of eight years died suddenly of AIDS in the early fall. The therapist, with whom he was deeply attached, had not told his client he was ill, nor was it certain whether the therapist himself knew he had an HIV infection. Mr. S. had known for several years that he was infected, had remained asymptomatic, but was aware through medical monitoring that his T-cell counts were gradually falling. The time of the therapist's memorial service was incorrectly printed in the local newspaper. Consequently, Mr. S. missed the service. Several months later, his T-cells had declined to the point where his physician recommended that he begin taking AZT. At this point he experienced a profound disorganization, terror and withdrawal that had persisted until he entered treatment with me. He acknowledged the fear that if his therapist could not manage his infection and died – what chances did he have? He had attempted to engage in a local seropositive organization but became anxious in large groups of people and withdrew. Mr. S. felt his death was imminent, and that he would die alone. He had not told any of his close friends or colleagues that he had begun taking AZT, let alone his response to the implications of this event.

Mr. S. related several other losses. His parents divorced when he was ten. When he was thirteen his mother committed suicide after a prolonged and intense depression. A series of housekeepers came into the home, only to leave as he became attached to them. Four years prior to entering treatment, his best friend had died of AIDS. Mr. S. had served as his primary caretaker. He related that he had not really "mourned" any of the losses, that his style was to "put things on the shelf – and get on with it." Now it was clear that with the loss of the therapist and his own medical symptomatology, the losses and associated affects had become merged – leaving him feeling acutely alone in the face of a terrifying illness. He related being aware of a great deal of sadness, but fearing that if he let himself experience it, he would fall into a "black hole" which would engulf him and from which he might never emerge.

Due to his extreme anxiety and depression, a medication consult was requested. He was initially medicated with an antidepressant with a good result. However, Mr. S.'s anxiety was so great that an anxiolytic medication was added several weeks later. With this medication combination and twice-a-week treatment he began to *relate his experience of each of the losses. Though he felt pulled to talk about these past relationships, he was initially terrified of the affect he feared he would experience. However, he quickly discovered that rather than being overwhelmed, he began to feel calmer, more stable and alive.*

As it was spring he began an extensive patio garden; he related that his mother was an avid gardener and his associations revealed that as a child he was enchanted by his mother's elaborate garden. He also related that he had accompanied his friend's body to a distant state for burial. However, due to the ground conditions, no graveside ceremony was held. He began to desire to see his friend's grave, to see his final resting place. Mr. S. did the necessary research, flew to the city one weekend, made several gravesight visits and settled several conflicts with his friend's mother that had left him guilt-ridden. As he prepared for the trip, he talked about the relationship. He was deeply attached to this individual. Mr. S. related that his friend made him feel very spontaneous, and they knew each other so well, they often anticipated each other's thoughts and spoke in "shorthand." The friend has also helped him to stop smoking, exercise regularly, and in general to get his "act together."

Mr. S. was curious about the disposition of his therapist's ashes. If they were interred, he wanted to visit that site as well. I did some investigating only to find that they had met the not uncommon fate of being consigned to a shelf in a relative's home. He was not distressed by this knowledge, rather satisfied that he at least knew where they were. As we discussed the relationship with the therapist, the transference aspects were highlighted. The relationship represented the first time he felt "special" with, and protected by, an adult male.

He then obtained copies of his mother's hospital records and brought them and copies of extensive correspondence between his mother and grandmother to several sessions. The documents painted a vivid picture of an exquisitely depressed and regressed woman who struggled for years with painful insecurity and doubt of her ability to mother her children. In reading the mother's correspondence, it was quite easy to empathize with her pain, sadness and insecurity. This was in sharp contrast to his father, whom he experienced as treating him and his sib like "things" that were more inconveniences than his children. Though he stopped his piercing activities and generally started taking considerably better care of himself, Mr. S. continued to periodically go on weekend binges of alcohol and cocaine. These binges are clearly related to his being flooded by rageful affect secondary to this experience of his father that has become the increasing focus of the treatment. The masochistic connection was made even clearer by his revelation that there were times when he had hoped he would die of AIDS as a revenge towards his father.

Concurrent to these activities and his work in the sessions, he began informing his immediate supervisor, with whom he has a long-standing, close relationship, exactly what he had been experiencing with HIV infection: the loss of his friend and therapist, his own need to go on AZT, and the terror, sadness and disorganization that had come to dominate his life. Consequently, the tension he was experiencing at work eased considerably as he offered an explanation for his recent behavior. He also related this information to several friends whom he had withdrawn from over the past several months. He had purchased a new home approximately 6 months earlier, but even though he had ample funds and was quite skilled, he had done little to decorate it to make it his own. Now he began painting and papering with a vengeance and was quite pleased with the result. Mr. S. also began meeting new people and engaged in a number of brief dating relationships. He became much more comfortable in revealing his antibody status, doing so initially in the course of conversations.

As Mr. S. began to feel better about himself, he became increasingly concerned about his use of cocaine and alcohol. Gradually he came to realize the extent of his dependency and was increasingly distraught by the masochistic sexual fantasies that accompanied his cravings and his highs. He eventually decided to seek inpatient treatment for his drug usage at a facility whose population was entirely gay men and lesbian women.

Discussion

Clearly this is a very complicated case. It serves to underscore a crucial point: that while the impact of losses and difficulty in mourning losses are often significant factors in an individual's experience of and adaptation to HIV infection, rarely do attempts at organizing the meaning of the loss constitute the entire treatment task. Rather it is but one—albeit often integral and very important—aspect of a larger therapeutic encounter.

Mr. S. had long-standing difficulties in negotiating the world in the face of chronic anxiety, painfully poor self-esteem and a pronounced sense of feeling "ungrounded." The successful clinical treatment of a man such as Mr. S. would be a long and complicated task even without the presence of HIV infection. Clearly a wide range of clinical skills is a necessary component. While the series of losses were a key factor in his current disorganization, his long-standing experience of himself as incompetent and incapable was equally important. As treatment progressed, strong idealizing and mirroring elements emerged in the transference. This allowed him to experience himself as capable and eager in his attempts to integrate the meaning of his losses, rather than "table them and go on." It has also provided access to his experience of his father and the severe self deficits secondary to the significant problems in the father/son dialogue.

The use of medication is often an integral aspect of working with individuals who have become acutely disorganized in their attempts to manage the impact of their own HIV infection in the face of the loss of central relationships to AIDS. When individuals are experiencing acute clinical symptomatology that is grossly interfering with their capacity to function, then a medication consult is indicated. Their lives have already been acutely disrupted. While the therapeutic dialogue may bring some relief, it will often take time, and in the meanwhile, the client is acutely distressed and disorganized. He may be risking the loss of his employment due to impaired performance and/or may be further jeopardizing his own health in maladaptive attempts to manage the affects he is experiencing. Appropriately administered and monitored antidepressant and anxiolytic medication will help to modulate the affects, provide more timely relief, and help support the client in his attempts to organize his experience.

As the therapeutic relationship solidified, transference elements emerged and the medication helped stabilize his affects, Mr. G. was able to approach the losses in his life and begin to organize the meaning the relationships had for him. This afforded him relief from the acute feeling of aloneness as well as providing him with the experience of being competent and capable of approaching painful aspects of his experience of self. As Mr. G.'s self-esteem continued to grow through these experiences and his experience of the transference, he began to acknowledge the extent of his reliance on substances to modulate his affects and self-esteem. The use of cocaine became increasingly abhorrent for Mr. G., and he also began to feel that perhaps he could overcome his dependence. After some discussion and a consult regarding his treatment options, he sought residential treatment for his dependency. His encounters at the treatment center provided radically new experiences of homosexual men and women. His many brief, frustrating and often woefully disappointing relationships had helped to build up a considerable degree of cynicism with regard to whether other gay men could be relied upon. At this point a return to outpatient treatment with the addition of the necessary elements to help sustain his sobriety is planned.

The Loss of a Friend

Mr. C. was 38 years of age when he was referred by a colleague. He was acutely distressed—depression, anxiety and labile mood states were prominent. He voiced a number of somatic complaints that he strongly felt were HIV-related, that after several years of struggling to fight disease progression, he was losing his battle. The beginning of the end was near; he was about to succumb to the disease and die. Bloodwork had been drawn six weeks earlier, but he had not returned or called for the results, fearing that his t-cell counts would only confirm his assumption. Though an accomplished professional, he was feeling alienated at work and painfully unsure of his skill.

Mr. C. focused a great deal on a current highly problematic relationship. All distortions aside, the boyfriend did sound like a very needy, depressed, naive and clingy young man. Mr. C. was acutely enraged with his boyfriend and at times was verbally and psychologically abusive. The crux of the problem appeared to be that Mr. C. desperately needed to idealize a partner-to feel that the partner could take care of him when, not if, he became ill. He was increasingly experiencing his friend as a drain on his attempts to manage his infection, rather than an asset, yet he was highly fearful of being alone.

Given his extreme distress, he was referred for medication and an antidepressant was initiated. Over the next few weeks, Mr. C.'s mood stabilized. With encouragement and exploration of his fears, he obtained his lab results to find that his counts were indeed stable, and his somatic preoccupation eased. In sessions he began to relate his experience of the illness and death of a friend approximately 18 months earlier, whose decline was slow, agonizing and gruesome.

It had been a ten-year ongoing soul-mate/sex buddy relationship, though they did not consider themselves partnered. They had seen each other through numerous ups and downs, had lived in the same building for a number of years, and there was a strong sense that each could rely on the other. The relationship had strong, clear boundaries, and he experienced it as very uncomplicated and sustaining. A strong sense of guilt now was associated with the previously uncomplicated experience of his friend. He felt that he had deceived him and let him down in his time of need. Mr. C. related that his friend had a "big mouth." He was concerned that if his friend knew of his being positive, the friend would tell others as well. Mr. C. felt his deception lay in that while he spent considerable time taking care of his friend during the illness, he did not tell him that he too was infected. Mr. C. was left feeling that he had potentially deprived his friend of comfort, by not sharing his own struggle and fear. Instead he had acted as an unaffected caretaker.

After relating his experience of his friend and the perceived deception, his condition began to improve and he stabilized rather quickly. He was able to arrive at a solution to the difficult relationship and began to once again experience himself as competent in his career. His fear that he was in the process of dying declined and he returned to experiencing himself as infected, but actively managing the infection and its psychological impact, not critically ill and depleted.

Several months into the relationship, Mr. C. moved to another building. The move was poorly planned and prompted a severe regression when people that he was counting on did not help him. The next few weeks were very difficult as he attempted to create a new home for himself, but felt unable to do so. Though reliable people

were at his disposal, he repeatedly called upon unreliable people
for assistance, only to be disappointed. He deeply missed his friend
whom he felt would be there for him and share his delight over a
new home. This led to a lengthy discussion of his experience of his
mother as unreliable and unhelpful, especially in times of acute
need. Gradually he was able to engage reliable people to help him
assemble his home. He hosted a small party and related that during
the evening he found himself looking at a picture of his friend and
smiling, rather than feeling acutely sad and alone.

Discussion

Depression in seropositive individuals is often expressed via the
fear that they are on the verge of or actually in the process of dying.
In the course of the clinical interview, when discrepancies emerge
between the individual's experience of himself and medical data,
then the clinician must turn their attention to factors that may be
contributing to a state of depression. Initially upon testing positive,
men often experience a period of feeling that they are dying and that
death is imminent. Gradually as coherence is restored, often
through encounters with other seropositive individuals, this often
terrifying state declines, and people experience themselves as infected, not critically ill.

When the self experience of terminal illness re-emerges (and it
often does), it is usually in response to a disruption in a sustaining
relationship. My experience with seropositive men has been that the
most disruptive experience is the illness and/or death of a friend. If
idealizing elements were an integral aspect of the dialogue, i.e., the
individual was experienced as role model, a guide for how to manage HIV infection, then the disorganization may be considerable.
The individual's private dialogue shifts from, "if he can stay on top
of it, so can I," to "if he can die, than surely I will as well."
Instead of being able to view his medical status via lab results or the
opinion of his physician, he views his status in relation to the lost
relationship and its sustaining aspects. Just as in surviving partners,
this complication may interfere with mourning the loss. Subsequently, seropositive men who have sustained a number of losses
may find that an increasing mass of grief comes to be an aspect of

their self experience. Unfortunately, this often serves to erode into their optimism and efforts to experience themselves as vitally involved in the world.

In the course of treatment, the clinician should help the client relate his experience of loss and the meaning of the loss. In the case of Mr. C., the complication in mourning the loss of his friend resulted in a "gap" in his experience of the relationship. Guilt and shame interfered with his ability to form and integrate a benign narrative of the relationship. Rather than be assured that he had indeed experienced an ongoing dialogue that was sustaining and meaningful, he was left feeling isolated and cut off from that experience. This was especially meaningful for him in that a central aspect of his personal narrative was that people will not be there in times of distress, but rather will abandon him.

The gradual focus on this aspect of the narrative resulted in attempts at understanding his experience of his mother. The relationship had been quite stormy, at times chaotic. During the period of treatment when he was recalling these experiences, a dialogue opened up between himself and his mother in which he was able to relate his experience of several key events in their lives and their subsequent impact. His mother was quite shocked at the extent of her son's fears secondary to his experience of her, but rather than defensively denying or minimizing his anxiety, she reassured him.

SUMMARY

This chapter has presented a brief overview of clinical intervention with men whose efforts at managing the impact of their own HIV infection have been disrupted by the experience of loss. As the epidemic continues, losses of central relationships to the same disease will most likely become integral factors in the difficulties clients present to us in our clinical practices. As clinicians we must understand theoretically the impact of loss on the experience of HIV infection and AIDS and include this knowledge in our clinical approach to and understanding of HIV impacted clients.

I am not proposing a narrow focus on losses, rather the meaning of loss in the context of the client's overall self structure. While each of the clients presented had sustained losses, in some cases a series of losses, the meaning, impact and relationship to their over-all self experience varied greatly. The loss must be viewed in the context of the client's larger experience, the nature of his difficulties, his medical status, and his experience of the clinician.

The majority of the individuals presented in this discussion were seen in intensive, usually twice weekly treatment over an extended period. Hence, managing, understanding and working within the transference was an integral component. Once established, sustaining selfobject transferences fueled and supported efforts at understanding the meaning of the loss, the personal meanings that infection represented, and longstanding meanings integral to the client's experience of self and served as a buffer against withdrawal from potentially sustaining relationships outside of the treatment relationship.

In closing, my ultimate hope is that this effort provides helpful knowledge to be added to the repertoire of clinicians working with HIV-related problems. I am well aware of the inherent stresses and strains on our own resiliency that accompanies work with this population. The epigraph that began this book, "You get to know their lovers and it all seems very real," gets at the heart of the matter. Examining AIDS in the context of the matrix of relationships in which it occurs conveys the depth of meaning that accompanies the illness and death of a person. Whether the person be a partner, friend, relative or client, the loss is felt. The drain on our own resiliency comes from the experience of the loss of our clients parallel to our efforts at sustaining others. Each client we have worked with has taught us something. Regarding the experience of the therapist at the conclusion of a successful treatment, Palombo (1990) states: "The therapist has gained in having succeeded in helping someone. What is gained is both knowledge and wisdom that has come from having participated and shared in the life of another being." Thus each loss has meaning for us as well.

I am equally aware of the dedication that a relatively small group of clinicians demonstrate in their work with the growing numbers of HIV impacted individuals. Throughout the country, small groups of physicians, nurses, social workers and other clinicians work with the majority of HIV patients. Far too often I have encountered the dedicated social worker of a medical facility reaching out to numerous HIV impacted individuals, offering a sustaining relationship and crucial help, yet doing so in isolation from colleagues who tend to avoid this population, and often the professionals who work with them. Again, I hope this work has provided a framework to understand the often complicated clinical situations we face, and ultimately, to make our work more meaningful, and less emotionally draining.

For partners who have read this book, I hope it has been a valuable aspect of managing the illness or your mourning process. Though I am sure it prompted the emergence of many painful memories, hopefully, it was ultimately reassuring and resulted in a more settled, affirming personal account of your experience. In closing I am reminded of one of the many titles proposed for this work, "Quiet Heros of the Plague." Partners rarely appear on the six o'clock news, are featured in print, or give invitational addresses at conferences, yet your contribution has been invaluable. You have taught me, and hopefully those who read this book, about the very human nature of AIDS.

References

Aldrich, C.N. (1974). Some dynamics of anticipatory grief. In B. Schoenberg (Ed.), *Anticipatory Grief* (pp. 143-156). New York: Columbia University Press.

Baker, H.S., & Baker, M.N. (1987). Heinz Kohut's self psychology: An overview. *American Journal of Psychiatry, 144* (1), 1-9.

Barbutto, J. (1984). Psychiatric care of seriously ill patients with acquired immune deficiency syndrome. In S.E. Nichols and D.G. Ostrow (Eds.), *Psychiatric Implications of the Acquired Immune Deficiency Syndrome* (pp. 71-82). Washington, DC: American Psychiatric Press.

Barton, D. (1977). The family of the dying person. In D. Barton (Ed.), *Dying and Death: A Clinical Guide for Caregivers*. Baltimore, MD: The Williams and Wilkens Company.

Basch, M. (1988). *Understanding Psychotherapy*. New York: Basic Books.

Bayer, R. (1965). *Homosexuality and American Psychiatry: The Politics of Diagnosis*. New York: Basic Books.

Bowlby, J. (1961). Processes of mourning. *International Journal of Psychoanalysis, 42,* 317-40.

Bowlby, J. (1980). *Attachment and Loss, Volume III, Loss: Sadness and Depression.* New York: Basic Books.

Buckingham, S. & Van Gorp, W. (1988). Essential knowledge about AIDS dementia. *Social Work, 3* (2), 112-115.

Burks, W. (1987, October 15) . Horizons conference workshop focuses on partners of gay men who get AIDS. *Chicago Outlines*, p. 7.

Christ, G., Wiener, L., & Moynihan, R. (1986). Psychosocial issues in AIDS. *Psychiatric Annals, 16* (3), 154-168.

Curtis, P. (Ed.). (1988). *Clinical Ethnography*. Manuscript submitted for publication.

Dilley, J.W. (1984). Treatment interventions and approaches to

care of patients wIth acquired immune deficiency syndrome. In
S.E. Nichols and D.G. Ostrow (Eds.), *Psychiatric Implications
of the Acquired Immune Deficiency Syndrome* (pp. 62-70).
Washington, DC: American Psychiatric Press.

Ferrara, A. (1984). My personal experience with AIDS. *American
Psychologist, 39* (11), 18-24.

Fosshage, J.L. (1988). Dream interpretation revisited. In A. Goldberg (Ed.), *Progress in Self Psychology Volume 7* (pp. 161-175).
Hillsdale, NJ: Analytic Press.

Freinhar, J. (1987). Oedipus or Odysseus: Developmental lines of
narcissism. *Psychiatric Annals, 16* (8), 477-485.

Freud, S. (1912-13). *Totem and Taboo.* Standard Edition *13,* 1-
162.

Freud, S. (1917). Mourning and Melancholia. Standard Edition 14:
243-58.

Geis, S., Fuller, R., & Rush, J. (1986). Lovers of AIDS victims:
Psychosocial stresses and counseling needs. *Death Studies, 10,*
43-53.

Glaser, B. (1978). *Theoretical sensitivity.* Mill Valley, CA: The
Free Press.

Glaser, B. & Strauss, A. (1967). *The discovery of grounded theory:
strategies for qualitative research.* Chicago: Aldine Publishing
Company.

Goldberg, A. (1990). *The Prisonhouse of Psychoanalysis.* Hillsdale, NJ: The Analytic Press.

Gonsiorek, J. (1982). The use of diagnostic concepts in working
with gay and lesbian populations. In J. Gonsiorek (Ed.), *Homosexuality and Psychotherapy: A Practitioner's Guide to Affirmative Models* (9-20). New York: The Haworth Press, Inc.

Helquist, M. (1987). Family, partners and friends. In M. Helquist
(Ed.), *Working with AIDS: A Resource Guide for Mental Health
Professionals* (pp. 225-247). San Francisco: AIDS Health Proj-
ect.

Isay, R. (1989). *Being Homosexual.* New York: Ferrar, Strauss,
Giroux.

Jacobsen, E. (1943). Depression: The oedipus conflict in the development of depressive mechanisms. *Psychoanalytic Quarterly,
12,* 541-60.

Jacobsen, E. (1946). The effect of disappointment on ego and super ego formation in normal and depressive development. *Psychoanalytic Review*, *33*, 129-147.

Kennedy, L. (1979). Generalizing from single case studies. *Evaluation quarterly*, *4*, 666-678.

Klein, M. (1935). A contribution to the psychogenesis of manic-depressive states. *Love, Guilt and Reparation and Other Papers*. London: Hogarth.

Klein, M. (1940). Mourning and its relation to manic depressive states. In *Love, Guilt and Reparation and Other Papers*. London: Hogarth.

Knapp, M. (1979). Ethnographic contributions to evaluation research. In M. Thomas, D. Cook, and C. Reichert (Eds.), *Qualitative and Quantitative Methods in Evaluation Research*. Beverly Hills, CA: Sage Publications.

Kohut, H. (1972). Thoughts on narcissism and narcissistic rage. *Psychoanalytic Study of the Child, 27*, 360-400.

Kohut, H. (1977), *The Restoration of the Self.* New York: International Universities Press.

Kohut, H. & Wolfe, E. (1978). The disorders of the self and their treatment: An outline. *International Journal of Psychoanalysis, 160*, 413-425.

Krystal, H. (1990). An information processing view of object-relations. *Psychoanalytic Inquiry, 10* (2), 221-251.

Lebow, G. (1976). Facilitating adaption in anticipatory mourning. *Social Casework*, *57* (7), 455-465.

Lewes, K. (1988). *The Psychoanalytic Theory of Male Homosexuality*. New York: Simon and Schuster.

Lincoln, Y. & Guba, 'E. (1985). *Naturalistic Inquiry*. Beverly Hills, CA: Sage Publications.

Lindeman, E. (1965). Symptomatology and management of acute grief. In H. Parad (Ed.). *Crises Intervention: Selected Readings* (7-21). New York: Family Service Association of America.

MacMahon, M. (1991). Selfobject experiences between men and women in intimate relationships. (Unpublished manuscript).

Martin, J. (1988). Psychological consequences of AIDS-related bereavement among gay men. *Journal of Consulting and Clinical Psychology*, *56* (6), 856-862.

Maylon, A.K. (1982). Psychotherapeutic implications of internalized homophobia in gay men. In J. Gonsiorek (Ed.), *Homosexuality and Psychotherapy* (pp. 59-70). New York: The Haworth Press, Inc.

Mendola, M. (1980). *The mendola report: New look at gay couples*. New York: Crown Publishers.

Morin, S. & Batchelor, W. (1984). Responding to the psychological threat of AIDS. *Public Health Reports, 99* (1), 1-4.

Muslin, H. (1985). Heinz Kohut: Beyond the pleasure principle, contributions to psychoanalysis. In J. Reppen (Ed.), *Beyond Freud: A Study in Modern Psychoanalytic Theorists* (pp. 203-230). Hillsdale, NJ: The Analytic Press.

Nichols, S. (1983). Psychiatric aspects of AIDS. *Psychosomatics, 24* (12), 1083-1089.

Nichols, S. (1984). Social and support groups for patients with acquired immune deficiency syndrome. In S.E. Nichols and D.G. Ostrow (Eds.), *Psychiatric Implications of the Acquired Immune Deficiency Syndrome* (pp. 89-98). Washington, DC: American Psychiatric Press.

Nichols, S. (1986). Psychotherapy and AIDS. In T. Stein, and C. Cohen, (Eds.), *Contemporary Perspectives on Psychotherapy with Lesbians and Gay Men* (pp. 209-240). New York: Plenum.

Palombo, J. (1981). Parent loss and childhood bereavement: Some theoretical considerations. *Clinical Social Work Journal, 9* (1), 3-33.

Palombo, J. (1982). The psychology of the self and the termination of treatment. *Clinical Social Work Journal, , 10* (1), 46-62.

Palombo, J. (Personal communication, February 24, 1989).

Palombo, J. (1990). Bridging the chasm between developmental theory and clinical theory: Part II. The bridge. In Press.

Parkes, C. (1972). *Bereavement: Studies of Grief in Adult Life*. New York: International Universities Press.

Perreten, D. (1989, February 9). AIDS statistics hew to predictions. *Windy City Times,* pp. 1, 12.

Pollock, G. (1961). Mourning and adaptation. *International Journal of Psychoanalysis, 42,* 341-361.

Rabins, P., Mace, N.L., & Lucas, M.J. (1982), The impact of

dementia on the family. *Journal of the American Medical Association,* *248* (3), 333-335.

Saari, C. (1986). *Clinical Social Work Treatment.* New York: Gardner Press.

Saghir, M. & Robbins, E. (1973), *Male and Female Homosexuality.* Baltimore, MD: Williams and Wilkins.

Schatzman, L. & Strauss, A. (1973). *Field Research Strategies for a Natural Sociology.* Englewood Cliffs, NJ: Prentice Hall.

Schwartz, H. & Jacobs, J. (1979). *Qualitative Sociology: A Method to the Madness* (pp. 37-61). New York: The Free Press.

Shane, M. & Shane, E. (1990). Object loss and selfobject loss: A consideration of self psychology's contribution to understanding mourning and the failure to mourn. In A. Goldberg (Ed.), *Progress In Self Psychology.* Volume 9. Hillsdale, NJ: Analytic Press.

Shearer, P. & McKusick, L. (1987). Counseling survivors. In M. Helquist (Ed.), *Working with AIDS: A Resource Guide for Mental Health Professionals* (pp. 225-247). AIDS Health Project: San Francisco.

Shelby, R.D. (1989). Internalized homophobia as narcissistic injury. (Unpublished paper.)

Siegal, R. & Hoeffer, D. (1981). Bereavement counseling for gay individuals. *American Journal of Psychotherapy,* *35* (4), 343-352.

Siegel, K. (1986). AIDS: The social dimension. *Psychiatric Annals,* *16* (3), 168-172.

Spiegel, D. (1989). *The Lancet,* October 14.

Stern, D. (1985). *The Interpersonal World of the Infant.* New York: Basic Books.

Stolorow, R., Brandchaft, B. & Atwood, G., (1987). *Psychoanalytic Treatment: An Intersubjective Approach.* Hillsdale, NJ: The Analytic Press.

Zarit, S.H., Reever, K.E. & Bach-Peterson, J. (1980). Relatives of the impaired elderly: Correlates of feelings of burden. *Gerontologist,* *20*, 649-655.

Index

Acquired immune deficiency
    syndrome. *See* AIDS
Affect
    experiential reorganization and,
      196,197,198,200
    selfobject functions and, 28
    therapeutic modulation, 225-226
AIDS. *See also* Human immune
    deficiency virus antibody
    testing; Human immune
    deficiency virus status
    clinical literature regarding, 15-20
    diagnosis. *See* Diagnosis, of
      AIDS
    disclosure of, 74,81-89
    to employer, 88,115
    to family, 81-88
    to friends, 81-83,87
    emotional reactions to, 16
    prevalence, 8,9
    psychological effects, 16-19
    psychosocial effects, 17-18
AIDS couple. *See also* partner;
    Surviving partner; Well
    partner
    clinical interventions with,
      226-237
    clinical literature regarding, 15-19
    discussion of AIDS by, 54-55
    interdependency, 127-128
    isolation, 201
    marriage, 102-103
    mutual illness, 99
AIDS organizations, volunteer work
    with, 102,153,158,212
AIDS quilt, 130,147-148,162,165,
    210,213
AIDS-related complex (ARC),
    56-58,61

Anger
    towards friends, 140-141
    of ill partner, 80
    of ill partner's family, 103
    of well/surviving partner, 79,80,
      244
Anniversary, of partner's death,
    135,155
Antidepressant drugs, 252,255,257
Anxiety
    HIV antibody testing-related,
      167-168
    of surviving partner, 19
Anxiolytic drugs, 252,255
Appetite loss, 79
Autonomy, of surviving partner, 19

Bereavement. *See also* Mourning;
    Mourning process
    AIDS-related, 12
    clinical literature regarding, 17
    psychological reactions of, 20
    as sleep disturbance cause, 20
    as stress cause, 20
Breast cancer patients, 223

Career plans, following partner's
    death, 176-177,183-185,
    216-217
Chaos experience, following
    partner's death, 47-48,49,
    123-128,205-206
    aloneness of, 124-126
    altered states of, 126-128
    calm and peace of, 47,124-125
Children

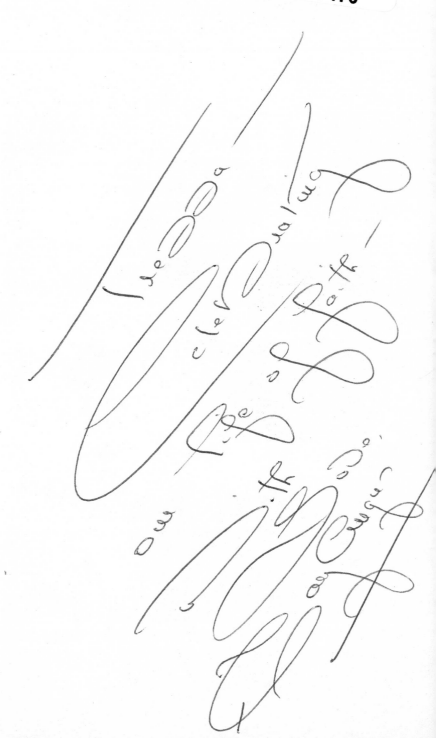

W9-CSX-176

ALSO BY FAY ANGUS

RUNNING AROUND IN SPIRITUAL CIRCLES

THE WHITE PAGODA

UP TO HEAVEN & DOWN TO EARTH

HOW TO DO EVERYTHING RIGHT
AND LIVE TO REGRET IT

How to Do Everything Right and Live to Regret It

FAY ANGUS

HARDCOVER EDITION
1983

HARPER & ROW, PUBLISHERS

San Francisco

Fifth Printing July 1993

Library of Congress Cataloging in Publication Data

Angus, Fay.
 HOW TO DO EVERYTHING RIGHT AND LIVE TO REGRET IT.
 1. Christian life - Anecdotes, facetiae, satire, etc.
2. Angus, Fay. I. Title
BV4157.A53 1983   248.4   82-48425
ISBN 0-9627269-0-7

85 86 87 10 9 8 7 6 5

To EVEN—
a most thoroughly misunderstood woman

Contents

Acknowledgments

Dr. Robert Vander Zaag, my pastor, who besides being marvelously good looking, taught me most of what I know about the sovereignty of God, the necessity of making midcourse corrections, and how to grow a choice cauliflower.

John Angus, my husband, who says *he* is the one who is marvelously good looking and, unless I acknowledge it, I may not live to regret it!

Anne and *Ian,* my children, who assure me that they are doing everything right, so I don't have to keep asking.

Roy M. Carlisle, my editor at Harper & Row San Francisco, who insisted that I write it right.

Lois Curley, my agent, who managed to tickle the muse in all the right places.

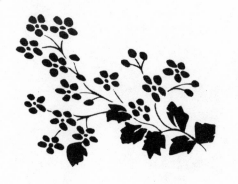

How to Do Everything Right & Live to Regret It

God knows, I tried!

To do everything right, that is. Whether I tried too hard, or not hard enough, depends upon whether you are me looking up at God, or God looking down at me, but whatever ... I ended up in a series of dithers that smudged themselves all over the best of my intentions, many of which blot their way through the ink in this book.

From the time I could talk, I tried to talk right. Elocution was stressed as a vital part of my education, and the sisters at the Convent of the Sacred Heart did their part by poking me every time I used "me" instead of "I," and said "seen" instead of "saw." They determined that the vowels and consonants of the rain in Spain fell very precisely on my plain with an articulation of the Queen's English that would have done Professor Higgins proud.

From the time I could walk, I tried to walk right. "Shoulders back, spine straight, and best foot forward." Nobody bothered, however, to tell me which was my best foot—which may be one of the reasons I had a tendency to trip over myself as well as other people. This led to my enrollment in ballet school, where the *maîtress de rigour* made very sure that both feet became my best.

From time to time she would also tap my rib cage and say, "Pull up, Fay, you're sagging!" All my vertebrae would snap to rigid attention, and I discovered at an early age that the backbone in developing quality of deportment began by developing quality of backbone.

For the first ten years of my life family snapshots show me looking as though, like Socrates, I had marbles in my mouth (actually, they were gum balls). The butterfly bows that held my curls in two knobs on the top of my head looked as though they were deliberately tied too tight in an effort to stretch me up an extra notch or two (which they were).

In my teenage years, Fair-try Ferris taught me mathematics. He was a large man with a raucous laugh, who handed out assignments and weekly tests with inordinate glee. He would peer over his wire-rimmed glasses and bellow, "Now give it a *fair-try*, that's all I ask!"

He was fond of saying such unsettling things as, "If at first you don't succeed, try, try again!" Whereas I was prone to say, "If at first you don't succeed, why bother?"

I soon found out that the problem with mathematics is that if everything is not done exactly right, it is done completely wrong. This means a *fair-try* is not fair at all, especially for anyone who is earnestly trying.

Fair-try's hero was Robert Bruce.

"Think of him," he would say, "battle weary and sick with discouragement, lying on a bed of straw as he watched a spider try to swing a web across the beams of the cottage ceiling. . . ." Six times the spider failed—on the seventh try he made it.

"I, too, will try again," said Bruce. He did, and trounced the English at the bloody battle of Bannockburn, which the English did not think was fair at all.

I was never quite sure what all that had to do with πr^2, but in mathematics, on both my seventh and eighth tries, I flunked.

"Fall in love with whomever you like," my mother told me, "but for heaven's sake marry right. It is just as easy to marry someone sensible as not, and you certainly don't want your children to be utter twits!"

I fell in love with a lot of people I liked, most of whom my mother didn't, and not many were sensible. But I did marry right—or so my husband likes to tell me.

From a bloodline remotely related to Robert Bruce, he makes a fetish of the seventh try, and tries hard enough for both of us. The problem is, I have to live through the first, second, and third through sixth tries, which usually means holding the flashlight under the kitchen sink while he tries to fix the plumbing, or steadying the ladder as he tinkers with the wiring in the attic.

At times like that, it is not so much that I regret his trying to do things right, but rather his insistence on trying to do *everything,* right or wrong! When we get the plumber's bill and the electrician's bill, having spent the weekend either without water or in total darkness, my regret turns to sobbing remorse.

I have now posted on our refrigerator door, "if at first you don't succeed, call an expert."

To further prove that I married right, my husband bought a plaque of the Angus coat of arms, which he proudly hung in a prominent place in our entry hall.

It shows a strong arm holding a bow, framed by a thick black belt with a gold buckle. Emblazoned across the top is written in Gaelic, "Fortitude is Virtue," which is a Scottish interpretation of "Bite the Bullet."

Every time we have a family row, my husband rubs this motto, like a talisman. He tells me that it does not ensure that our children won't be twits, but it does ensure that at least his bloodline (if not mine) will give him (if not me) the endurance to cope with them if they are.

In trying to do everything right, this time by upholding the traditions of the family crest, I decided to build some fortitude into my son's virtue that would help give him a feeling for his heritage. On his tenth birthday I bought him an Angus tartan tie, a thick black belt with a gold buckle, and a bow and arrow. I told him to go outside and develop a strong arm.

Now it might have been perfectly all right for Henry Wadsworth Longfellow to shoot an arrow into the air and have it fall to earth he knew not where, but in our neighborhood people are very sticky about accountability, especially when it comes to arrows and other airborne projectiles.

"Under no circumstances are you to shoot it outside our yard, or up into the trees," I cautioned.

"But then we won't have enough range," my son grumbled, as his friend Bobby twanged the bow.

"Well . . ." I said thoughtfully, "I suppose you can stand in our driveway and aim towards the bushes, but only in our own wilderness area."

We live in a wilderness area. This is a nice way of saying that the frontage along our street has not been weeded, trimmed, or husbanded by the various husbands on our street for years and years, which gives it the look of the Garden of Eden after the curse.

I brought in the cat and dog and stayed safely under the protective covering of my own roof as the arrows went whizzing by.

Within a few minutes, a police car pulled into the driveway.

Bobby, being somewhat streetwise and knowing the ramifications of being caught with the evidence, handed my son all the arrows, put his hands in his pockets, looked down demurely, and whistled.

"Do you know that you are in possession of dangerous weapons?" asked the cop, counting the arrows my son was holding and pulling out his little yellow pad.

"Nope," said my son.

"Where did you get these?" asked the cop.

"From my Mom," said my son.

"I want to talk to your mother," said the cop.

"Sure—come on up," said my son.

"You tell her to come on down," snapped the cop.

What followed was ten minutes of verbal fortitude on the part of the cop, the like of which was enough to crumble the virtue of Robert Bruce himself. This gave me a disposition to thumb my nose at heraldry as I passed it hanging in our entry hall, and mutter unspeakable things under my breath, in neoclassical Gaelic.

That night at dinner I suggested that we augment the family coat of arms with a biblical motto—perhaps a scriptural version of "Fortitude is Virtue," where the only dangerous weapon would be the sword of the Spirit which is the word of God, and I would like to see any cop tangle with that!

At the time, our adult Sunday School class was studying an excellent exposé of Dungeons and Dragons—the book of Revelation. Coming complete with candlesticks, seals that needed breaking, Gog, Magog, Leviathan, and a beast with seven heads rising up out of the sea, its prophetic forebodings are enough to curdle the most fortitudinous of virtuous blood.

Fortunately, good triumphs over evil and the faithful get to rejoice at the marriage feast of the Lamb, which is a great relief.

Angelic choirs sing, "Blessings and glory, and wisdom and thanksgiving, and honor, and power, and might, be unto our God for ever and ever . . ." to which we all can shout an enthusiastic *amen!*

It is heraldry that heralds the most magnificent of all—Maranatha, the Lord cometh!

Having long considered wishy-washy to be one of the cardinal sins, I suggested that we take as our spiritual motto, "Hot or cold, but never lukewarm!" (Revelation 3:15–16).

"Just think," I said, "it is applicable to tea, lemonade, porridge, meat and potatoes, political opinions, spiritual convictions, and showers—all inclusive!"

"Harumph," said my husband, "we're liable to burn our tongues, get hot under the collar, be called a bunch of hotheads, and have someone slam us into the cooler."

Then, giving a pathetic little sigh, he added, "Isn't there something like, 'In peace and quietness is my strength'?"

"Nope," I said. "There is, 'Thou shalt keep him in perfect peace whose mind is stayed on thee' (Isaiah 26:3), and, 'In quietness and in confidence shall be your strength' (Isaiah 30:15), but not peace and quietness together."

"Well, then there should be!" he said impatiently.

"Harumph!" I said.

To push my point, several days later I served up a lukewarm meal. The water was lukewarm, the soup lukewarm, the mashed potatoes, fried chicken, vegetables, and even the jello cubes, sloshing disgustingly around the bowl, were lukewarm.

"Ptui!" spluttered my son, dribbling a mouthful of water all over the lace tablecloth, "I need an ice cube."

"Ah-ha," I gloated, now you know what God feels

like: 'I would that thou wert cold or hot—so then, because thou art lukewarm, and neither cold nor hot, I will spew thee out of my mouth.'"

Red hot is the commitment that sparks the derring-do of faith lived in the active tense.

It pulls us out of the lethargy of casual complacency, and although it occasionally takes us where angels fear to tread, nevertheless, it takes us.

Faith is a verb—it moves.

Sometimes agonizingly slowly!

"My spiritual life advances with all the alacrity of an arthritic snail," a friend wrote. "I crawl onwards, inch by inch, blinking in unaccustomed light."

I thought of C. S. Lewis. "Now that I am a Christian," he said, "I do have moods in which the whole thing looks very improbable, but when I was an atheist I had moods in which Christianity looked terribly probable."

"Keep on crawling along," I wrote my friend. He did, through the quagmire of doubt and depression, until at last he was astonished by the powerful response of God to his stuttered confession, "Lord, I believe—help thou my unbelief!"

Heaven moved.

It moved him out of a hospital bed and into a reconstructed life.

Faith may not do everything right, but it dares to do.

It dares to ask the controversial question, "Why?" It dares to admit the equally controversial answer, "I don't know!" It sallies forth with a determination to slice truth from error; it wrestles down the elusive and the enigmatic ... until it flames the soul in a red-hot passion of conviction that burns away immobile, insipid indifference.

In my poetry writing days, I attended monthly meetings with a group of local poets. We deliberately chose to ruffle one another's creative feathers and we went through many a molting process in order to plume the qualitative productivity of trying to write things right.

I was the youngest in the bunch, which was rather a nice feeling. It is a considerable shock to find that nowadays I am frequently among the oldest in the bunch! I am finding out with some relief, however, that this too can be rather a nice feeling, especially when the youngest in the bunch turns to me and says, "What do *you* think?"

We met in the basement of the library, around a table pushed to one side in a labyrinth of books and stacks of outdated magazines. We talked over our work as the ghosts of writers past listened from their dusty shelves. Every once in a while, caught up with a burst of nostalgia, we would pick up an old book and quote a few lines. We realized with pertinent self-application that even the best pass through prime-time popularity and are all too soon gathering dust with yesterday.

The poet's pen probes deep into caverns of the heart—it scrapes away at the very bedrock of human emotions and writes in life-blood. Poets are never wishy-washy, seldom cold, and nearly always red hot! Esther Webb was a red-hot poet.

She had spent most of her career as a Professor of English at Iowa Wesleyan College. She retired into the snug, almost obscure foothills of Sierra Madre, California, affectionately referred to by canyon folk as our oasis from insanity.

Esther may have nestled into our oasis, but in no way would she put up with snug obscurity. A spry seventy-five, with a mind sharp as a nettle, she continued to be a prolific writer. Her pen had a pitch that frequently rocked our boat.

Tall and gangly, she wore sweaters, even through much of the sweltering California heat. Her hands rustled papers with quick familiarity and her eye was trained to dart through pages searching for that special twist of words that puts excitement into the English language. When she found them, she would tilt back her head, rock on the hind legs of her chair, and smile with satisfaction, "Now, *that* is good!"

Esther never settled for a *fair-try*, she went for only the best!

The clarity of her thoughts had an impact on my life. She gave me many a "word in due season." They cling, like barnacles firmly attached to the hull of memory.

"Dare to discuss, dare to dispute. Dare to develop a different point of view. Dare to try—dare to fail. Dare to put a courage to your convictions that will raise you above the dead level of average."

"One man (woman) with courage makes a majority," she would say, quoting Andrew Jackson. "Make your life that majority of one, because strangely soon, life stops!"

I was just over the hump of thirty, grappling with toddlers and prey to the tyranny of chronic exhaustion. Far from thinking about the possibility of life stopping, the mundane routines that pilfered my time made me wonder if and when life would ever really start!

Esther was just what I needed—me, she probably could have done without.

One day she read aloud her "Portrait of a Woman." It changed my life.

It still haunts me, like Scrooge and his Ghost of Christmas Yet to Come, and apprehension wrings my heart. I use it, like a mirror, to see if year by passing year in any way it is beginning to reflect my face. Then it drives me on to renewed vigor.

> She has walked circumspectly all her days
> cautioned her feet against snow-hidden ice
> clutched guard-rails, dared no dangerous roads
> avoided climbing rocks toward mountain tops.
>
> She has walked circumspectly all her days
> thwarted the impulse to crash chairs to bits
> kept tongue from lashing men's stupidity
> restrained caresses, whispered no fervent words.
>
> Now, old, she sits in her one-windowed room
> piecing together blocks for patchwork quilts
> measuring time, her careful days stretched out
> a waste of sterile, cold serenity.

A one-windowed room may have a pleasant view, patchwork is pretty, and serenity stretched out sounds exactly right, but . . .

"Please, O God, not cold and sterile wasted days!" "Flame my soul red-hot with the courage of a conviction that will make my life a majority of one," I prayed. "Help me whisper fervent words, unleash my caresses. Let me stumble over the rocks on mountain paths, and slip and skid, but pick me up and push me on. Redeem my time, and let me risk the dare to do, in derring-do. Infect my sterile days with a rage to live, and a rage to give . . . my utmost . . . and then more."

I have never crashed a chair to bits.

"At $69.95 each, please don't," my husband said; but he added that it would be perfectly all right to bash my fist down on the dining room table once in a while, provided I did it very carefully so as not to rattle the cups and slop his tea.

My tongue has all too often lashed stupidity— most frequently my own! Now I search for fervent words.

"What is your most fervent word?" I asked my husband, as we watched the evening news.

"Chocolate, as in chocolate pudding," he said, as he finished off the last in his bowl and licked the spoon.

"Good heavens," I replied. "Mine is ecstasy, as in 'you are my ecstasy!'"

"Good heavens," he said, as he turned off the set.

That portrait of a woman moved me out from a

tap-polishing, drawer-lining, tissue-folding circumspection, to the accelerated pace of ring-around-the-bathtub and the comfortable clutter of ordered chaos that is often the fallout of faith lived in the active tense.

Red-hot conviction does not necessarily mean that we become foot-stomping, back-whomping, Bible-thumping believers (though God knows, I am!).

It does mean that we become the glove into which the hand of God will fit—passively available to do his active will.

It does mean obedience.

When I was in my early twenties, I applied for a job at a rather prestigious organization. The personnel questionnaire was long, and my experience was short.

Finally, I made it up through a series of interviews to one with the man who was vice-president, whose assistant I would become.

"Are you any good with figures?" he asked.

"No," I had to admit, somewhat shakily, and he looked disappointed.

"But," I added brightly, "I am rather good at doing *exactly* what I'm told!"

He smiled. I got the job! Obedience paid off.

Faith in the active tense is singing through the doldrums, or cheerfully tackling a humdrum task to bathe the commonplace with the radiance of a job well done.

It may even mean stifling a moan in the middle of the night, and a pillow wet with loneliness as soggy prayers palpate a heart numb with desperation. For some, faith lived in the active tense is simply fear that has the courage to keep moving forward.

Mother Angelica, the Roman Catholic nun who responded to what she calls the miracles of opportunity that God placed in her life and founded the Eternal Word Television Network, describes her faith as "... one foot on the ground and one foot in the air, and that queasy feeling in your stomach."

Called a woman of great faith, she says, "No. I'm not a woman of great faith; I'm a coward that keeps moving."

At age fifty-nine she is moving a monthly budget of $2.5 million through the RCA satellite Satcom, which budget she holds together by her dependence on divine guidance and providence.

"Do anything but just sit there and be a sponge," she says.

Hot or cold, but never lukewarm?

Make mine hot!

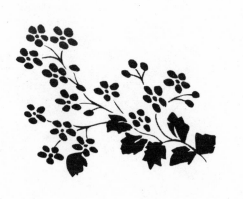

Adam & EveN, God's Complement to Man

EveN in Eden

In the beginning, God created man. He took a long hard look and said, "Boy, this guy sure could use some help!"

Enter Eve, God's complement to man. She was a new and improved model of creation, with no whiskers, more curves, and, best of all, indoor plumbing.

Posturing an early narcissus complex, man promptly appropriated the complement toward himself and named her "wo-man." This gives rise to a lot of speculation as to what might have happened to the course of history had he named her something else—"aspidistra," for example. As it was, she had no choice in the matter but to tag along as the prefix to his ego, not only as the *"wo"* in *wo*man, but also as the *"fe"* in *fe*male.

Her first impulse was to go home to mother, but then she realized that she had no mother to go home to.

"Adam," she said, "I have a bone to pick with you!"

"Madam," said Adam, rubbing his ribs, "you already have!"

That became the first of many bones of contention between them, and was the root of such ominous expressions as, "I feel it in my bones," "Make no bones about it," and "You're nothing but a bone-head."

As the bone of his bone and flesh of his flesh, woman was made from man, for man. God could have made a man from man, for man and thus developed a totally hu*man* race . . . Adam and *B*ruce, followed perhaps by *C*harles, *D*aniel, *E*gbert, *F*rederick, and so on and so forth through all the letters of the alphabet.

Of course, just how Adam and Bruce would have birthed their genealogy is a matter for serious scientific conjecture, but it would have eliminated such sticky wickets as "discrimination on account of sex." For that matter, it would have eliminated the word "sex" altogether, as well as such controversial phrases as *vive la difference,* which would have been a terrible bore.

Instead, God paraded all the animals, two by two, in front of Adam until it dawned on him that there was a boy lion and a girl lion, a boy giraffe and a girl giraffe, and he began to put two and two together and said, "I seem to be missing somebody."

"By Jove, you've got it!" shouted God. "I thought you'd never notice . . . it is not good that man should be alone."

Then God got busy and set about putting together a special somebody just for Adam.

She would out-mane the lion, out-plume the peacock, and out-fox the fox. She would be so well put together that from then till Kingdom come, men would be apt to nudge one another, whistle, and gasp, "I say—is she well put together!"

Realizing that one earthy person was quite enough (and at times one too many), God decided that woman should not be made from the dust of the ground, but from a somewhat higher form of life. As Adam was the highest living form (being formed after the image and likeness of God himself), he was put to sleep with what was the first recorded use of anesthetic. Without so much as getting his signature on a medical release, God removed one of Adam's ribs and from it whittled Eve. She came complete with the designer label, "Adam's Rib." This turned her into a very designing woman.

Because of his dusty origins, man was predisposed to be a dusty person. To balance this, woman was programmed with an aversion to dust (and dirt and grime) that has had her shaking a duster in man's direction ever since . . . as well as asking him such things as, "Did you remember to wipe your feet before coming into the house?" and, "Are those your black finger marks all over the clean towels?"

In order that she would be the perfect complement to man, woman was built to fit. Where he stuck out, she didn't. Where she stuck out, he didn't. He had massive doses of testosterone, and she had massive doses of estrogen. He had hair on his face and chest, and she had a peaches and cream complexion, and a chest plus a chest.

Man had the ability to calculate figures, and woman had the figure worth calculating.

When all her checks and balances were made, God brought her to Adam.

He could have placed her in the middle of a petunia patch and had Adam stumble over her while walking through the garden. Or he could have had her kiss Adam awake in a reverse role-play of Sleeping Beauty. But he didn't.

God wanted to make it perfectly clear that he had specifically designed woman for man. He must have had exquisite pleasure in anticipating the gleam in Adam's eye when first he saw Eve. That glorious moment when all of creation sang, "Who giveth this woman to be united with this man?" and God, as both Father of the bride and Father of the groom (which, under normal circumstances, would have been recorded as a conflict of interest), said, "I do!"

What artist would dare to capture the mystery of that first long, lingering look! No awkward shyness, no posturing, no intimidation, no self-doubt, no fear of rejection . . . but the radiance of the perfection of man and woman mirrored in each other.

That moment holds eternity enthralled.

Details dazzle the imagination. Did they start from the bottom and look up, or did they start from the top and look down? Did Adam reach out to first stroke her hair, or did he first touch her lips in wonder? Did Eve take his hand in hers and hold it pressed against her heart?

They instigated life's supreme adventure. One

poet called it "the Divinest gift of fate ... to discover at a glance, the heart's true friend, the soul's true mate!"

The honeymoon was never meant to be over.

Adam was kicking up the dust somewhere, probably in a preliminary trial run to inventing the wheel, and Eve was polishing the fruit on the various trees in the garden, making effective use of her duster even then.

The apples on the tree of knowledge of good and evil looked as though they could use some polishing. Sitting under the branches was a gorgeous creature. As he saw Eve approach, he rose and bowed.

"EveN," he hissed, "How beguiling to see you here! In the name of liberté, fraternité, and equalité ... come sit, and talk a while."

Adam had never told her, "Don't sit under the apple tree with anyone else but me." At best he was a terrible communicator whose vocabulary was heavily weighted with, "Yup," "Nope," and "Uh-huh," so she supposed it would be all right. (As it turned out, it was all wrong.)

"Have an apple?" offered the serpent.

"Thanks, but no thanks," declined Eve.

She was trying to remember her Sunday School verse for the week. In the divine chain of command, God had taught it to Adam, and Adam had taught it to her (but not well enough): "Of every tree of the garden thou mayest freely eat; but of the tree of the knowledge of good and evil, thou shalt not eat of it; for in the day that thou eatest thereof thou shalt surely die" (Genesis 2:16–18).

"What is 'die'?" she had asked Adam.

"How should I know?" Adam replied with his customary insight. "God said it, we believe it, and that settles it!"

He made a mental note that as an extra precaution, he really should put a fence of barbed wire around the tree, with a flashing neon light to warn, "Trespassers will be prosecuted."

"Next Saturday morning, for sure," he thought, setting a trend of procrastination that man has lived to regret ever since.

"Did you know that an apple a day keeps the doctor away?" hissed the serpent.

"It's not on my diet," said Eve.

"Only 80 calories . . ."

"But the Surgeon General says that eating apples may be dangerous to our health."

"Balderdash!" hissed the serpent. "It's all hearsay! Test the facts for yourself. Try it, you might like it. Besides, can't you make even one solitary decision on your own? Haven't you ever thought of being EveN?"

Eve's eyes lit up!

"If you eat this fruit," continued the serpent, "you won't die—why, you will know the difference between good and evil and that will make you equal with God himself. You will be the founding mother of the equal rights movement—think of what that will mean to the National Organization for *Wo-men.*"

"Hum-m-m," said Eve, picking a large red apple and crunching into it. "When you put it that way—it might be fun to know the difference between good and evil, and to make my mark in history, and I especially like the sound of EveN!"

"Eve ..." called Adam.

"EveN," she corrected him immediately, surprised at the domineering snap to her voice. Feeling a new authority, she handed him the apple with the terse comment, "Eat!"

Adam paused a moment and thought, "This woman has been deceived, but I am not being deceived. I am doing this with my eyes open, not beguiled, in full command of all my faculties, with all clarity, come what may, so help me God" (1 Timothy 2:14).

"Delicious," he said as he munched it all the way down to the core.

"Adam, I don't have a thing to wear," whined EveN.

"So I've noticed," snickered Adam, handing her a bunch of fig leaves as he hid behind a bush.

"Now look what you've gone and done!" boomed the voice of God.

The lion started snarling at the lamb, and thorns and thistles sprung up from the ground.

"She made me do it," groaned Adam, pointing his finger at EveN, while beads of sweat formed on his brow.

"He made me do it," sobbed EveN, pointing her

finger at the serpent, and she noticed that she had a headache.

"The buck stops here," hissed the serpent, "but hiss-ss-tory will set the record straight," and he pointed the tip of his tail back to Adam and slithered off.

At Odds with EveN

> Blessed art thou, O Lord our God,
> King of the Universe,
> who has not made me
> a heathen,
> a bondman,
> a *woman.*

The jaundiced eye of the patriarchial society that grew like a thorn out of Eden was epitomized in this old Jewish prayer. It set Adam on a collision course with EveN.

The shining glory that was her role as complement to man corroded. Through the centuries, all that she was meant to be became instead all that man would let her be.

The gospel of Jesus Christ became her liberating force.

Moving out from under the stigma she carried as Eve of the forbidden fruit of Eden, she was anointed as Mary of the blessed fruit of Advent. Divinity affirmed her in his grace, cast himself dependent on her care, stooped to grow himself within her—then suckled at her breast.

From that point on, women forever more could

sing with Mary her hymn of restoration and praise:

"My soul doth magnify the Lord, and my spirit hath rejoiced in God my Saviour. For he hath regarded the low estate of his handmaiden; for, behold from henceforth all generations shall call me blessed ..." (Luke 1:46–48).

What love but that of woman would demonstrate itself by the extravagance of costly perfume poured over the feet of the one she held beloved—then drying them with her hair!

After the crucifixion, the power of that same love stretched far beyond the constraints of logic. Before daybreak, notwithstanding the formidable security of armed guards on duty, and a heavy stone sealing the entrance to the tomb, Mary Magdalene (together with other women) took unguents with which to once again anoint the body of Jesus—this time in death.

This was the complement of a love that did not cower frightened, hidden in a room, but moved forward, determined to breach the barriers of separation from one beloved.

Heart-tearing astonishment and a flood of tears at seeing the empty tomb was but a prelude to the indescribable joy of the resurrection.

"Woman, why weepest thou?"

"Because they have taken away my Lord and I know not where they have laid him."

"Mary ... " the simple endearment of her name.

"Rabboni!" soaring recognition.

Returning the compliment of her love, Jesus spoke the name "woman" as his *first* word of resurrection—he showed himself *first* to her—and he gave her the commission to be the *first* evangel, the bearer of the good news of his victory over death.

The men could not believe it!

As the women ran in, hearts bursting with excitement and jubilation, they were met with a wall of skepticism: "... Their words seemed to them [the disciples] as idle tales and they believed them not" (Luke 24:11).

They had to believe it! They saw for themselves—the sepulcher was empty, the linen burial cloths folded. They shouted with the women, "Hallelujah, Jesus Christ is risen indeed!"

At the turn of the century, scaffolds were scattered throughout the Chinese countryside. They hung like gallows against the tranquil landscape of rolling hills and paddies brilliant green with sprouting rice. These were "baby towers," monuments of death where step by laddered step women could climb to throw down their unwanted baby girls.

The Chinese people have, as one of their culture's prime characteristics, a love of children. But for the poorest of the poor, when there was yet another mouth to feed and not enough food, the boy took preference over the girl.

So gutted by oppression and superstition was the image of women in the old Chinese culture that baby boys were frequently dressed as little girls, complete with earrings and ribbons in their hair. This was to deceive the evil spirits, who would not bother to attack a girl.

The feet of little girls were cruelly bound with tapes that pulled the ball at one end of the arch towards the heel at the other. This was tightened regularly, and the so-called beauty of the "tiny feet" of the women of China was laid on a foundation of pain and grotesque deformity.

The liberating love of Jesus Christ sent missionaries to China. They unbound the feet of the women, and rescued the abandoned babies.

All around the world, the Christian gospel has delivered women from tribal rituals and atrocities that had led many of them to suicide as the only acceptable alternative.

Jesus Christ replaced oppression and despair with the promise of an equality of salvation and an equal inheritance of the Kingdom of God, regardless of sex, age, ethnic origin, or avowed political party!

In Christ there is no East or West, and there is neither male nor female (Galatians 3:28) but we are all one in the spirit.

Fortunately, we are not all one in the body.

Celebrating our equality as men and women in Christ does not preclude celebrating our differences as men and women. Therein lies the rub in the perils of the Pauline Epistles.

Plowing through all the interpretations, misinterpretations, appropriations, inappropriations, designations, connotations, quotes, and misquotes of the Apostle Paul is enough to grow hair on the chest of the most feminine of women!

It is indeed a puzzlement.

If the patriarchal society was bad, the matriarchal society may be worse.

In the book *The Coming Matriarchy,* co-authored with Laura Ashcraft, Elizabeth Nickles writes, "Women are changing in ways that will collide with and forever alter the comfortable contours of our social and economic topography. They are assuming characteristics associated with leadership—becoming more aggressive, independent, authoritative, decisive and goal-oriented."

With many seminaries reporting that between 30 and 40 percent of students enrolled are now women, the comfortable contours of our theological topography may also be forever altered.

Walking across the high-tension wire of controversy, we take the balance pole that has at one end the chauvinistic parody of Paul shouting, "Put a woman in to preach? They're an emotional sort—they'll speak up for women's choices with their shrill and squeaky voices, if we ever put a woman in to preach!" (1 Corinthians 14:34–35).

At the other end, liturgical feminism pushes its demands for a sexual textual revolution throughout the scriptures. A "she for a he," and a "he for a she," that castrates out of the book of Psalms alone more than two hundred pronouns, neuters the Fatherhood of God to a suggested "Heavenly Parent," "Eternal One," or "Divine Providence," and androgynizes the *son*ship of Christ to a male/female inclusive as "child" of God. We teeter on the edge of Matthew, Mark, Luke, and Joan, and the possibility of a God and Goddess translation of the Bible that raises as its flag Galatians 3:28.

The one end spells sudden death to the ordination of women, and the other to the credibility of biblical feminism.

Somewhere in the middle is the right place to grip, but where?

Being a rather tolerant sort, anxious to understand alternative points of view, I read *Let Me Be a Woman,* by Elizabeth Eliot, and *I Am a Woman by God's Design,* by Beverly LaHaye, and I say "You're absolutely right!"

Then I read *Our Struggle to Serve,* by Virginia Hearn, and *The Apostle Paul and Women in the Church,* by Don Williams, and I say, "You're absolutely right!"

Then the party of the first part says to the party of the second part that I must be a dolt to agree with such diverse attitudes, and I say, "You're absolutely right!"

It all boils down to the fact that there is a little bit of good in the worst of what has been written, and a little bit of bad in the best of what has been written, and it makes me shudder to think of what next might be written.

I am somewhat abashed to say that my own personal struggle has not been so much to serve, but more frequently to find some loophole out through which I could wiggle my way not to serve!

Having a disposition that enjoys "elevenses," and four o'clock with crumpets and hot tea, as well as flower arranging, classical ballet, and lolling on my backside watching the clouds go by, whenever I am asked if I could serve, I am inclined to blanch and ask the person doing the asking if they really think I am the one that should; and then God reminds me that I told him that I would ... however, whenever, wherever and in whatever way he may choose, come what may. I remember that I started my day that morning, with the first open wink of an eye, as I do every morning—by emptying myself of myself and asking the Holy Spirit to fill me to overflowing, and to live his life through mine.

Suddenly, the applicable opportunity of my commitment whomps me. I say, "Oh, bother!" and leave my flowers, and my tea, and the glorious music of "Les Sylphides," and go to my knees with the resolution that I should if I could ... so I would.

As a result of a commitment to obedience that prays never to quench the flow of the Holy Spirit through my life, and asks forgiveness for being perverse in wanting to do only that which I want to do, rather than that which the Lord wants me to do, I have ended up serving where a lot of people, myself included, would prefer not to serve ... such as in the horrid research necessary to stand against the degeneracy of pornography.

It is one thing to serve in the glorious experience of sharing the speaker's platform at Christian women's retreats and conferences, where the joy of the Lord flows to strengthen the ties that bind us first to him, then to each other.

It is another to serve in the traumatizing experience of entering the cross-cultures that are the tap roots of moral erosion. Yet, where more necessary to shine the light of the redemptive love of Jesus Christ?

As I tearfully struggled to find an excuse by which I could avoid serving in that arena, I prayed, "Lord, here am I—please send someone else," and I very efficiently rattled off some half-dozen names of spiritual giants in the faith who would be highly qualified as having the intestinal fortitude with which to cope with human depravity.

The Lord replied, "But Fay—YOU are my someone else."

Without compromising my commitment, what could I say but a shaky, "Yes."

Taking Philippians 4:8, "Finally brethren, whatsoever things are true, whatsoever things are honest, whatsoever things are just—pure—lovely—of *GOOD REPORT*, think on these things," as the windshield wiper to cleanse my mind (moment by moment) of the filth being put into it; and strengthened by my pastor, who stood by my side and prayerfully pledged his full support, I went out to slay the giants of organized crime.

In my struggle not to serve, I found heartache that had no ease as I entered the world of the sexually abused child. Suddenly I saw Jesus weeping over Jerusalem, only Jerusalem was Los Angeles, San Francisco, Chicago, New York, Dallas, and the trickle down to the little towns of America where depravity tries to hide as it twists and misuses the lives of these his little ones.

I discovered that a day in the life of an ordinary housewife may include picketing a porno store; a radio or television interview; debating the explosive and anguished homosexual issue on many college platforms; being called a "fundamental fascist" and seeing your name written up with those of your colleagues in a hard-core magazine opposite the picture of a naked bride with flowers in her groin.

In my struggle not to serve, I found my equilibrium balanced by Wedgwood china, Waterford crystal, and East Indian curry served piping hot with exotic condiments on a rotating tray. I found friends who did not shunt me off as a social hazard, or try to change the conversation when someone asked what I had been doing lately, but who said, "Decorum be damned—tell it as it is!" and cared enough to join their breaking hearts with mine as our tears dripped over the cherries flambé.

I learned that although the doors of opportunity that the Lord opens for us are not always the doors of our preference, the faithfulness in our call to obedience, "come what may," taps the grace of God's strength as our all sufficiency.

I also learned that by being willing to stick my neck out, I ended up seeing a lot more of the world!

In confronting the serious moral and ethical questions of reproductive manipulation—the holocaust of abortion, wombs for rent, gender selection, among many others, I entered the fascinating science of genetics.

Instead of spending endless hours caught up in the coffee klatch, I spent endless hours in research libraries and listening to lectures by some of the nation's top scientists, assimilating data on all the awesome possibilities and ramifications of the recreation of life.

By breaking out of the comfortable cloister of merely watering my own spiritual rose garden, I learned that the expanded dimensions of the Christian witness are exciting, exhilarating, at times very entertaining, and exhausting!

In celebrating our differences as men and women, somewhere in time the domestic woman has been sold down the river as an addle-headed nitwit.

She is anything but!

Conscious of her alternatives and vulnerable to the contrast of accolades poured on women of achievement in education, finance, and the arts, she winces at this sociological squint.

The diversity of her role as a generalist, maneuvering the multitransitions of her own life, as well as those in her family, coupled with the opportunities of her community involvement, make hers one of the most demanding of all careers.

In a long overdue tribute, the *Wall Street Journal* published an ad from United Technologies Corporation of Hartford, Connecticut:

THE MOST CREATIVE JOB IN THE WORLD . . .

It involves taste, fashion, decorating, recreation, education, transportation, psychology, romance, cuisine, designing, literature, medicine, handicraft, art, horticulture, economics, government, community relations, pediatrics, entertainment, maintenance, purchasing, direct mail, law, accounting, religion, energy and management.

Anyone who can handle all those has to be somebody special. She is. She's a homemaker!

A positive from all the negatives in the demise of the dollar, and high interest rates that make negotiating a home mortgage comparable to the most complicated of corporate wheeling and dealing, is that owning a *house* has now become an apex of achievement. Concurrently, the traditional woman, pivoting as housewife in that house, is worth her weight in gold. When I scrub my kitchen walls and floor, I consider in awe, "Aye, now—there alone is $10,000 of spit and polish gleaming!" I chalk up my doctorate in domesticity which, in today's economy, is worth probably considerably more than a Ford Foundation Grant to keep bugs jumping under a microscope!

Reinforcing the worth of the woman in the home is a first step to removing her from the endangered species list, and a primary requirement in stabilizing the shaking foundations of the family, the backbone of the country and the church.

With all the hullabaloo over the ordination of women, there is a tendency to elevate the pulpit above the pew.

Pity.

I find the pew diverse, flexible, and far more liberating. No power play with the board of deacons; no reassignment on the Bishop's whim to the Archdiocese of Antarctica; no passing the plate for a pay raise; and, instead of Hebrew, Greek, and homiletics, the Sunday funnies and several long, slow cups of coffee before ambling down to church!

When I read of the anger of a woman who said that when she was served communion by twenty-five "males" and no "females," she reached a point of resentment where she felt she could not even take communion, I was crushed by sadness—to see, much less count, twenty-five "males" instead of Christ!

I am usually passed communion by the person sitting next to me in the pew. In some churches, the message is whispered from one to the other, "This do in remembrance of Me." Sometimes it is a little child who carefully tries to steady the tray with its tiny wobbling cups of wine. Sometimes it is my own dear daughter, or son, or husband, or favorite friend. Sometimes it is age, whose vein-lined shaking hand I want to kiss as I take the broken bread.

I think the spirit of the love of Christ would be enhanced if, during the communion service, we would deliberately choose to sit next to someone who had irritated us, or hurt us, or annoyed us, so that in the sharing of the cup we may be cleansed by enacting the words of the Carmelite priest St. John of the Cross, "Where there is no love, put love and you will find love...."

Not frequently, but at very special times, we share communion here at home—with new friends or old friends, or maybe just ourselves. Then each one present has the joy of saying a special word of remembrance of him as we serve one another.

As *kamikaze* pilots shouted, "Tora! Tora! Tora!" and struck at Pearl Harbor, the guns of war sailed down the Whangpoo River into the Chinese port of Shanghai. Together with 600 others, my mother and I were taken as POWs and shipped up the Grand Canal made famous by Marco Polo, to a camp at Yangchow. Perhaps the most significant communion services in my memory were those we shared there during our 2½ years of internment.

This was the most leveling experience of my life; the common denominator of starvation and suffering is the most equalizing factor in the human condition.

Woman has stood as a very necessary complement to man through the bloodbath of many wars. She loaded muskets and fought by his side with the Minutemen; as a nurse she died in foreign fields where her cross, too, marks a place, row on row. She drove ambulances in the Battle of Britain, and shared the equal right of torture and death in the gas chambers of Auschwitz.

Rosie the Riveter kept the assembly lines rolling and, best of all, the home fires burning.

Lest we forget, women also served who only stood to wait ... all too often their hands clutching little fingers as caskets were unloaded. The brightly folded flag her recompense, the waiting woman held it tightly to her heart and drew from its strength courage in the darkness of the lonely night—she carried on alone and grew the family through those war-filled years.

In the shabbiest of circumstances in that prison camp, man and woman rose to new heights of dignity in their complement one to the other. Roots of beauty were dug in the simplicity of caring and sharing exchanged in the common cause—survival. It was not unusual to see a woman break in half the ration of her slice of bread and share it with a man whose larger frame hung the more gaunt from hunger. He in turn would see that her pail was filled with water from the well, a woman's aching arms-distance away.

There, too, we shared communion. We saved our rationed bread to break and pass. We had no wine, but just as sweet was the pale tea, diluted, almost colorless. We were a shabby, raggy crew, suddenly gowned in glory by his grace, as we remembered ... the washing of the feet, the crown of thorns, the scourge, the cross and spear-pierced side.

Remembrance of the Easter dawn, the empty tomb, and the power of the resurrected life transfused us with new courage. We could look to the guards marching atop the walls that imprisoned us, and say with Paul, "Neither death nor life, neither messenger of Heaven nor monarch of earth, neither what happens today nor what may happen tomorrow, neither a power from high nor a power from below, nor anything else in God's whole world has any power to separate us from the love of God in Christ Jesus our Lord!" (Romans 8:38, Phillips translation).

I take communion as a lover's moment, secluded with my Lord.

At that time I pray no intercessory prayer—I shut out the world and the people around me so that I may better remember *only him*. It is an act of love and worship that I would seek to orchestrate only by the throbbing of my prostrate heart. . . .

Father, I adore you, lay my life before you, how I

love you! Jesus, I adore you. . . . Spirit, I adore you. . . .

Twenty-five men could not serve me communion, nor could twenty-five women, not even twenty-five angels. Only Christ can serve me communion!

It was thrilling to me, as a Christian woman, when Mother Teresa won the Nobel Peace Prize.

It is spiritually significant to note that it was not awarded to the Pope, or to Dr. Billy Graham, or to Dr. Anybody Else, but to a simple serving *woman,* who went where others did not want to go.

As a complement to all mankind, she holds both men and women, dying in her arms; she serves—the cup of cold water in his name, and lets the love of Jesus flow through the channel of her life.

She wears a *woman's veil,* as bride of Christ. She has no pulpit, nor parish, but she has spoken in pulpits and parishes around the world. Her prayer of equal rights?

> Dear Jesus—help me to spread thy fragrance everywhere I go. Flood my soul with thy Spirit and life. Penetrate and possess my whole being so utterly that all my life may only be a radiance of thine. Shine through me and be so in me that every soul I come in contact with may feel thy presence. Let them look up and see no longer me, but only Christ. . . . Let me preach thee without preaching. Not by words, but by my example. By the catching force, the sympathetic influence of what I do—the evident fullness of the love my heart bears to thee. . . ."

The cartoonist CONRAD paid her tribute in the *Los Angeles Times* with a simple line drawing of her weathered face, and a caption that is more eloquent than volumes of words: *"Why be a priest when you can be a saint!"*

Science, building a bridge over the troubled waters of biological destiny, is at last on the threshold of solving the feminine mystique and the gusto behind the macho man.

There is a difference between the male and female brain. Testosterone, which develops the male genitalia, also masculinizes brain tissue; estrogen, produced by the female ovaries, feminizes brain tissue.

Writing for *Discover* magazine in April 1981, Pamela Weintraub says, "Yes, male and female brains do differ." She goes on to affirm that "behavioral and intellectual differences between the sexes are partly rooted in the structure of the brain." That women are inherently superior in some areas of endeavor, and men in others, is a fact that she maintains "would in no way undermine legitimate demands for social equality," but would result in a better understanding between the sexes.

Dr. Eleanor Maccoby of Stanford stresses the enormous "overlap" of male/female characteristics, yet she states that boys have certain things going for them, and girls have certain things going for them— the differences complement and compensate for each other, and it is "fortunate that we're both together in the same world co-operating!"

It is in that cooperation that we find the essence of our complement, one to the other.

During my elementary school days, we used to tease each other with the ditty, "Adam and Eve and Pinch-Me went down to the river to swim. Adam and

Eve jumped in—who do you think was left?"

After several doses of "Pinch-Me's," both on the receiving and the giving end, I decided to change the wording to, "Adam and Eve and Hug-Me-Tight went down to the river to swim. . . ."

Early, I discovered that it was far more complimentary and comfortable to be hugged than to be pinched, and the popularity of the tease then increased not only among the student body, but among the teachers as well.

God gave us arms to wrap around each other.

In the intoxicating lure of the arts, the one that epitomizes our tandem role as man and woman is the showcase of the *grand pas de deux* in classical ballet.

During my studio years, I learned the necessity of strong, sensitive partnering. The slightest touch can hold a balance, missed timing can wreak disaster.

At a dress rehearsal of the "Aurora's Wedding" *pas de deux* from the ballet *Sleeping Beauty,* I ran across the stage, rose *en pointe* to take a *penche* (bending) arabesque against the hands of my kneeling partner, and . . . he was not there! He had paused, for the fraction of a moment, to adjust a shoe—he missed a beat, and I fell flat on my face. Of course in performance he would have let the shoe fall off rather than miss a beat, but the flaw became a touchstone of remembrance between us.

The exquisite line of the ballerina that flows from her fingertips through the lyrical curve of her leg, to reach for infinity in the stretch of arch and pointed toe, is held aloft in breathless wonder as woman places her confidence in the strength of man. He

holds her with the illusion that if he were to let go
she would fly out of his grasp. He has timed her every turn, or leap. He is there to balance her, to
steady her, and to catch her.

He is the enabler and enhancer of her grace. He
pulls from her impossibilities of interpretation and
technique. He revels in the fragile glory of her form,
yet knows the ramrod of her endurance and her
strength.

As they perform their individual solo divertisse-
ment, the ballerina feathers her steps across the
stage with ethereal lightness. She spins in pirouettes
and holds, seemingly forever, the line that reaches
up to heaven. She is Eve—enchanting and elusive.

The *danceur* fairly boils up from the wings with a
series of *grande jete* leaps that brings out bursts of
applause. His vigor, elevation, and power defy gravity. He crouches and pounces to beat his legs against
a quickening tempo set to match his muscle. He is
Adam, subduing the earth.

In the grande finale, they dance together to cele-
brate the perfect harmony of their love—one has a
glimpse of Paradise revisited.

As they bow in curtain calls, he presents her
proudly to the audience, then offers a bouquet, from
which she takes a rose, kisses it, and gives it back to
him.

She is EveN—God's complement to man.

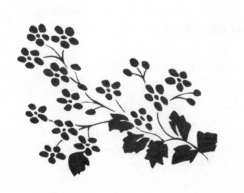

For Good, Better, & Best—
Marriage, That Is!

The weight of John's arm was crushing my ribs, and his rhythmic breathing was blowing hot air all over my face—it was like sleeping with a blast furnace.

"Romance befuddled," I thought. "There are times when it is downright uncomfortable!"

I had been awake for over an hour, jolted by a subliminal alert that stems from the core of restless thought.

Now when you are wide awake in the middle of the night, thinking, and the person next to you is sound asleep, that person frequently becomes the focus of your thinking. The fact that he is sound asleep, and you are wide awake when you would prefer to be sound asleep, colors your waking thoughts towards him—and many cases of slander have gone through the docket to prove the point.

As an out-and-out romanticist, I have always felt that life should be orchestrated with a sound track comparable to that of a Cecil B. deMille extravaganza; and that love should have as its prelude a rapture like that caught by the promoters of Tabu perfume. Their ad, enduring through the years and hidden in the fantasies of generations of women, shows a pause in the melody as a tuxedo-clad violinist clutches his startled pianist in unrestrained desire. His arm embraces her wasplike waist, and the gossamer of her skirt billows provocatively over the piano bench. We never do see her face, but his is the chiseled answer to a maiden's prayer.

Projecting myself into the ad, I imagine a continuum of desperate courtship to the marriage bed, the passionate climax of which would rise with a crescendo of strings playing, "Ah, Sweet Mystery of Life, at Last I've Found You!" The morning after would be kissed into awareness with breathless moans of lyrical ecstasy, followed by a breakfast of peaches and cream served on a rose-bedecked tray. Languid and alluring, all I would ever have to worry about is buying satin sheets, and the regular use of Oil of Olay for a silken skin he would yearn to touch.

As it was, the luminous dial on the digital clock in our bedroom spun over to 3:57 A.M. The night sounds of my wedded bliss were the steady drip of a faucet that had needed a new washer for several months and the guttural wheezes that came from my husband's grotesquely contorted face as he struggled to breathe through one nostril. The other was smothered against bunches of blue forget-me-nots printed on the pillow case.

I sat up and stared at him.

Heart of my heart, light of my eyes, and the total

resource of any romantic image I might try to conjure up in our marriage; after twenty-five years I was buffeted between the double tension of knowing him too well, and wondering whether I really knew him at all.

A far cry from the violin strings of Brahms, Beethoven, and Bach, his music was Benny Goodman through the Swinging Years. Instead of chiseled poetry, his rugged features were strictly High Noon at the O.K. Corral.

We did have gossamer—once. On our honeymoon, four layers of beribboned nylon, in the best of my trousseau white, tangled round about us. Far from languid and alluring, I giggled hysterically, and he cursed, "Where does the bloody stuff end!"

There were no morning-after peaches and cream, but there were runs hand-in-hand along the shore, and mystery walks through pine-scented forest paths. There was a touch of morning madness when, caught within the spell of pungent earth and blackberries, ripe along a mossy bank, we shed our clothes and frolicked in the seclusion of a mountain stream. The bed stones were slippery and the current bumped bruises on our bottoms, through waters cold as ice. We dressed slowly, in the warmth of a sunbeam, intoxicated by what we called our Eden adventure.

In British tradition, I had preceded my bridesmaids down the aisle, and our vows came out of the Episcopal Book of Common Prayer. "The Form of Solemnization of Matrimony," from good King

James' Royal Days, with thee's and thou's and here-
tofores . . .

John stirred.

"Are you awake? I asked.

"No," he sniffed.

"Wake up," I nudged. "I've been lying here thinking . . ."

"Careful," he interrupted. "It might become a
habit!"

"Seriously," I said. "I've been thinking over our
marriage vows. Give me a ten-point outline of your
'worse.'"

"My what?"

"Your 'worse.' You know—the love and the cher-
ish, the in sickness and in health, the for richer or for
poorer. I've been thinking about the for better or for
worse and it's the 'worse' that's got me worried! I
need to know exactly what I took you for, until death
us do part."

"Good heavens," he yawned, "couldn't it wait 'till
morning?"

Then he chuckled, winked, and pulled me down to
snuggle on his chest.

"Forget the 'worse,' honey. I'll never get tired of
holding your hand. You and I are going to make it
for good, better, and best!"

Three words, uttered in the middle of the night,
caught an ultimate in the directional for marriage as
it's meant to be.

The richer or poorer is circumstantial, the sickness
and health is providential, the better is alluring, but

plighting one's troth to a "worse" is nothing less than reinforcing bad behavior. It is giving witness before all the dearly beloved gathered together that we can be as rotten as we like to each other and we will still stick it through.

With all the criminal elements worsening up the world, who needs it at the altar? It is the worse, worser, and worst in each of us that is filling our divorce courts.

Someone once said that if marriage is the seventh sacrament, divorce might now be considered the eighth.

Half the people I know are not married and wish that they were; 80 percent of the other half are married and wish that they weren't. One constant that does not change is the agonizing hurt of shattered relationships.

As devastating as it is, loneliness without a partner may not be as abrasive as loneliness with a partner who does not understand, who does not communicate, and who long since stopped caring.

By temperament, the average man checks out as a cross between Winnie-the-Pooh and Hitler. He is either full of honey and cozies up with the warm fuzzies, or he is a violent explosion that sets the home fires blazing—frequently out of control.

The average woman fluctuates on a slightly broader base (especially when she sits down). She is Little Mary Sunshine, and the glad game of Pollyanna; the manipulative tactics of Mata Hari; or the broom-riding finesse of the Wicked Witch from the West.

Given these factors, we mull them together and come up with a love quotient that thrusts us into what Peter Marshall called the Halls of Highest Human Happiness.

We are an imperfect people, looking for the perfect partner with whom to live out our perfect romantic dream. The static of our diversities interrupt that dream and we find ourselves with the lights turned off, alone in the dark.

Hearts ice up in a resistance to intimacy, and freeze-frame in a holding pattern of "worse."

There are marriages that never should have been. They are mutations bred of human error, and God forgives us.

But most are born in crested love and spirits full of hope. Yet they, too, teeter through the years, held in fragile balance of all that is good, or "worse," in man and wife.

We *can* move up from sliding scales of "worse." There is a *good,* there is an even *better,* and always, there is the ultimate *best!*

We lost a towering oak during last winter's rains. It stood and canopied our home. It nested jays and caught a kite entangled in its heights. It brushed the stars at night and shimmered in the eerie light of many crescent moons. It weathered lightning, thunder, and the frequent tremors of California's quaking earth. Pruned by the fury of a Santa Ana wind, it snapped its branches and warmed our hearth with slow, long burning logs.

I loved that oak.

It fell. We counted rings and aged it at three hundred years or more. Having stood fast through centuries of stormy onslaught, it died, eroded at the root by tiny borer bugs and rot that hollowed out its strength.

Those little things that grate, and chafe, and dig, and pick, and nag.

Love seldom dies. It tarnishes and, lacking luster, dulls and sometimes simply fades away.

Little things help keep it shining bright. Small acts of kindness warm and joy our hearts; gentle words stroke fears and say, *"I* believe in *you!"* Bits of fun break the tension of a stress.

As I race around the country speaking at various conferences, getting ready to bed down for the night is often a lonely time. What a comfort it is to open up my suitcase and find a note from my husband pinned to my nightie, that says "Wish I were here!"

During one midwinter freeze, my son threw a pair of his red and white striped long-johns into my case, and said, "Here Mom, it's cold in Minneapolis, you'd better sleep in these." When I went to pull them on that night, my husband's note read, "Thank God, I'm not!"

Nothing is so small as to be insignificant. Jesus numbers each hair on our heads.

Ruskin said, "In mortals there is a care for trifles which proceeds from love and conscience, and is most holy; and a care for trifles which comes of idleness and frivolity, and is most base."

The wisdom lies in sifting through the difference.

During a radio interview with Dr. James Dobson, I teased him about his book *What Wives Wished Their Husbands Knew About Women.*

"My disposition," I said, "bends towards what wives thank God their husbands *don't know* about women, and pray they never find out!"

He threw back his head and howled.

Some things we confront head on, others we can walk around. By our response, or lack of it, we set the limit beyond which we will not go without direct, and sometimes painful, confrontation. We program attitudes towards ourselves and inherit the behavioral patterns we have reinforced.

I heard one woman hiss, *"Love* is just another four letter word."

She had been subjected to eight years of verbal battering and physical abuse. At last she went for help. Through therapy the bullying tactics stopped and mutual changepoints were established. Her marriage is not yet good, but she has moved it out of "worse."

The patterns of our live-and-let-live are cut in mutual tolerance; a perspective that sees first the beam in our own eye, before the splinter in another.

My own glaring flaws humble me to tolerant reciprocity, like the girl who listed endless qualities she would demand in any man she married, and then was asked, "And what have you to offer in return?"

There are facets of my nature I try to hide from everyone, my husband most of all. He does not need to know the many times I smoulder with resentment and would like to konk him over the head with the proverbial rolling pin. It is called restraint and biting my tongue, lest I blurt out barbs that prick and hurt and find myself impaled on petty trifles.

A Chinese philosopher urged, "Think three times before you speak." Confucius said, "Twice is enough."

Mary "pondered all these things within her heart" (Luke 2:19); she quietly thought things through.

I used to rant and rave a lot. I majored in the minors.

I have a tendency to think that there is only one way to do anything, and it is my way. I like quick efficiency and lose patience with those who just plod through a task, especially if it is a task concerning me. This gives me a disposition to steamroller through and take over.

After one appalling family confrontation that involved not only my husband, son, and daughter, but had me cracking the whip even at the cat and dog, my husband snarled, "You remind me of the woman on the can of Old Dutch cleanser—rushing around, waving a big stick, stirring up even the air around you!"

"Rubbish!" I reacted. "I'm getting things done! You remind me of a butt-inski, cranky Old Goat!"

We stopped in our tracks, took stock, and burst out laughing.

The hurtful truth is, he was right. I frequently am that Old Dutch cleanser woman, charging around

with my apron flying. I have had to pause, and ask
God to develop in me the "ornament of a meek and
quiet spirit, which is in the sight of God, great price"
(1 Peter 3:4). This modifies my bombastic nature
and gives the rest of the family a chance to function
on their own level without my bossy interference.

Now when we rub each other the wrong way, all
John and I have to say is, "*O.D.*" (Old Dutch) or
"*O.G.*" (Old Goat) and we both shift gears.

Or—instead of ranting and raving over petty trifles, when I get irritated with some of his peculiari-
ties (and he is the first to deny he has any), I just
work out my frustrations by scrubbing down the
grout in the shower stall . . . with his toothbrush!
(One of the things I thank God my husband does not
know, and I pray he never finds out!) The spin-off is
that I feel vindicated, we have a spotless shower, and
he sports a bright Old Dutch smile.

Ruth Graham was asked if she had ever thought of
divorcing Billy. She hesitated a moment, then said,
"Divorce? No. Murder—yes!" Hopefully, Billy does
not know.

Miss Piggy has it right. "Can a woman ever really
know what is in the heart of a man?" she asks. "No,
never—she can only guess. That is life. The good
news is, men can only guess what is in the heart of a
woman. And they are lousy guessers."

I opt to keep 'em guessing.

Paul says, "Esteem each other more highly than
yourselves" (Philippians 2:3). This is the keynote of
respect that stretches the dimensions of our love
with the heart attitude, "You are more important to

me, than me—your happiness is more important to me, than mine."

In developing a comfortable intimacy, we so frequently tend to put everything but each other first.

Pity.

It is dazzling to be first in someone's life, whether we are the ones doing the putting, or we are the ones being put. Preferably both.

Looking beyond all that we are not, and moving all that we are under the potential of all that we can become together in Christ: that is the encouraging, the enabling, and the ennobling of our commitment.

As television cameras around the world beamed the splendor and pageantry of the royal wedding into millions of homes, what an inspiration it was to hear the Archbishop of Canterbury give Prince Charles and Lady Diana the undergirding of spiritual commitment and direction:

> To know God more clearly.
> To follow him more nearly.
> To love him more dearly.

My husband and I chose to have engraved within our wedding rings a line from William Carey: "One for the other, and both for God."

After the assassination attempt on the life of the President, Nancy Reagan was interviewed by *Parade* magazine. "It's a particular kind of trauma that never leaves you once you've known it," she said. "It makes your times together so much more precious and your priorities are changed."

She went on to say that she did not think that

people worked at marriage as hard as they should. "It certainly isn't all 50-50. *Ever.* Sometimes it's 90-10. And you have to be willing to give the 90 percent. Or he to give the 90."

She struck a syncopated beat of mutual give and take.

She maintained that marriages often fail because the moment something goes wrong, one or the other partner gives up and says, "That's it! I'm leaving!" instead of communicating and trying to work things through.

She should know—she has "worked" her marriage through for thirty years.

In his book *Mortal Lessons,* Dr. Richard Selzer uses his pen to perform surgery on the human spirit as effectively as he uses his scalpel on the human body.

In order to remove a tumor from the cheek of a young woman, he had to cut a small facial nerve. It left her mouth twisted—"clownish," he said.

As he stood in the hospital room he watched the exchange between the young husband and wife.

"Who are they, I ask myself, he and this wry-mouth I have made, who gaze at and touch each other so generously, greedily?"

The young woman asks him if her mouth will always be twisted, and the surgeon has to tell her, "Yes, it will. It is because the nerve was cut."

"She nods and is silent," Selzer writes, "But the young man smiles. 'I like it,' he says, 'It is kind of cute.' All at once I *know* who he is. I understand, and

I lower my gaze. One is not bold in an encounter with a god. Unmindful, he bends to kiss her crooked mouth, and I so close I can see how he twists his own lips to accommodate to hers, to show her that their kiss still works. . . ."

Selzer lowers his gaze to "let the wonder in."

We bend, and twist ourselves to fit—that stirs in us divinity!

Some marriages need miracles. It is significant that Jesus performed his first miracle at a marriage. He has been performing miracles there ever since.

He worked a miracle for Margaret. Her marriage not only survived, but moved out of the safety zone of mediocrity and into the exciting potential that makes her every day a challenging new adventure of faith.

If anyone knew anything about women, it should have been Solomon. As kids we used to quip:

King David and King Solomon led very merry lives,
With many, many lady friends, and many, many wives.
When old age came upon them, with many, many qualms,
King Solomon wrote the Proverbs, and King David wrote the Psalms!

Yet Solomon tells us, "There be three things which are too wonderful for me, yea four which I know not: The way of an eagle in the air; the way of a serpent upon a rock; the way of a ship in the midst of the sea; and *the way of a man with a maid*" (Proverbs 30:18–19).

Centuries later, through countless volumes of ana-
lytical words, *the way of a man with a maid* is still
too wonderful for us.

The awesome power of human sexuality that
makes us one in the flesh so often is the force that
drives us asunder. Statistics show approximately 62
percent of the couples seeking therapy do so because
of sexual dissatisfaction. One therapist estimates
that 85 percent of married couples "have failed to
utilize their God-given sexual potential."

Most often the man feels that if their sex life were
better, the marriage would be happier; and the woman feels that if their marriage were happier, their sex
life would be better!

She feels that a comfortable intimacy should lead
the way to sex, and he feels that sex is what leads the
way to comfortable intimacy.

Margaret's marriage had fallen into frustrated
confusion. Her miracle took a balance of divine intervention, a teachable spirit, and her own willingness to let the miracle begin in her.

In each of us, there is a bit of Margaret.

We sat on the edge of a bubbling hot jacuzzi, and
took turns running our feet across the power jets.
Bunches of tawny curls were caught at the nape of
her neck and twisted through a tortoise shell comb.
A few wisps straggled down her forehead and teased
eyebrows tilted to accent a face arranged with pi-
quant curiosity. Her lithe figure paid tribute to the
disciplines of diet and exercise.

"She must have been stunning in her prime," I

thought, and bristled at the warp of time. It had set her jaw in a grim contrast to gentle eyes, now brimming with tears.

"There is no doubt," she said, *"I* drove him into the arms of another woman."

It was an unusual admission. I gave her a quizzical look.

"He was a silent lover. The only way he could communicate his affection for me was through his body. He never said a word—no endearments, no verbal flirtations, just a fierce sexual appetite. It was completely one-sided; I was never gratified. After a few limp tries at talking things through, I quit. The whole experience, which was never good, went down the skids to bad, then on to progressive stages of worse. I was frigid."

"Did you consider therapy?" I asked.

"Yes," she said, "but he wouldn't go. Even to suggest it was an affront to his pride. But I went. I didn't like what I was told . . . you know, the old story of relief through various techniques of self-gratification. But one thing I did learn, and that was, if my marriage needed help, and he was unwilling to seek it, *I* was the only one able to do anything about it— provided, of course, that I still cared enough to want to try.

"I did care. That was the brutal hurt."

She paused and carefully dried each toe. I noticed polish chipping off the nails, and brown age spots dappling her hands.

"I decided to compromise. There was a lot that

was good in our marriage. We had three lovely kids, my husband was a decent father and a good provider, it was *just* our sex life that stank. That is the galling part. My *just* was his *most!* With that kind of a guy, I don't care how good a woman is in the kitchen, how trim, slim, or sleek an image she maintains, if she can't keep him happy in bed, she stands the risk of losing him."

"Yeah?" I countered, "But what about him keeping her happy in bed? Don't you think it's a two-way street?"

"In my case, no." She wagged a finger to emphasize the point. "I don't think I'm unique. I'll bet most women are satisfied to coast along in the warm security of the 'good-Buddy, I'll thank God for what I've got' partnership. I could have gone on, probably indefinitely, but he couldn't."

I thought of a friend whose husband had gone through the Battle of Britain. His body had been hit by shrapnel, and he was impotent. Yet they seemed to have an intimacy and love in their marriage that stretched beyond the sexual dimension.

Another woman wrote to Dear Abby that, despite the bungled operation which resulted in the loss of her husband's sexual desire, their love for each other did not lessen. "When we cuddle up in each other's arms on a cold winter night," she wrote, "we achieve a more lasting closeness than those couples who make love for three minutes, then leave each other to go to sleep in separate beds."

The ying and the yang of our options!

Margaret caught her husband in his office in the arms of his secretary—a girl young enough to be his daughter. In the two seconds it took her to open the door, her world blew away.

That night, she confronted him—to be faithful or not? He chose not. The irony was, he held her tenderly for most of the night. In the morning he packed and left.

The 4 Ds of marriage are depression, despair, drink, and divorce.

Margaret hit the bottle—heavily.

Her husband had walked out on her for another woman, so she felt that she had failed as a wife. Her friends were getting sick and tired of listening to her cries of loneliness, so she felt that she was failing even them. There was no light at the end of her tunnel; she could not see through the darkness, so she gave up.

Fortunately, God didn't.

One night, just as she was about to pour another vodka, the phone rang. It was a neighbor who had been trying for months to get her to a weekly Bible study. She was a sweet girl, but Margaret had written her off.

"She didn't come across with an intellectual snap," she said. "I figured she was just another dogooder, mesmerized into the escape mechanism of religion. The fact that I was escaping through booze didn't enter my rationale."

Who calendars our hearts and marks the moment of our greatest need? At what particular point does

heaven reach down and let the glory in? Angels, unaware, who intersect our lives, may live next door.

Margaret's voice broke, "She cared enough to drop
everything and come right over. She perked some
fresh coffee and, taking my hands in hers, with tears
running down her face, she told me how much God
loved me."

"It seemed so trite—but, God knows, I needed
someone to tell me somebody loved me! I had nothing to lose. I no longer wanted my life, my husband
no longer wanted my life, if God wanted it, He could
have it."

That night Margaret stumbled through a prayer of
desperation and laid the tattered remnants of her
life in the hands of a Savior who said, simply,
"Come . . . to me." Then she passed out on the living
room sofa.

The next day she went to the Bible study. It became a weekly commitment.

"The word of God became my therapist," she said.

She spent hours pouring over the concordance in
her Bible. She looked up every reference she could
find to wives, husbands, and marriage. She could not
do anything to change her husband's attitude, he
was not even around. But she could search her own
heart, and she did.

Through the women in her small discussion group,
Margaret found support, encouragement, and intercessory prayer. They taught her to pray, and that
she needed not only to look up for divine intervention, but that she needed to look down and seek out

practical applications of the scriptures that could be used as change agents in her life.

"I cried out to God to do something . . . and he did, *in me!*" she said.

This was a dimension that she had not bargained for. It was a humiliating experience. She asked God to pinpoint her faults—the areas where she was responsible for creating many of her own problems, not only with her husband, but in the totality of her family relationships. Then she had to allow him to develop in her the attitudes that would lead to the eventual healing of her marriage.

Within a few months, Margaret's husband returned. Without the consistency of commitment, the magic of his moments of conquest faded and irritations led to a series of spats that dumped his whole affair. He returned to the creature comforts that he had spent half a lifetime building into a hearth and home.

There is a love unique to reconciliation that draws us deeper to the heart of God. Perhaps it is the tremor of self-doubt that builds our confidence only in his strength, and kneads us in the faith.

Margaret did not know how she would react to a second whack at the marriage bed.

"I put my trust in 1 Corinthians 7," she said. "Do not cheat each other of normal sexual intercourse, unless of course you both decide to abstain temporarily to make special opportunity for fasting and prayer. But afterwards you should resume relations as before, or you will expose yourselves to the obvi-

62 / How to Do Everything Right & Live to Regret It

ous temptations of the devil" (Phillips translation).

Margaret abandoned her body to the ownership of her husband. Not only did she determine never again to deny him sexual intercourse, but she went a step further and initiated it frequently. It was a surprise to him. Her surprise was that she began to enjoy it.

"Three children into marriage," she said, "in the middle of the menopause, I learned how much fun sex can be when you actively go after it!"

"What about your husband's fidelity?" I asked. "He is an attractive man, in the swim of opportunity, aren't you concerned that he might have other affairs?"

"Yes," she frowned, "to be perfectly honest, I'm scared stiff. But I am learning to discipline my mind, rejecting what Paul calls vain imaginations. Instead of acting on my own fears and feelings, I have learned to set the priority of first acting on what I know and believe, through the scriptures, to be God's will for my marriage."

Margaret's husband is self-centered, body-proud, and goal-oriented. What he wants, he wants *now* and he works hard to get it. This means that sometimes she is pushed aside. He is not a Christian, which puts even more flexibility and spiritual focus on her.

She is learning how to love him differently. Her love has moved from *taker* to *giver*.

"I care for him and value his happiness to the point where, not just theoretically, but factually, through deliberate choice, it has become far more important to me than my own."

Her love is a growing, living, active, moving force.

What began in desperation is now building in confidence and mutual trust. Her marriage has moved up and out of *worse,* it is pushing through to *good,* and is getting *better* all the time.

The Spanish have a proverb, *"El prescuezo da vuelta a la cabeza":* "It is the neck that turns the head." In Margaret's case, she turned her husband's 180 degrees.

Love thrives on love. Love withers for want of love. Paul defines it with only active verbs. Love tolerates, is kind, is not jealous, nor self-centered. It is modest, good mannered, thinks the best, celebrates truth, believes, hopes, endures, never fails (1 Corinthians 13).

Love actively participates. It is sequential and progressive. It does not sit on its haunches and passively twiddle it's thumbs.

It has an environmental impact that can change any landscape.

On the occasion of his twentieth wedding anniversary, Jon Roe of the *Wichita Eagle & Beacon* wrote a tribute to his wife:

> Perfect marriages can't stand the strain of imperfect people. That's why you don't see any of them around for long. Had we sought the perfect marriage, we should have married people more fitting, and settled into one of those marriages that run on their own momentum.
>
> The "Let's Watch the Bulls Run at Pamploma" marriage in which the participants are constantly partying so they won't ever have to be alone together. Or the

"Old Dog Tray" marriage, in which each asks but one thing of the other—Don't ever surprise me.

But we fell into neither of those safe marriages, nor into the fatal "Push-Pull" type in which one partner grows while the other doesn't. Instead, we both had an awful lot of growing to do . . . so much that we've been growing ever since, going through such changes that each of those 20 years has found us very different persons, and given us scores of opportunities to divorce. Luckily, each day of those 20 years, we've chosen each other all over again. That's 7,300 affirmative choices. Not a bad record.

But, had we started out perfect, we'd have had nothing to work on, nowhere to go and no one to be constantly fascinated by. You see, I may not know for certain just who you'll be from day to day . . . but I know I'll be fascinated. Because I was lucky enough 20 years back to respond to some quality in you that I guessed would grow stronger over the years. Maybe that quality was simply your capacity for growth. Whatever it was, I've found that new person in my life each day at least as interesting, intriguing, charming and compelling as the one she replaces. I'm constantly fascinated."

Now that's *good*, that's the growing edge of *better*, that's moving up towards the very *best!*

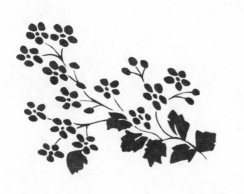

Motherhood, Apple Pie, & Other Irritations

Motherhood announces itself with a sinking feeling in the pit of the stomach and a craving for pickles. The craving for pickles eventually leaves, but the sinking feeling never quite goes away.

It is significant that our first biological response to being with child is the urge to throw up. It is also significant that shortly after delivery, some nine months later, the urge is to cry nonstop for several days, with the baby blues!

Obviously, our body knows something that we don't—namely, that on and off we will continue to have one or the other (or at times both) of these urges for much of our mothering lives.

This is confirmed all too soon as we pass through the terrible twos, the traumatic teens, and move along to the temperamental twenties . . . sometimes known as the "you've come a long way baby" blues.

Fathers operate on a delayed reaction. They experience the urge to throw up the moment they change their first diaper, and the urge to cry nonstop when they get the obstetrician's bill, the pediatrician's bill, and the hospital bill. This gives many of them a disposition to name their baby "Bill" (or "Billie") with the same flourish of the pen that signs their checks. Little do they know that the orthodontist's bill and the college tuition bill are just around the corner, and that while one little hand is clutching their finger, the other little hand is reaching for their wallet.

The nesting instinct that woos us into the nursery pulls in tension against the stark terror of the responsibility to grow, mold, and finance another human being. We develop a worry-worry, stew-stew syndrome that comes from wondering whether we are doing all that we should as parents, and whether they are doing all that they should, or shouldn't (which is worse) as children.

The stress intensifies when we mirror our performance in Proverbs 22:6, "Train up a child in the way he should go and when he is old, he will not depart from it."

Although Solomon dug this thorn into our parental flesh, there is comfort in the fact that he does not say how old is "old."

Furthermore, as he was to find out with his son Rehoboam (who pranced through the pages of 1 Kings, and 2 Chronicles, with antics that made his name synonymous with folly, apostasy, and evil), training up a child in the way that he should go is easier said than done. And seeking divine intervention that he will not depart from it is what keeps parents on their knees and running to and from the confessional with furrows on their brows.

Solomon had seven hundred wives and three hundred concubines. This gives us the awesome statistic that, averaging one a night, it would have taken him nearly three years to make the rounds of all his women. In between, he managed to write three thousand proverbs and 1,005 songs. With proverbs outnumbering songs three to one, this goes to show he did not have quite as much to sing about as he did to warn and instruct about as a result of all his connubial bliss.

Missing the mark of much of his God-given spiritual wisdom, and having tragically departed from the training up of his own childhood, Solomon died at the relatively young biblical age of sixty-two, probably from sheer exhaustion and an overdose of ginseng.

There is no record of just how many children he had. Counting them, much less training them up, would have in itself been a laudable feat.

We do know that Rehoboam had twenty-eight sons and sixty daughters, and the scriptures tell us that he "dealt wisely with them," dispersing them throughout many countries. This seems practical and certainly far easier than keeping all eighty-eight of them at home and underfoot.

Coping with only two or three sons and daughters, there are many times when today's parents would like to deal wisely with their children by dispersing them throughout many countries ... far away places, with strange-sounding names like Timbuktu and Lower Slobovia.

Instead of which they grit their teeth, pull out their Bibles, and memorize such verses as, "Spare the rod and spoil the child" (Proverbs 13:24), and, "This too shall pass" (Revelation 21:1).

The first test of training up a child comes on the toilet—the throne before which every mother kneels, cajoles, begs, whistles through her teeth, threatens, bribes, and wipes up.

Then, having spent two years of her baby's life in trying to get him to focus his attention on the performance of his private parts, she spends the next twenty-two years of his life trying to get him not to.

Unfortunately, one never knows in what likely or unlikely places training, or lack of it, may show up. When it does it inevitably reverts back to, "For goodness sake, didn't his *mother* teach him anything!"

This is one reason why so many mothers wear sunglasses and mumble a lot.

When our son was six years old we pushed him into the youth choir in the church. He wore a blue robe with a gold bow and stood in the front row. He had dark curly hair, large hazel eyes, and a toothless grin.

We called him "our pride and joy"—that is, until one memorable Sunday, during the singing of the second stanza of "All Things Bright and Beautiful." He developed an itch and decided to scratch. He scratched vigorously. The whole congregation averted their eyes and blushed, and the choir director turned pale.

Four hundred people buzzed the same thought, and it swarmed directly around my head: "Whose child is this?"

He was mine.

Suddenly, it did not seem to matter that he knew all ten of the commandments, or that he could recite John 3:16. Obviously, his training up had not included, "When you itch in public, don't scratch."

I have been wearing sunglasses and mumbling around the Sunday School ever since . . . so have his teachers.

As God's crisis intervention center, motherhood winces every time Dennis the Menace prays, "I got in a good fight with Tommy, Mr. Wilson chased me home again, and Margaret said she hates me. Thank you, Lord, for a perfect day!"

Teenage is a disease that only age will cure. From acne to algebra, it is the pit at the bottom of the rainbow, and the main cause of Excedrin headache numbers thirteen, fourteen, fifteen, and sixteen (years).

I was sitting in one of the off-studio waiting rooms discussing with the other members of the panel the various points each of us would make during an upcoming TV interview, when a young man walked in.

He was stunningly good looking, nicely dressed complete with the detail of every mother's fantasy—a shirt and tie. He was introduced to us as the teenage representative from one of the area high schools. His qualifications were a grade point average of 4.0, he was an Eagle Scout, and he had won several scholastic as well as Service Club awards. He was well-mannered and articulate.

He was the sort of son I had always imagined that *I* would have.

Instead, I had left mine that morning wearing a pair of his Dad's oversized trousers hitched up with suspenders, a white doctor's smock that he had picked up at a rummage sale, and with his naturally curly hair frizzed in an Afro to give him the Harpo Marx look.

It was "Spirit Day" at school and he was in top form. He would not talk, which could have been rather nice for a change, except that in reply to everything I said, he went "honk-honk" in my face with a large motor horn.

His room was clutter wall-to-wall and chances were that he had not quite finished his homework. That would mean yet another confrontation when his midterm grades came out. Expending only enough effort necessary to squeak him through the minimum required to stay on the football team, his major was pizza and girls, not necessarily in that order—a lot depended on the girl.

Had I taken him on the talk show that morning, he would have rolled his eyes and honk-honked his way through the interview. This would probably have won us a lot more points for our side than did our dialogue, and would have undoubtedly upped the ratings by at least 200 percent, but Little Lord Fauntleroy he was not!

The eleventh commandment is, "Thou shalt not covet thy neighbor's child."

As I mulled over the contrast between the desires of my mother's heart and the reality of the flesh of my flesh, I flipped through the pages of my Bible. Stuck opposite Proverbs 22 was a hand-drawn birthday card done when Ian was eight. It was a cartoon of Super-Mom, swinging from a trapeze—his scrawled greeting read, "MOM upside down is wow!"

Guilt misted my heart and I whispered, "Harpo Marx frizz, 2.0 grade point average, pizza and girls not withstanding . . . you're a little bit of all right, son!"

When it comes down to the nitty-gritty (and motherhood has more gritty in it than anything else, especially when she lives by the beach), MOM is the wow that melts the human heart.

Between the agony that is Howard Cosell and Monday Night Football is the ecstasy when the camera zooms in to a close up of a 250-pound tackle sipping Gatorade from a straw. He may belch and spit, and be the crunch of the defense, but when he looks into the TV lens, waves and says, "Hi Mom!" he is Little Boy Blue, and a time-out back to diaper pins, measles, detentions, and building the Alamo with toothpicks. Across the nation motherhood smiles, wipes a tear from her eyes, sits up a little straighter, and says, "Go for it, son!"

The fact of the matter is that the greatest national resource of a country is not the bullion in its banks, nor the trees in its forests, but the children in its homes.

Today's toddler wiping his nose on the living room drapes and sending his mother climbing the walls may be tomorrow's judge, pounding the gavel on the Supreme Court.

Whatever we may begin, or accomplish, our children will have the option to continue or destroy. The control of our political process, corporate power, education, church, and home, all pass into their hands. They will keep the peace or wage the war.

An investment in a child is an investment in tomorrow.

With human life as her product, and an estimated budget between $85,000 and $134,000 (from birth to age eighteen), motherhood comes into focus as an all-time high in professional calling.

Her options are many.

She may be part of the dwindling elite still able to stay within the confines of her traditional role, planting pansies and pushing the pram around suburbia. This gives her a full and flexible time span and is an ideal environment in which to grow and train up a child. Battling an inflation that makes the American dream of owning a home almost a two-income necessity, she may have to bite the economic bullet and tighten her family's belt, but this is a small trade-off against two little arms around her neck, hearing the first word, watching the first step, drying a tear-stained cheek, and building memories into every hour.

"After years in the work force I never thought I could endure just being at home with the baby," one mother told me, "but I love it! Who could guess that ten pink baby toes could be so alluring ... or nap time such a welcome relief! I don't want to miss a moment of these growing years and I'll sacrifice a lot rather than have to go back to work."

On the other hand, breaking the tie that has too long bound her to the kitchen sink, motherhood is emerging with a new image and proving that she can cope with the executive suite.

With a child on one hip and a career on the other, a generation of tiny tots are the new breed spoon-fed in the board rooms of major corporations or nursed in the family atmosphere of business facilities that have been specifically designed and staffed to accommodate the on-the-job-child. There is space for coffee break cuddles, nursing mothers, and lunchtime togetherness.

Her training him up may call for creative innovations that emphasize quality rather than quantity of time commitment, remote-control supervision, or manipulating her hours in the work force to coincide with his in school. But she is rising to the occasion and is effectively balancing her priorities.

Sometimes she has no choice, she has to—and with God's help, she can.

Kudos to fathers who respond positively to the custodial care of their children. One who was left with three ranging in age from twelve to three, said, "Problems? I prefer to think of them as the greatest opportunity of my life!" He rearranged his business hours, shuffled priorities, and did not merely cope— he enjoyed! So did his kids.

The *be*-attitudes of effective parenting are *be fair, be firm,* and *be fun.*

These are the guidelines used by Barbara Woodhouse, the international authority on the training of dogs. Not only will the dogs under her instruction go and fetch a stick or a ball, they will also *joyfully* go and fetch the choke collar with which she restrains and disciplines them.

If she can do it with Bowser, we can do it with Buster!

Be Fair

When my daughter was sixteen, after a family fracas, she stomped out of the room, tossed her head, and snapped, "The only reason I am still living at home is because of adolescence and poverty!"

I could not take credit for the adolescence, but thank heavens I had done something right in keeping her poor!

The golden rule around our house is, "He who has the gold makes the rule." Disbursing financial aid by way of weekly allowances, car keys, tanks full of gas, as well as the basic necessities of shelter, clothing, and food—our parental premise is, "As long as you are living under our roof and we are paying your bills, we will set the rules and you will need to keep them." Believing in the democratic process and fair play, we give our children the opportunity of sitting on the home-rule committee, and voting on final decisions. We keep the power of parental veto.

I grew up under the adage that children were to be seen and not heard, and I cannot remember the adults around me asking my opinion on anything apart from perhaps the color of a party dress. It was strictly, "Be quiet, sit down, and do as I say because

I say so with no questions asked." Or it was *the glare*—the evil eye that withered me on the spot!

I can still taste the bile of resentment and remember the tears of anger as I seethed, pounded my pillow at night and groaned, "It's not fair!"

As a result, I vowed that if ever I had children I would afford them the dignity of asking their opinion, and seriously considering their point of view in an open two-way communication.

One of the greatest gifts to a child is an ear, eager to listen. When stock broker E. F. Hutton speaks, the world may stop and listen, but when my kids speak, I stop and listen. Because I have very chatty kids, I have become a very good listener. I even listen when they don't know I'm listening . . . and that makes *them* seethe with anger, pound their pillows at night, and groan, "It's not fair!"

Conversely, when I talk I expect them to listen—not only with an eager ear, but with a focused eye. That way I can be sure that what I say is not going in one ear and out the other, but is taking at least a moment, however fleeting, to buzz around their heads.

Eye contact is one of the requirements in effective communication. Occasionally we stare each other down in silence, eyes blazing with anger, but . . . the first one who cracks up and smiles, wins!

For twelve years of their lives I was able to look down at them. Now in varying degrees, commensurate with their spurts of growth, they are able to look down at me—but whether it is up or down, even if we don't quite *see* eye to eye, at least we make the contact.

"Just because I say so" is not fair.

When a child is old enough to ask, he is old enough to know—on *any* subject. Perhaps not in full detail, but with sufficient explanation to make sense. If he does not get his answers from his parents, he will get them from someone else, and they may be the wrong answers.

My mothering services offer the short-form explanation, the come-and-sit-on-the-couch detailed explanation, or the deferred explanation ("We don't have time right now, but I will explain later.") Through the years I have become so expert in explanations that now in their behavior negotiations my children are apt to say, "Aw Mom, pleeze, I'm in a hurry—no explanations. Gimme a straight yes or no answer, or, 'just because you say so!'"

This is a foul aimed directly at my soap box.

When they are old enough to ask and they haven't, I do.

At sixteen my daughter started dating and I asked, "Have you set your sexual limits yet?"

"My what?" she squawked.

"How can you possibly go out," I said, "without knowing just what you will or will not let him do? He may touch you here, he may touch you there, he may try to touch you everywhere!"

She thought about it . . . for nearly two weeks. Then we talked about it for another two weeks, and on and off for another two years.

Considering her alternatives on her own, then talking them over in open (sometimes graphic) discussion, she eventually arrived at vital conclusions compatible with her Christian commitment. She now moves with confidence in the decisions that make her very much her own person, and not the pawn of her peers.

We tend to wear our children as badges of accomplishment—and that is not fair.

We glow at the thought of Stanford or Yale, and forget that Jesus went to Trade Tech—he was a carpenter.

We rate our children a spiritual ten if they stay in our faith, and marry in our faith, and twice times ten if they end up in the ministry or on the mission field. I spoke at a church once where, listed across the top of the Sunday bulletin, was the statement: "Pastor—every member of this church!" As ambassadors of Christ, every step that we take and every hand that we shake becomes our mission field.

If we are fundamental and our children turn ecumenical, or if we are ecumenical and they turn fundamental; or if they are charismatic, and we are not, and vice versa, we try to remember to say "Praise the Lord" in their church services, and hope they will remember not to say "Praise the Lord" in our church services, all of which is very hard on our spiritual arteries and keeps us balanced precariously on the edge of our Blessed Assurance.

If they smoke pot or "live in sin," their life scripts embarrass us; and if our church structure is built around 1 Timothy 3, we worry because we may get thrown off the board of deacons for not having our "children in subjection with all gravity." Obviously, Timothy forgot that Adam had Cain, David (who wrote the Psalms) had Absolom, and Jacob had ten raunchy sons who tried to kill their brother by throwing him down a well.

Far from doing everything right and living to regret it, the track record of many of the Patriarchs knocks them off their parental pedestal, and is a far cry from the admonition to be "sober, vigilant, the husband of one wife, and blameless."

Sorry Abraham, you flunked!

If, in spite of all our training up, our children end up marrying nonbelievers, we have a spiritual hot-flash and mutter things like "unequally yoked."

Some years ago, my life was touched during a lecture by Marianne Alireza, the first American woman to marry an Arabian prince and to be admitted to a harem.

She was not a Moslem and the Prince's family could have been devastated by the choice of their son to take an American bride—not of their race and not of their creed. As Marianne arrived at her new home and stepped out of the limousine in front of the palace, instead of being cold and haughty, her mother-in-law came flying down the steps, flung her arms around her, and said, "*Because my son loves you, I will love you too!*"

That is what God the Father says to me.

That is what I pray I will be able to say to whoever my children chose to marry, and I intend to mean it and live it with all my heart.

We love, but on whose terms?

We hope it will be with the unconditional love that wrote in the sand, "Let he that is without sin among you cast the first stone."

Be Firm

Maureen was fifteen. She was what my husband called a "spirited child." That was a nice way of saying she was stubborn, self-willed and a holy terror who wreaked havoc in her family circle. She was very pretty and had a charming coyness when she chose, which I suspect is why my husband was so kindly disposed towards her. Had she been ugly, he probably would have called her a spoiled brat.

Having been something of a spoiled brat myself, I liked Maureen. She had taught my daughter how to "sex" a guinea pig (tell the difference between male and female—no easy task!), and she had given us her three hens, Tasha, Rhoda, and Hilda, when her interest advanced from collecting eggs as a daily hobby to collecting boys as a weekly hobby. Whether she could distinguish the good eggs from the rotten eggs in the boys as easily as she could in the hens remained to be seen. Reports had it that she couldn't, and that was what was making her family very queasy.

After years of loneliness, her mother was getting married again. We were thrilled. But who would keep Maureen during the honeymoon? She had a reputation of climbing out of her bedroom window in order to keep a forbidden nocturnal rendezvous—she certainly could not be trusted to stay by herself. Her aunts and uncles were all somewhat intimidated by her, and were very nervously disposed towards her.

We volunteered, and invited her to move in with us for the ten-day period.

"Give us her schedule and a list of her dos and don'ts." we asked. "Set the ground rules with her, and let *her* set the penalty for breaking them ... then have her sign the list!"

Maureen arrived like a lamb and we expected that within twenty-four hours she would be a roaring lion.

We posted her list on the refrigerator door, and the children, several years younger than she was, had eyes as round as saucers as they helped drag in her stereo and speakers. She won them over immediately by letting them take turns in listening through the earphones. When I asked for a turn, she took great delight at my grimace and scream of pain as I felt my brains being blasted out of the top of my head. Without the earphones, we could not have made it through the week; with earphones, I felt we had a chance.

Monday, Wednesday, Friday, and Saturday nights were her nights out—she had a curfew of midnight. Monday night we watched her primp and blow-dry her hair, then shook the hand of the gawky boy who came to pick her up.

"I'm going to sleep," I told her, "but I will set the alarm to wake me at 11:45 just so I can be sure you're home on time."

"You don't have to do that," she said sweetly.

"Oh yes I do," I said sweetly.

"What do you care?" she challenged.

"I do care," I said. "Enough to check that you made it home safely and on time. Besides, maybe we can even have a late-night cup of tea together!"

Both Monday and Wednesday she was home in good time. Friday night the alarm went off at 11:45—I put the kettle on and waited. At 11:55, still no Maureen. I peered through the drapes, clock in hand, and prayed with every ticking second, "Hurry her home, Lord." More than anything, I didn't want to have to punish her. Grounding her would probably set her off in such bad temper that it would be harder on me than on her!

At 11:59, Maureen's clock started to bong a countdown in the last minute to midnight. I was pacing the floor—suddenly, headlights screeched into the driveway, a slight girl with her long hair flying like a thoroughbred straining to the finish line dashed up the front steps, turned the key in the lock and fell into my waiting arms. We hugged and I giggled, "Where is your glass slipper, Cinderella?"

I told her how tempted I was to turn back the clock to get her off the hook.

The tears came into her eyes. "Would you do that just for me?" she asked.

"Yes," I said, "I would do practically anything just not to have to punish you. I'm for you, not against you, but we must keep the rules."

We talked a lot that week. I learned about the rotten egg boys and the good egg boys. We had pizza for breakfast, or leftover curry stuffed into pita bread pockets. Every morning she would rush in and say, "What's for breakfast today?"

We out-outraged each other, and tried to out-love each other.

We broke a few traditional molds and ran our imaginations along the hours of that week to burst joy into every bright new day.

John was right, she was a "spirited child," bored with the commonplace, fired by the adventure of the new.

Some rules are fixed, immovable, where parents stand back-to-back so that the child cannot squeeze in between them like the stuffing in a sandwich, and use one as lever against the other. These rules are kept and the penalty firmly exercised, come hell or high water, despite howls and yowls, or slamming doors, or biting words.

Some rules are made for stretching.

We have programmed into our family disciplines a "way of escape."

Paul tells us, "There hath no temptation taken you but such as is common to man; but God is faithful, who will not suffer you to be tempted above that ye are able; but will with the temptation also make a way to escape, that ye may be able to bear it" (1 Corinthians 10:13).

Reacting rather than responding, may God forgive me for the many times I have punished my children as a result of my own short temper and frustration, rather than in proportion to their transgression.

The cardinal sin of parenting is expecting our children to be adults. Some penalties, seemingly simple, are just too much for them to bear.

John and I decided that when our children needed a firm discipline, we would offer them a choice of alternatives, or an opportunity to "earn" their way out, as a way of escape.

We have a "redemption" bottle with chores written on slips of paper folded up inside—these may be pulled and done to modify a punishment.

When the children were little, so were the chores—as they grew, so did the tasks. Sometimes I would drop in an assignment such as, "Write an essay on why obscenity is socially unacceptable," or "Table manners are necessary—agree, or disagree?" Got them thinking! My son would generally stick with the punishment after pulling one of those, but my daughter would usually opt for the essay. Once she wrote a marvelous piece on "The Value of Housework, as it relates to God's order in the universe." Made even me want to pick up the broom and get busy!

Occasionally I would put in a slip that read, "Surprise! You're off the hook for free. One kiss will clear the slate—and see that it doesn't happen again." Like the dad who made a way of escape by rolling up his newspaper, taking junior to his room, then whispering, "Now you yell, while I wallop the chair."

All too often *firm* becomes *harsh*—that bitter root with its bitter fruit.

We push away in anger instead of pull towards in love.

Betsy was on heroin. She was prostituting herself in order to get the money for her fix, and she was caught in the worst of all possible worlds.

"If only I could go home," she wept.

She could not. Her family had thrown her out and slammed the door shut.

"Oh God," I prayed, "no matter what they do, please help me to always keep an open heart and an open home to our kids." The alternative is pushing them in to the street.

As the young prostitutes, some of them just eleven or twelve years old, go through Covenant House in the middle of New York City, Father Bruce Ritter calls their parents.

He twists up in grief as, all too frequently, he hears, "We don't want her home—you can keep her there!" He tries to modify the hurt as he translates, "Your parents say it's OK for you to stay here with me for a while." The child knows . . . she is not fooled.

My heart broke as I watched a TV special that showed a young man phoning home from the streets of Hollywood.

"Mom, I want to come home," he said.

"No," she said stoically, "you can't."

"Lady," I screamed at the television, "don't send

him back on the street! Do you know what it is like for a boy to turn ten tricks a night?" I wanted to shout, "Come here, son!"

Father Ritter says that for the kids on the street, the saddest day in the year is not Christmas, Thanksgiving, or Easter . . . it is Mother's Day.

Be Fun

Each New Year the members of our immediate family exchange resolutions—that means I give three and I get three. Correction, I only get two. . . . My husband usually kisses me and says, "I wouldn't dare improve on perfection!" And that makes me tear up the one I had prepared for him, which is very aggravating, as I have usually spent the entire year plotting just what I would give him.

My son is liable to get, "Improve your grades this year without being nagged." And he is liable to give, "Don't nag me to improve my grades this year."

My daughter gives hers out in a sealed envelope with little green unicorns stamped all over it. Mine generally reads, "Dear Mom, I love you, but . . ." there follows not one, but some fifteen possible resolutions that are her way of saying, "These are the things you do that bug me half to death."

Imagine my delight the year her note read:

Dear Mother:

In the past I have been frustrated with you. Now I want to commend you.

You have been much more comfortable when I practice my driving, and I have noticed that. You are not critical and are very accepting of my friends. You have been kind to them, and I am beginning to believe those nice things they say about you behind your back.

I realize that mothering is very difficult, and I just want to commend you on the excellent progress you have made during this past year.

I love you very much.

Anne

And that made me tear up the one I had for her!

Humor is the tilt of the soul that keeps us looking up even though we may be feeling down.

Using family fun as a safety valve through which to blow off steam, we work out the kinks that tend to stiffen up the joints linking us together. We have learned to laugh at ourselves and with each other, and to develop family jokes and traditions that will probably carry on through many generations.

We went through a siege of chicken pox with two balls of green yarn. I suggested to the children that they web their rooms and when they were through, they could entice me in, like the spider to the fly, and see whether I could meander through the maze. From the bedpost, through the loops in the wagon-wheel lamp, on to the latch on the window, back to the doorknob . . . I do not think there was a drawer or cupboard pull that escaped their innovative spin. We climbed our way in and out for days and ended up shooting paper airplanes into the webbing. Chicken pox was fun!

Summertime is for eating strawberries dripping with cream, and wind-whipped walks along the shore.

I slam my typewriter shut, put my brain on hold, and tie on an apron. I become Little Red Hen, packing picnic baskets and washing thousands of towels.

"Who will dust the living room?" I ask.

"Not I," says the son, "I have a part-time job."

"Not I," says the daughter, "I have a date."

"I will, I will," says the Little Red Hen, and she does.

"Who will fold the laundry?" asks the Little Red Hen.

"Not I," says the son, "I am completely bushed."

"Not I," says the daughter, "my nails are still wet."

"I will, I will," says the Little Red Hen, and she does.

When Little Red Hen gets to the Pearly Gates, Saint Peter will take her by her worn-out feathery wing and say, "Well done, my good and faithful Little Red Momma Hen, come and sit in the eternally clean room I have prepared for you where there is no more dusting, or folding, and you may eat strawberries and cream for the next two thousand years!"

"Nonsense!" says a friend of mine. "Saint Peter will take you by the wing and say, 'Stupid Little Red Momma Hen, you did not train up your children in the way that they should go, to help you with the chores. Go and dust the halos and fold the angel wings for the next two thousand years!'"

Traditions are the pearls that space the beads of memory and ornament our lives.

Not having much luck with apple pie (apples irritatingly undercooked, piecrust irritatingly overcooked!) the sweet-smelling savor that comes out of our kitchen is Christmas cake.

As legend has it, it all began in the little town of Tisdale, Saskatchewan, when great-grandfather Angus came over from Scotland and great-grandmother Collins came over from Ireland. They met and they married and they began to propagate the earth, as many of their kith and kin across the Canadian prairies will testify. But whether it was because of his Scottish thrift and they did not go out and spend much, or because of her Irish temper and they did not sit down and talk much, or whether it was just because it was forty degrees below zero in Tisdale, Saskatchewan and there was not much else to do but shiver, they decided to bake a Christmas cake.

Some 3,640 walnuts, 10,112 raisins, and several other thousands of ingredients of fruit and nuts later, to say nothing of the spices and cups of brandy (both in the cake and in great-grandfather, which is probably why he suggested it in the first place) later, the famous Angus fruitcake recipe was perfected.

It became part of the tradition of their clan to pass along the recipe for the cake to every new bride, together with one for haggis, cock-a-leekie, and Irish soda bread. I received mine, neatly packaged in a tartan recipe box, with the motto, "What food these morsels be!"

In the first year of our marriage, the genes from his great-grandfather started jumping in my husband, and with one eye on the brandy bottle and the other on the recipe box, he decided that we should establish our own tradition by making the famous cake. Had he chosen the haggis (cooked in a sheep's paunch), he would not have enjoyed a second year of marriage.

Not having a bowl big enough in which to mix the fifteen pounds of assorted fruit and nuts, we decided to mix it in the kitchen sink. Unfortunately, the sink was not stopped up well enough and most of the brandy was lost down the drain, which made ours the driest fruitcake this side of Carrie Nation—a terrible hardship on any Scot, but obviously the nemesis of God.

After our babies were born we immediately decided to include them in our Christmas cake tradition by mixing it in their plastic bath tub. This worked wonders for retaining all the moisture, but lent a distinct flavor of Johnson's baby soap to the cake. It also lent a distinct aroma of brandy to the babies' bathwater, which is probably one of the reasons they smiled so much during early infancy.

As the children grew, it was their part of the continuing tradition to collect all ten eggs needed for the cake from Tasha, Rhoda, and Hilda, so that we could say that they were fresh-laid from Angus hens.

We said "fresh" based, of course, on the day that they were found, not necessarily on the day that they were laid. As the hens changed their nest from day to day, it sometimes took the children several weeks to find the fresh-laid eggs—and by that time they were piled so high it was impossible to miss them.

Running free and nourished with the best slugs, snails, worms, earwigs, and sow bugs that our garden could produce, our hens lay organic eggs, which we then process into our organic cake. However, we would prefer the organisms found in the cake not be examined under a microscope as the Department of Health might abort our family Christmas tradition.

Sometimes we encourage the children to put lucky dimes into the cake. This means you are especially lucky if they don't crack a bicuspid crown, or gum up the works in the garbage disposal. As it is part of the tradition to make a wish with the first bite of cake every Christmas, we ask our guests to make the wish before they bite, as after they bite they may wish they had never bitten, thus wasting a perfectly good wish.

When we raise our children on a lap full of laughter, we program into them the merry heart that Solomon says is a "continual feast" (Proverbs 15:15).

It will nourish them all their lives.

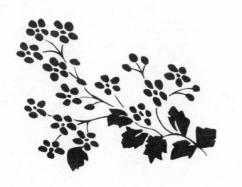

How to Get Up on Your Down Days

I have enough trouble trying to get up on my *up* days, much less on my *down* days! Most days I'd rather not get up at all. As the first glimmer of light breaks through the fuzz of morning, I search frantically for my pulse, just to be sure I'm still alive. I roll out of bed, stagger to the bathroom mirror, take one look at the puffy eyes, tousled hair, bleak pallor of my natural self, and gasp, "Good grief, do I have to depend on *you* to get me through another day?"

The fact of the matter is, yes I do, and the motivational question is *how*?

Hubert Humphrey knew how.

His father taught him step one of affirmative action: *get up!* "Stay out of bed as long as you can. Most people die there. You are only alive when you are awake."

Humphrey went on to develop a zest for life that never left him. It won him the reputation of being an evangelist of benevolence, and a chronic enthusiast. When he died, his colleagues eulogized: "He taught us how to win, how to lose, how to live, and now he has taught us how to die."

Humphrey won, lost, lived, and died enthusiastically! It was not only chronic, it was contagious—it reached out to infect those with whom he came in contact.

Enthusiasm was the buoyancy that tossed him up and floated him over the storms in his life. It was the glue that held together the shattered pieces of his varied experiences, and enabled him to carry on with fortitude and vigor.

Now the tah-rah-rah-boom-dee-ay of "everything's going my way," is an anthem easy to toot. It is the win syndrome of successful living. But when the chips are down, in this case even to the point of death itself, the ability to maintain an unmitigated enthusiasm reflects an essence of being that stretches far beyond the norm of human capacity.

"I have done my best. I have lost. Mr. Nixon has won. The democratic process has worked its will, so now let's get on with the urgent task of uniting our country."

Humphrey wrote that, "In a lifetime of thousands of speeches and millions of words, those were the hardest ones I have ever had to speak."

Yet his sense of national priority lifted him *up* and over the disappointment of personal defeat. His "let's get on with it . . ." stirred a motivational enthusiasm that fired him up for what he called the "art of the possible."

Poignantly, on the final Christmas day that tolled his coming death, his thoughts went to the man who beat him out of the White House.

Nixon sat exiled in the post-Watergate loneliness

of San Clemente. Cognizant of his own rundown on the clock, Humphrey phoned, and dipping into the reservoirs of his magnanimous heart he extended, with compassionate memory, his warm seasonal greetings. Although bitter antagonists on the political platform, he broke through the veneer of Nixon's cold personality to clasp him in the grip of the most equalizing of human need—mutual suffering.

This parting tribute embodied his philosophy that, "no matter how high a man may rise in this democracy, he functions with the human emotions and limitations that we all share."

In his final days, those limitations wracked Humphrey's body and pinioned him as a monument to his own articulate truth.

During one particularly difficult bout with chemotherapy, his liver was injected, directly.

"I just wanted it all to end .... The pain was just too much to bear. I couldn't catch my breath. Every bone in my body ached," he confided to his doctor, Edgar Berman, "but ... a man just has to count his blessings!"

At the tag end of his battle with cancer, those blessings had dwindled down to gratitude for the ability to digest one spoonful of cereal—a taste of Special K.

"But ..." Humphrey said cheerfully, "a week ago I couldn't even face a cracker."

The word enthusiasm has as its root the Greek *en theos*, meaning "in God." Humphrey's enthusiasm was rooted in his faith in God, in America, and the political process, and in the intense commitment of his life. A gut-level confidence that enabled him to be "an optimist—without apology!"

His directionals revolved around a simple slogan: "Life is to be enjoyed, not merely endured."

Jesus Christ said the same thing. He told us that he came that we might have life, and that we might have it "more abundantly" (John 10:10).

If our life is a dull shade of tattle-tale grey, Jesus came to brighten it up. If our life is shattered, he came to put it back together again. If our life is empty, he came to fill it. And if our life is bountiful, he came to bring it even more abundance.

He points us to the crux: "These things have I told you, so that *my joy* might remain in you, and that *your joy* might be full" (John 15:11).

How full is our joy?

In making the clear differential between his joy and ours, Jesus zeros in on the essential priority—first his, before ours can ever be full.

Our joy, which has its frustrating dependence on all that we are, on the interaction of our relationships with those around us, and on the circumstances of our environment, weighed in counterpoint perspective against God's joy, dependent on all that Jesus is. This is the differential that transcends the limitations of our finite capacity with the infinite resource of the Godhead to translate and empower our lives.

In the back of my Bible, I have written these words:

If I look at myself I am depressed.
If I look at those around me I am often disappointed.
If I look at my circumstances I am discouraged.
If I look at Jesus Christ, I am constantly, consistently, and eternally fulfilled.

Years ago, a friend used that little verse to develop in me a tunnel-vision to Jesus Christ.

If We Look at Ourselves ...

Our bookshelves are lined with all that we are, all that we aren't, and all that somebody else thinks we should be. *How to Be Your Own Best Friend, I'm OK—You're OK,* or *I'm OK—You're Not So Hot!*

With psychologists pumping self-images into us, with theologians translating concepts at us, with all the information we have at our fingertips, somehow we still do not seem to be able to live up to our own, much less anyone else's, expectations. We are part of the "I blew it again" consequence of finite performance.

When Ian was seven years old, I came into the house one day and found him reading a magazine he had no business looking at nor bringing into our home.

He was born one hot August night under the smoggy light of the full California moon. This gave him a predisposition to yowl long and hard until he was blue in the face, or until he got his own way, whichever came first (usually blue in the face).

He greeted the world "butts-up" in a breech delivery, and one look at his mass of dark hair creeping half way down his neck told me that his hormones would be jumping long before puberty.

We thought about calling him Esau (the hairy one), but were afraid it might predict the selling of his birthright for a bowl of porridge; a natural temptation, porridge being the birthright and yen of any good Scot by the name of Angus.

Instead, we called him Ian—the classic, Gaelic form of John, "the beloved."

He was a winsome lad, with a merry heart and a twinkle in his eye. He had a smile that could sell snow to the Eskimos, and a wanderlust that took him on escapades around the neighborhood—enough to put patience and long-suffering into any mother's life. Whether there was too much lust to his wander, or too much wander to his lust, we have yet to find out; but at age three, after spending the afternoon with one of his playmates, I got a call from her mother.

"My daughter is in the bathtub, and I want you to know that your son has drawn a happy face on her bare bottom!"

"Hold on a jiff," I squeaked in panic, as I rushed to take a look at Ian, splashing around in our tub. "Sure 'nuff," I breathed in hilarious relief, "your daughter has drawn a happy face on my son's bare bottom."

The grin-and-share-it of a camaraderie sealed with the mark of childhood innocence.

Fortunately, the happy faces were both smiling. Unfortunately, they were drawn in indelible ink.

Now, four years later, I was not smiling as I confronted him, caught with the graphic evidence of a *Playboy* centerfold.

He put his hands over his ears and said, "Hear no evil . . ." his hands over his mouth and said, "Speak no evil . . ." then he grinned sheepishly, shrugged his shoulders and said, "Two out of three ain't bad!"

He hit the mark to pinpoint where most of us are. It is not that we go about serializing sin through our lives (although some of us do!). It is just our simple failure to measure up to all that we know we should be. For the most part, we are a "two out of three ain't bad" people.

We get depressed.

The fact of the matter is that life is only as good as our disposition—that is what sold Carter's Little Liver Pills in the forties, and that is what has our national statistic at 3.2 *billion* valium tablets consumed annually.

We are a hurting people.

What generally hurts us are other people.

Lack of other people sometimes hurts us more. It is called the stark terror of loneliness. Lonely is one of the few words in our language that does not have a word to express its opposite. We are either lonely, or we are not.

An experience that intersected the complacency of my status quo and enlarged the peripheral vision of my heart was the day I held in my arms the sobbed-out anguish of a woman devastated by loneliness.

She was parched for affection and the simple milk

of human kindness. She had reached a breaking point.

"Sometimes I go into my hall closet," she cried in desperation, "and I tug on the coats and jackets hanging thère—'Talk to me,' I beg them, 'please, talk to me!'"

"Oh God," I prayed, "put our arms into those empty sleeves and teach us how to wrap them around each other!"

I have always felt a strange affinity for those who move on the fringes of our culture. Drifting in and out of our lives are "angels of opportunity."

Sophie walked around the town in white ankle socks, sandals and a short knitted cape that turned whatever dress she may choose to wear into a uniform. She dyed her hair, but not often enough, so that dark roots streaked through garish red. She lived alone, with no one to talk to, and no one to care. She was arrogantly loquacious, which gave one the tendency to cross the street rather than become entrapped in one of her long conversations. She sniffed a lot.

When she started coming to church I sought her out, and sat next to her, delighted with the opportunity to let the outrage of her style rub me with a new dimension.

When she sniffed and people looked back, I handed her a kleenex. "Thanks," she'd say, and blow her nose. One day I didn't have a kleenex, so I just started sniffing with her. If people were going to scowl and stare, they could—at both of us!

After the service, she generally walked to the local market, bought a sandwich from the deli, and sat on the bench outside, watching cars full of family and friends drive home. I had the odd feeling that she was an observer from some strange galaxy, sent to analyze our hearts.

As we drove past, Sunday after Sunday, on our way home to a dinner, ample to share, I wanted to invite her to come . . . but I never did, and I wish I had. She's gone now. God alone knows where. She left my horizon, and I feel the pain of an empty sleeve into which I never put my arm.

Depression is not to be taken lightly. Frequently, it is the symptom of what might be a severe illness, and needs clinical diagnosis and treatment.

But sometimes all it calls for is a good shot of estrogen, or a run around the block, or several slams on the tennis court to work out a stress. For the most part, our depression stems from a bad case of the blahs. The saggy, baggy, down-in-the-mouth feeling that has us dive under the bedclothes, pull the covers up over our heads, and whine, "Pass me by, world, I don't want to get on!"

One emotionally drenched day, when I was caught in the ebb tide of my own frustrations, I sat wrapped in the colorful squares of an heirloom afghan, watching an interview with Golda Meir over Public Broadcasting.

"Do you ever feel depressed about the State of Israel?" she was asked, "Do you get pessimistic?"

She had seen six million Jews march to Hitler's

crematoriums, many chanting the anthem of their faith, *Ani ma'amin be'emuna shlema beviat ha-Mashiah* ("I believe with perfect faith in the coming of the Messiah"). She had groaned in agony at reports of the atrocities. She had wrestled for a lifetime with the right of her nation to exist.

Yet in retrospect, she noted, "Emotional stamina is mostly a matter of habit, and whatever else we lacked, we did not lack opportunities for testing ourselves in times of crisis. . . . One can always push oneself a little bit beyond what only yesterday was thought to be the absolute limit of one's endurance."

Now her dark eyes were flashing at mine through the television camera. Her answer whipped my spirit.

"The State of Israel, the Israeli people," she said, "cannot afford to take the time to feel pessimistic or depressed about anything, because the Israeli people have too much to do!"

So do we.

Each of us has been curiously and carefully made (some more curiously than others!). We have been individually programmed and finely tuned for the specific opportunity of God working in and through our lives. We are his instruments of purpose.

Stradivari made instruments—among the finest in the world. George Eliot wrote:

> When any master holds
> 'Twixt chin and hand a violin of mine,
> He will be glad that Stradivari lived,
> Made violins and made them of the best.

For while God gives them skill
I give them instruments to play upon,
God choosing me to help Him . . .
If my hand slacked
I should rob God—since He is fullest good—
Leaving a blank instead of violins.
He could not make Antonio Stradivari's violins
Without Antonio!

If our hands slack, they should rob God. He puts purpose into our lives when our lives are committed to his purpose.

A young son was asked to give the blessing at the dinner table one night. He thanked God for the food, then paused, and added, "And thank you, God, for the neat little brother you gave this family."

"Neat little brother?" his father asked, "Where?"

"Right here," said the son, pointing to himself, "I mean me!"

He was on target—we need to thank God for ourselves. Not for the flubs that we make, nor for the flabs that we might be becoming, but for all the possibilities he has in working through our lives. We all come tagged: "With the compliments of your Creator!"

If I Look at Those Around Me . . .

Been disappointed lately? By a spouse? A child? Children, plural? Or perhaps a close friend unintentially breaking a confidence? A mother-in-law?

Or maybe you and I, as that close friend or mother-in-law, have disappointed someone else. What is worse than someone disappointing us is the awful, anguished realization that we have been the source of someone else's disappointment.

After speaking at a retreat in California, a beautiful white-haired lady came to the foot of the podium. There were tears in her eyes and on her face was a twisted expression of grief.

"I am the pastor's mother-in-law," she said. "And I have been such a terrible disappointment to him and to my family. I have been a complainer, a meddler, and a trouble-maker. I have been disruptive. I have made his ministry difficult, and . . . oh, I am so sorry!"

As she broke down and sobbed, her daughter, the pastor's wife, stepped down from the platform where she had been standing beside me. She reached out, and with the tears welling up in her own eyes, she hugged her mother and cried, "Oh Momma, I forgive you!"

The magic words—two of the most healing words in our vocabulary, "I'm *sorry*," and "I *forgive* you."

A few years ago, this saying made the rounds; "Love is never having to say you're sorry."

Baloney.

Love is saying you're sorry—love is saying you're sorry over and over again, and then one more time, just to make sure. Love is saying you're sorry even when it is not your fault.

That is what Jesus did. He hung there on the cross . . . "I'm sorry, my Father. I'm sorry for the sins of the world. I'm sorry for all those things that Fay does that she shouldn't do. For all those things that she thinks that she shouldn't think. For all those things that she says that she shouldn't say. I'm sorry!"

He was sorry unto death.

Some of the most tension-filled times in our family occur during the dinner hour. What I call the "jowl and scowl" time. These lead to knots in our tummies and massive cases of indigestion. They frequently occur because no one is willing to say "I'm sorry." No one is willing to take the blame.

"I'm not going to say 'I'm sorry,'" snorts my son; "it's all her fault, she started it!"

"Huh—listen to Mr. Big over there," snarls my daughter, "why should I say I'm sorry for something I didn't do!"

I see the muscles in my husband's face twitching, and his jaws moving faster and faster as he bolts down his food. I think, "Good grief, he's changing from Winnie-the-Pooh into Hitler, and we're going to have an explosion!"

"Now listen here," I say, "I don't care whose fault it is. *I* will take the blame, *I* will say 'I'm sorry' for both of you. Just see to it that you've learned a lesson and that it doesn't happen again."

Oh the bumbles of our bitter pride that snuffs out the joy in each other when all the while our hearts are lonely to be loved.

The second most healing word in our vocabulary is, "I *forgive* you."

"Father, forgive them . . ." Jesus prayed.

Billy Graham once said that he believed in patting a kid on the back if the pat was low enough and hard enough to do some good.

When my daughter was eight I had a rare occasion to pat her on the back, good and low and hard!

She developed the art of plea bargaining at an early age, and became adroit at negotiating her options. If threatened with a punishment, she would want to know exactly what kind, for how long, and if she had the choice of substitute timing, or redemption.

If I caught her doing something she shouldn't, I'd say, "Stop it, or I'll swat you!"

"Where?" she would ask, and "how hard?" to weigh, not whether the punishment fit the crime, but rather whether the crime was worth the punishment. By the time she got through a manipulative dialogue, chances were I'd lost track of what it was all about. A strategy that should qualify her for a career in politics, or as an investigator for the IRS.

On this occasion, I bent her over my knee. With every whack she yelled, "I forgive you! I forgive you! I forgive you!" (The things they teach those kids in Sunday school.)

Now one doesn't paddle hard nor long when a child is yelling, "I forgive you!" with every whack. I don't remember her transgression, but maybe I did need her forgiveness, and she gave it immediately, without even waiting for me to say, "I'm sorry!"

I have a friend who wrestled with a very severe option of forgiveness when her beautiful daughter was brutally murdered.

The young husband returned home from work at

about four in the afternoon and found the body of his wife lying in a pool of blood at the foot of their baby's cot. Her last moments in life were the desperate effort of trying to reach her baby.

The authorities estimated that she died at about ten in the morning, which meant that the little child lay unattended in his crib for some six hours—surrounded, I'm sure, by the angels of mercy.

The funeral of that young girl was an inspiring celebration of placing her eternal life in the arms of Jesus.

Some weeks later, her mother and I were at a Bible study together, talking about forgiveness.

"I can accept the fact that my daughter is dead, and is with the Lord," she said, "but I cannot accept the way in which she died. I wake up sobbing, with nightmares—graphic dreams of brutality. Don't ask me to forgive her murderer."

"No," I replied. "I don't have the right to ask you to forgive anybody. All I can do is show you the alternatives of nonforgiveness—the development of a root of bitterness springing up in your life; resentment, depression, anger, perhaps even revenge. These will hurt you and could grow in intensity to eat their way through your disposition."

She chose to forgive the murderer, and she prayed for him. It is not very difficult to forgive people when you are praying for them. The healing of her memories began, and her nightmares stopped.

More difficult than forgiving others is the ability to forgive ourselves. But if Jesus forgives us, the least we can do is forgive ourselves.

After I spoke at a conference on this message, a pretty young woman sought me out. Tearfully, she told the story of her young husband's tragic illness and death.

"A year ago, I was attending a retreat at this very same spot. My husband phoned to tell me that he wasn't feeling well and pleaded with me to come home."

She took a deep breath, "I needed to get away so badly. It seemed that I was the one being buried, day after day, coping with the physical and emotional drain of his illness—it was wearing me out. When he called, I exploded with resentment and pent-up anger, to think that he couldn't even spare me one weekend in which to restore my spirit and strengthen my soul."

"I'm not going to tell you the mean things I said to him," she sobbed, "but I didn't drop everything and run home. I even hung up on him. A few weeks later, he died. I have never been able to forgive myself."

She took forgiveness, and as we prayed together she entered into the blessed peace and joy of casting off a burden she had no need to carry.

If I Look at My Circumstances . . .

Shortly after my first book was published, I had a letter from a girl in Arizona. She had come to the end of her rope—she was at a point of despair and discouragement where she felt it would be a lot easier to die rather than to live.

She had been through a traumatic divorce and had three small children. She was a born-again Christian, and attended an evangelical church.

She met a charming man at Sunday school, who professed to be a Christian. She felt that he was an answer to her loneliness and to her prayers. They were married.

Within one year, he had taken her financially for all that she had, and had left. She came down with a debilitating illness and was flat on her back for months, struggling to keep her small family going. She was so down, she could not even look up, much less get up!

Together, we went to the twenty-third Psalm.

"Yea, though I go through the valley of the shadow of death . . ."

Sometimes the valley of the shadow of life is more difficult than the valley of the shadow of death.

The key word in that psalm is "through." David did not say, Yea, though I *live* in the valley of the shadow. . . ." The going *through* is a moving, walking experience.

That girl had been ambushed in a valley; she pitched her tent there and stayed—trapped by the steep slopes of her own discouragement.

Slowly, with the help of the people from her church, she started moving. She would take two steps forward, and slip one step backward. She crept and crawled her way *through* the devastating circumstances of her life. Her brethren in Christ roped themselves together, like mountain climbers, to pull and tug her up and out. The cords binding them were not only prayer, but the practical gift of help.

It is a gift that we do not hear talked about much,

yet it is a gift that none of us can do without. A cup of cold water, a warm dinner, a $5 bill tucked into a cheery note, a drive to the doctor's office, children kept for a few hours. Lights shining through the end of a tunnel when everything within it is dark and gloomy.

That girl not only got up when she was flat down, but the last I heard from her she was working in a special facility, using her experience to help disturbed young women "make it *through*."

How I thank God that there is not a bleak experience in our lives that he cannot use for his purposes and glory!

An executive from World Vision taught me a marvelous definition of the word "experience."

A young man who was impressed with the efficiency of that outstanding organization, and the way the executive handled an international staff whose purpose was to ease the suffering of hurting people around the world, asked, "How did you manage to pull all this together and get it running smoothly?"

"Two words," said the executive. "Right decisions."

"Ah," said the young man, "but how did you come to make the right decisions?"

"One word," thundered the executive, "EXPERI-ENCE."

"How did you get the experience?"

"Two words," said the executive, "Wrong decisions!"

The wrong decisions that clobber us *down*, processed through our experience and the commitment of our faith, can be the turning points that pull us *up* and over the humps in our lives.

When I Look to Jesus Christ . . .

. . . I am constantly, consistently, and eternally fulfilled.

We have the promise of *his presence* that will never leave us, nor forsake us, but will be with us, always.

We have the promise of *his love,* that no power, terrestrial, nor extraterrestrial; no event in the past nor yet to come; life, nor even death itself, will ever be able to separate us from.

We have the promise of *his joy*—that spiritual condition that may not change the circumstances, but changes us, and fills us with a calm beyond our understanding. A peace that puts its confidence in the sovereignty of God to superintend our lives, and work "all things" together for our good, so that though the tears may be streaming down our faces and our hearts may be shattering into a thousand pieces, we are still able to look *up* and sing, "Great is Thy Faithfulness, O God, My Father!"

We enter into that supernatural joy by abiding in Christ. Jesus set the priority, "Abide in me"—first— then, "I in you" (John 15:4).

When we abide in someone, we live within their environment. We move into their home, so to speak. One of the first things we do when we live with someone is communicate, we talk; if we don't, chances are we won't be living with them much longer.

How many anguished nights have John and I

spent, clinging by our toenails to the separate edges of our double bed because we have had a tiff and are "not speaking!"

One ghastly night I ended up on the living room couch. John insisted that the bed was the sanctification of our marriage, and come injured feelings, harsh words, or whatever—we belonged there. He would not budge, which I thought was very ungentlemanly, so I did. It was rotten. I didn't sleep a wink that night.

We now have a new rule in our family relations— all differences are to be talked through before we go to bed. Of course, that sometimes means that we are still hassling, come 2 A.M., and sheer emotional exhaustion leads us to reconciliation, which is probably God's way of saying, "Make it up, you two!"

When it comes to talking, God's line is never busy and he will never hang up on us. He will never say, "Can't you wait till half time!" He will not scowl and grouch, "Heavens, woman, it is third down on the five yard line with only 37 seconds left in the game and the score tied!"

He is always available, waiting as anxiously as a courting lover, to hear our voice . . . we call it prayer.

When we live with someone, we eat and we drink with them. No matter how much we talk, if we don't eat we will starve to death.

I feast on the word of God—it has no calories and is full of energy. The scriptures are my stress tabs for the day, and I wear the garment of praise—it is always in style.

In my purse I carry around a little blue booklet

called *The Bible When You Want It*. It is small and flat and has indexed scriptures under the headings, "doubt, loneliness, sorrow, fear, illness, anger, joy, love, confidence," and many more.

When I need a shot of spiritual adrenalin I flip to the relative heading and read such comforting words as, "The Lord is the strength of my life, why should I be afraid?" (Psalm 27:1).

One of the most challenging is, "Ye have not because ye ask not." I don't want to get to heaven, face my Lord, and have Him say, "But Fay . . . you never asked me for that!"

I ask for joy.

For the fullness of all that Jesus is to radiate in and through all that I can become in him. Then I practice my joy. Practice makes perfect.

When Ian was ten, he came whistling into the kitchen one day, threw his school books down on the counter, and said, "Hey Mom, can I practice my kissing on you?"

Reeling with astonishment, I said, "Certainly not! And furthermore, I don't want you practicing your kissing on anyone."

But the boy had a point. He was not about to venture forth into the scarey world of girls an inexperienced kisser.

I can remember my first kiss—I could have used some practice!

The kids have tacked up on my refrigerator door: "Be happy, or shut up!" Most times we can deliberately choose to develop a cheerful disposition.

During a tour through Europe an evangelist and

his young aide registered at a hotel after a heavy day of meetings. Late that night as they were getting ready for bed, the young man heard gales of laughter coming from the evangelist's adjoining room.

"Oh," he thought, "the preacher must have visitors."

The laughter continued and his curiosity got the better of him. Determined not to be left out of the fun, he pulled on a robe and knocked on the door.

The evangelist opened it, dressed in his pajamas.

"Yes?" he asked.

"Have you got company?" asked the young man, "I heard laughter and I thought I'd come over."

"Ha-ha," chuckled the evangelist, "what you heard was me. Every night, the last thing before I turn in, I practice my laughing. Then I practice it again first thing in the morning. It shakes up my liver and keeps me fit."

Norman Cousins says much the same thing and he has written *Anatomy of an Illness* to prove his point. While critically ill, Cousins found, "If I watched Marx Brothers movies and had ten minutes of solid laughter, I could have a night of pain free sleep without any medication. Humor provides the essential vitamin of the soul."

He made the correlation that if negative emotions such as fear, pain, stress, suppressed rage, and hate cause secretions in the brain to dry up so that it cannot do its job well, then the positive emotions of faith, hope, love, laughter, and the will to live must have a role in the stimulation of those secretions.

"The tragedy of life is not death but what dies inside us while we live," he says. "We can be programmed to live, or programmed to die."

My husband and I decided to practice our laughter for one week. Last thing at night and first thing in the morning, we would sit bolt upright in bed and force ourselves to roar with laughter. Once we started we did not have to force—the sheer absurdity took over and we could not stop.

You never saw two children come running into a bedroom so fast! We had a whale of a good time, and it did shake up our livers and make us feel fit, but our children nearly had nervous breakdowns!

Like the Confederate soldier who asked for "all things" that he might enjoy life, but instead was "given life" that he might enjoy all things—we take life and enjoy it.

Now I leap out of bed in the morning with the joy of the Lord as my promise and my strength. I rush to the bathroom mirror and make eye contact, not with the phantom pallor I see reflected there, but with God the Father, God the Son, and God the Holy Spirit living in and through the commitment of my life, and I say, "Good morning, Lord, what have you got planned for us today?"

William Carey tells us, "Expect great things from God—attempt great things for God."

When our get up and go has got up and gone, *his* get up and go will give us a shove!

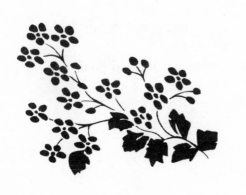

Passing Through the Middle Ages

I know exactly when it happened. The very moment I stepped out of the fountain of youth and plunged, bottoms-up, into the murky waters of middle age.

The scenario seems fitting.

The crimson and gold trappings of the Pasadena Huntington-Sheraton Hotel have a turn-of-the-century elegance, conjuring up an era when the clatter of dapple-greys pulled flower-bedecked buggies through the portico of its long circular driveway. Ivy vines, digging roots of memory through cracks in a stone foundation, rise thick tentacles to cling around the beams of a covered wooden promenade. The boards creak underfoot and tell of lovers' knots tied in the magic of its filtered moonlight.

Through the midnight hours, bridal suites whisper secrets in the walls and the sweet murmurs of ecstasy trap in echo chambers drifting down the halls. In its massive ballroom ghosts of frolics past, dressed in long flowing chiffon and pearls, tails and white silk ties, pop champagne corks and dance, mingling with the spiked heels and short swaying fringes that shimmy to the music of the Boopity-Boop girl.

Moods and tempos change, but through the decades the Huntington-Sheraton sparkles consistently as one of the brightest jewels in the crown city of Pasadena.

As snowflakes twirl the first breath of winter, and most of the nation digs in for a deep freeze, the California sun breaks morning rays across its sweeping lawns to set the dew on fire. Here, at the poolside patio, for many years the Tournament of Roses chose its royal court. Studied grace and fluttering hearts glided many a young girl's hopes and dreams past the fancy of the judges on the reviewing stand.

In 1927 Francesca Falk Miller caught the magic of the moments:

> Oh the crimson of each sunset
> And the glowing pink of dawn,
> Royal colors of the roses
> Holding court upon the lawn.
> Oh the joy, the smiles, the fragrance
> Of a land that knows no gloom,
> Just a peaceful sun-kissed heaven
> When the roses are in bloom.

With each New Year comes a bustling crowd to trample the lush carpets. Pleasure and ambition mull with romance and excitement—they bubble in and focus on the parade of all parades . . . Mary Pickford, Charlie McCarthy and Edgar Bergen, Shirley Temple, Bob Hope, and Billy Graham have all participated in the overnight celebrations preliminary to leading the way as Grand Marshals to the granddaddy of the football games—the Rose Bowl.

There traditions of Stanford, Notre Dame, Michigan, Alabama, USC thunder over the turf. The crowd roars as statistics tumble. Wrong-way Riegels, running the ball back to his own one yard line in a turnabout that still dumbfounds sports history; the upsets in the last few seconds of play—they liven up the archives of the Huntington-Sheraton Hotel.

Sitting at my desk in the main lobby, I looked out on a tranquil scene. A white lattice gazebo joined a horseshoe of flowers. Poppies and snapdragons spaced with clumps of yellow daisies garnished the rose garden with a rainbow of brilliant color.

It seemed innocent enough. I was filling in for a friend who had established a relocation service, networking through major hotels in the United States. I was a point of information and hospitality, and was to exude a warm charm that would win goodwill and influence clients in the direction of our major accounts.

Under the glass across the front of my desk was a map detailing the complex freeway system that joins the cities of Southern California—always a web of confusion to the visiting motorist. A small rack held complimentary copies, stamped with our logo, and available "For Your Convenience."

He was from the *Paris Match*. Debonair, taller than the average Frenchman, with cornflower-blue eyes that burst springtime through dark, long lashes.

There was purpose in his stride. Pausing just long enough to light up a fresh cigarette, he nodded a quick greeting and bent over the map on my desk.

Thinking that I could better assist him by reading directions right-side-up, I walked around and cheerily smiled, "Can I help you?"

He straightened, took a short deliberate step backward, and inhaled. He looked first at my ankles, then spiraled a slow, discriminatory gaze, like a barley twist, around my legs, up past my hips and waist, to linger for a moment at my bust. He burned a tantalizing second on my lips, circled my hair, then, in a moment of poignant truth, those springtime eyes met mine and turned to winter.

He flicked the ash from his cigarette onto the crimson carpet, and said abruptly, "No."

Taking a "For Your Convenience" map from the rack, he spun on his heel and walked off.

I was left standing in the aftershock of faded glory.

One word, casually tossed, intersected the complacency of my status quo.

It was not a "No–!" nor a "No–?" Not even a "No ..." which may have held the tinge of regret. The finality of his "No" period was match point from *Paris Match!*

He had found a nerve ending, like the elusive tip on a spool of thread, and unraveled me. I crumpled in a tangled heap, fuming with a combination of rage, insult, hurt, rejection, and the awful realization that I was no longer stimuli to a man's libido.

I had grown up with the hubba-hubba generation, when long loud wolf whistles were not considered sexual harassment, but a compliment to a well-turned curve. I would blush, or scowl in mock annoyance, but secretly I was very pleased that I had what it took to get "the look."

My face fell like a mudslide. I sat down hard and bit my bottom lip.

I doodled a picture of Marie Antoinette getting her head chopped off by Robespierre. Then I thought of Napoleon and the Duke of Wellington at the Battle of Waterloo, and I gloated, "Jolly good—one for our side!"

I made up my mind to thoroughly dislike the French with their can-can girls, Folies Bergere, escargot, and naughty thoughts. But then I remembered bon ami, bon appetit, Pouilly-Fuisse, deja vu, the lilting delight of Maurice Chevalier, and blossoms on the Champs-Elysees. These smoothed out the creases on my psyche and I had to love them in spite of my encounter with their gauche journalist. When I had mustered up enough courage I went sniveling into the ladies lounge to confront my image in the long mirror.

(Some years ago I visited Garden Grove Community Church. The Crystal Cathedral was still under construction, but even then the church was an impressive structure. I used a rest room in the Sunday School building. Whether or not it was part of Robert Schuller's projection of "possibility thinking" I don't know, but in that rest room—and maybe even in all his rest rooms, men's included, which would be a good idea—was a mirror that made one look slimmer and taller. Never have I spent so much time twirling and swirling, "oohing" and "ahhing."

Afraid that I had slid down the drain, my companion came looking for me. She caught her reflection in that mirror, and Garden Grove had captivated one more recruit.

Forget the theology, forget the impact of the preaching, forget the voices of heavenly choirs, the television program, the chandelier elegance of glittering glass ... ditch the church growth programs and outreach ministries, all we need are possibility mirrors throughout our facilities to double, triple, or even quadruple attendance each Sunday. Add glasses of cranberry juice, served during the coffee hour, and the flood tide of the flush will pull people to the reflected regeneration of their new image of loveliness that will immediately sign them up on the roster of church membership!

Those mirrors should be mandatory—everywhere.)

As it was, the image I confronted was ten pounds overweight, the gathered skirt of my pastel sun dress was not only not flattering, it made me look like a barrel, and I noticed flab on my underarms.

I burst into tears!

The elixir of youth is spelled THIN.

When I was carrying our first baby, my husband put his arms around me and said, "Well honey, your anchor's dragging, and your cargo's shifting, but you're still my dream boat!"

Eighteen years later I was no longer with child, but my anchor was still dragging and my cargo was still shifting—I had entered middle age.

There is a navigational term called "midcourse correction." This is a point on the chart when directions need checking, the compass needs verifying, and adjustments need to be made in order to maintain a "steady as she goes," or the ship may flounder on a very unsteady course.

My ship was floundering and it was time, long overdue, for a series of midcourse corrections.

I ran home and smeared egg white all over my face. Every wrinkle disappeared. I looked twenty years younger, only better.

"Quick," I shouted, "somebody take my picture!"

Nobody was there to hear me. Trouble with egg white is that it is effective for only twenty minutes at a time.

That night I faced the family. I had a triangular "frown-eraser" plaster in between my eyes, and Elastin cream coating my face and neck. Porcelana glistened on the age spots on my hands.

"Holy baloney!" said my son when he saw me.

"I am tired of looking like a frump," I said.

"So, what else is new?" he sniped.

"You can't talk about my wife that way!" said my husband.

"Aw . . . Mom!" said my daughter as she gave me a hug.

"Now hear this," I continued. "Our bodies are being destroyed by inertia. I think we should join a health spa."

"Right on!" said my son, his eyes lighting up. "Let's go to one with all the machines."

"Aw . . . Mom!" said my daughter.

"How much will it cost?" said my husband suspiciously.

That Christmas I gave John a membership to the local spa, with me tacked on as a rider at a specially reduced rate. The children could come once in a while as guests, but on our pinched budget they would have to wait for full-fledged membership until they could help pay their own way.

"It's a bummer," said my son.

"Aw . . . Mom!" said my daughter.

"Men and women mixed?" asked my husband, picking up an astonishing enthusiasm as he sucked in his stomach. "Or men and women separate?"

Straightening to my full height (5'1"), I took a short step backward, and inhaled (my breath only, as at an early age I decided hot fudge sundaes were a lot tastier than cigarettes). I looked first at his ankles (those French have their priorities right), then I deliberately spiraled a slow, discriminatory gaze, like a barley twist, around his legs, up past his bulging torso, until my eyes met his in a moment of poignant truth . . .

"No." I said.

"For the sake of the women, dahling," I explained, "better make it men and women, separate."

He let his tummy pop out and said, "Rats!"

My daughter waved in front of me a magazine ad for a digital computer scale. "Here, this is what we need," she said.

It claimed an electronic breakthrough that would:

"Memorize your weight and the weights of three other family members, so you can compare previous weights with present weights to keep fit, look good, feel healthy."

"Yeah," I groaned, "just what we need . . . to have every Tom, Dick, and Harry or Sally, Jill, and Jane that comes into this house and uses the bathroom pushing my own personalized 'Individual Memory Assignment Button.' Then have my past weight compared with my present weight flashed in red on the digital display readout! When high technology starts publicizing my vital statistics, it has gone too far! Next thing we know, they will add a synthesizer audio circuit that will give us a computerized voice tittering, 'Ha-ha-ha, Mrs. Angus, you cheated on your diet this week—naughty, naughty . . . three pounds gained!' "

I pulled on the black leotard and tights from my ballet days. Every bump of cellulite showed. Years back, I remembered looking at my mother's figure slowly changing and thinking, "My bottom is *never* going to look like that!"

My bottom looked exactly like that.

It was hard to believe that at one time I had every muscle ramrod tight and under disciplined control. It was harder to believe I had ever had any muscle at all.

For the sake of propriety I added a cover-up sweatshirt. All in all, thanks to my legs which were still pretty good, I looked quite professional.

Early in the new year I presented myself at the

registration desk of the spa. The manager was named Abdul. He had a dark receding hairline, pitch black eyes, and a shiny skin that glistened rippling muscles through the mesh of his workout shirt. He looked down at me and flashed a broad, bright smile.

"Trim n'tone," he said, and he took me over to one of the chrome machines. It was a twentieth-century replica of the medieval rack. Suddenly I felt a camaraderie with the victims of the Spanish Inquisition— an omen of things yet to come.

"Easy warmup," he said, "five minutes bicycle, ten times for each leg on the lifts, ten times for each arm on the weights, here on the slant for the sit-ups, aerobics to oxygenate . . . we get you in shape real good!"

He wrote the program down on my chart, just under the depressing figures of my weight and the measurements of my hips and upper thighs.

A chubby woman with a sweet face came in. I decided that she looked a sympathetic sort, so I sheepishly followed alongside her.

Looks are deceiving.

She was Atilla the Hen, pushing steel and tyrannizing the stress in every mechanical device that confronted us. By comparison, I was Chicken Little with the sky falling in.

"You should have seen me when I first came in," she chortled, lifting thirty pounds with one arm.

My eyes got bigger, my spirits got lower, my body got breathless, and my mind got boggled!

My ship was not only floundering, there was the

strong possibility it would sink from sheer exhaustion in the process, but I was determined to make the midcourse correction in the navigational chart of my physical fitness.

(Wanna see me lift thirty pounds with one arm?)

Satchel Paige said, "How old would you be if you didn't know how old you was?" Twaddle! There comes a time in the biological time clock when a woman's estrogen count and her hot flashes tell her *exactly* how old she is—she's middle-aged, that's how old!

When a man's stress levels blink stop lights through the fast lane of his high blood pressure, and his cholesterol count puts a roadblock in his arteries, he's midlife crisis, that's how old!

Suddenly you find yourself telling the kids, "Go easy on your Dad, he is under a lot of pressure these days, y'know." You tell your husband, "Go easy on the kids, they are going through puberty, y'know." And then, when your back is turned you find that your husband has been telling them, "Go easy on your Mom, she is at that time of life, y'know." Only he does not know how to go easy on her himself and says things like, "For goodness sake, what are you sniffling about now . . ." or, "Why are all the windows wide open when it's freezing cold in here?" and he slams them shut and turns the furnace up.

One day your twelve-year-old son phones from school and you say, "Hello there, Janet!" which makes him scowl at you for the next two years, or until his voice drops, whichever comes first.

Your daughter has her first broken romance, and cries nonstop for three weeks, refusing to eat. She loses ten pounds in the process while you put on fifteen by eating all her refusals so as not to waste them.

Grandma whispers, "I don't know what to do with your father, he has been retired for only one month, and already he's moping about the house and driving me nuts."

Grandpa gets you in a corner and says, "Your mother sure is edgy these days!"

It all adds up to a huge conspiracy with everyone in the family tippy-toeing around everyone else and smiling knowing smiles at each other, which does not fool anyone, but only aggravates the condition of the people involved.

Welcome to the middle ages!

Although at times we may feel as skittish as we did at seventeen, and at others as senile as we probably will at 117, it is time to admit that at fifty we are not the people we were at twenty-five, which generally speaking is good news.

Passing through the middle ages takes strategic planning and sailing under the flag called *cope.*

It is an opportunity to redefine our values; to intercept our attitudes and analyze our alternatives; to make whatever midcourse corrections are necessary to keep us on an even keel; and to reset our directives for the future.

It is the determination to live on the *forward urge* rather than on the backward skid.

We cannot change the past, but we can learn from

it. We can influence the present, and we can move confidently ahead. Like the soldier who led a charge up a hill with the bullets whizzing around about him—"Come back," yelled his comrades. "I can't come back," he shouted, "you come on!"

With Paul, "forgetting those things which are behind, and reaching forth unto those things which are before," we press on, "toward the mark for the prize of the high calling of God in Christ Jesus" (Philippians 3:13–14).

My husband tends to be a backward-looking person. An avid historian, he sits up in bed with twenty volumes of the works of Washington Irving in his nightstand, and immerses himself in the past.

I, on the other hand, tend to be a futurist. I sit up in bed with the works of Alvin Toffler, Vance Packard, and Isaac Asimov in my nightstand.

Between us, there is a danger of missing the present altogether!

So we make appointments with each other, "I say, do you suppose we could fit in a little romance at 10:15?" (Middle age synchronizes its time clock to the fact that 10 p.m. is tired, 11 p.m. is utterly exhausted!)

He is always willing, and I am always willing, and most times we are early for the appointment, which goes to show that basic urges are far more motivational than backward urges or forward urges.

To keep in touch with the present, middle age makes appointments and writes notes to itself constantly.

"Pay the utility bills," or, "I am parked in D-2 on

the lower level." Or, "My telephone number is
_____."

Ever since a fellow middle-ager passed me a note that said, "If you haven't thought a new thought, read something interesting, or developed a point of view in the last forty-eight hours, check your pulse, you may be dead!" I make appointments with myself to check my pulse regularly, and to take time to think.

I keep a list of "Thoughts Worth Thinking." These are gleaned from what I have been reading, or from a sermon here and there. Occasionally (very) a provocative television program. Sometimes (rare) a clever thought from my husband, and once in a while (startling) one of my own original thoughts, all of which give enormous momentum to my thinking process.

When my mind feels sluggish and dull, I just pull out my "Thoughts Worth Thinking" list and I am immediately plugged into a fascinating conversation with myself.

Considering that psychologists tell us that subconsciously we talk to ourselves at the rate of 1,300 words per minute, the vital question is: what are we saying? What we are saying originates with what we are thinking.

On learning about the list that I keep, well-meaning friends frequently clip and send me things that they think I should be thinking about. I am very cordial and nice, but deep down inside, instead of putting my thinking apparatus on overload, I wish they would think about these things themselves and then tell me what they thought. In the olden days, before television, this used to be called cultivating the art of conversation.

I also keep a list of "Thoughts *Not* Worth Thinking." The Bible calls these "vain imaginations" that should be cast down. I cast them down by writing them down.

Regrets such as, "Why did I say that, when I should have said this . . ." or resentments such as, "Why did he say that, when he could have said this . . ." I index under the headings of mean, nasty, deadly (watch out for those), silly, and utterly useless. After I have written them down, which is a good catharsis for getting them out of my system, I cross them out. They are still there, as documentation of my own time-wasting folly, but negated as thoughts not worth thinking.

When my not worth thinking list gets longer than my worth thinking list, I realize that I am on the backward skid rather than on the *forward urge*, and it is time for another midcourse correction.

One difficulty is in sorting out what thoughts to place on which list. Such as, what would happen if the *National Enquirer* got a hold of the thoughts I have listed under mean, nasty, deadly, silly, and utterly useless.

My husband checks my lists periodically just to make sure his name does not show up under "Thoughts Not Worth Thinking."

As a precaution, and probably in self-defense, he

purchased a 7 pound, 2,174 page, 1929 edition of the *Lincoln Library of Essential Information*, from a yard sale. It has quizzes behind each of its subject sections and when I get a bit uppity, he throws these at me (the questions, not the 7 pound book, which is fortunate).

"Where and when was the first recorded raising of the American flag over a school?" he asks smugly. "What is the Dawes Plan designed to accomplish— tell how it aims to secure this result. What is the salary of the vice president of the United States?"

It turns out that my intelligence quotient on essential information is sub-zero. This is very intimidating. I live with the apprehension that one day my husband will compile his own list of essential information and that I may not be on it!

What we think about is tremendously important to keep us moving on the *forward urge*.

Statistics tell us that approximately 50 percent of what we worry about never comes to pass. Another 40 percent does not amount to much if and when it does come to pass. And 5 percent we cannot do anything about anyway, which leaves us with a mere 5 percent about which we may have a legitimate reason to worry. Most of our worries belong on our "Thoughts *Not* Worth Thinking" list.

"To think" is the key to staying mentally alive, alert, informed, and involved. In the late 1930s, several great theologians and philosophers were asked to look back in retrospect and choose what specific discipline they would cultivate if they had their youth to live over.

One said, "At the age of ten we wonder, at twenty we imagine, at thirty we cogitate, at forty we think, at fifty we have 'an idea or two,' at sixty we have two ideas, and at seventy we are working on 'one idea.' The sooner you get to that one idea the better." He concluded that he would strive to be an original thinker.

The blasphemy of middle age is, "I can't be bothered!" It clouds our vision, cancels our options, and catapults us down the backward skid.

A few years ago, Gail Sheehy (the author of *Passages*) took a survey through the readers of *Redbook Magazine*. The results were startling. Analyzing the replies of some 52,000 women, from assorted age levels, she found that listed as top priority were the values of "mature love, family security, and inner harmony."

The middle-aged woman, in her mid-fifties or up, was the happiest. These were overcomers!

Earlier than most men, generally at thirty-five or forty, many women face midlife crises. This is not to be confused with the menopause.

She may suddenly see her life as mediocrity, her dreams unrealized or shattered. She may be enduring marital strains or she may be traumatized by a sequence of broken relationships that have fractured her self-worth. She feels as though she has been pulled through a hedge backwards and is emotionally and physically disheveled in the process.

"I am nothing but a zero!" one woman told me. "Marvelous," I said. "Now let's figure out a way to put a one in front of it and you'll become a 10!"

We did, and she may not be quite a 10, but maybe—7½?

The overcomer switches her gears and makes the midcourse corrections necessary to move her in a new direction.

Another woman told me that midlife crisis was the exact time in her life when she came to a conviction of faith. She simply could not endure the thought of death as the final solution to life, and floundered about in search of meaning. The promise of "*everlasting life*" put zest and courage into what had been dismal days.

Sheehy found that by the time she has reached the big 5-0 the mature woman has established a "seasoned" happiness. Such women have, as she puts it, "validated themselves by overcoming dependency on other people's approval and reached a new tolerance and satisfaction with their mates."

She assures us that "each stage ahead holds the promise of a new beginning in which it is possible to throw off old fears and conflicts, leave behind outlived roles and release a more certain, valid self who is capable of loving more richly and living more fiercely."

If only we will bother to do so!

We need to remember the promise, "To him that overcometh will I grant to sit with me in my throne, even as I also overcame and am set down with my Father in his throne . . ." (Revelation 3:21).

Men who most successfully survive passage through the middle ages are those who do not fret and stew about the things not accomplished in their lives, but grab a firm hold on the present, thankful for the simple pleasures of love, laughter, and an honest day's work well done. The affirmation of a support group of friends and family puts the baseline at "having someone who cares whether you come home or not."

The average man has not climbed the pinnacle on the corporate peaks of success, but does that really matter? Many who have may have lost their happiness in the process. Success, as defined by the world's hype, is most often achieved at enormous price, and sometimes with devastating consequence. This does not mean that we shrug off healthy ambition. We are programmed for productivity, and thumb-twiddling inertia leads to hardening of the arteries.

When we moderate the tyranny of the immediate by carefully and prayerfully set priorities, well-cut patterns for living balanced by realistic goals, we crumble the walls of life on the treadmill of the Skinner box. This maintains the thrust of the *forward urge* while eliminating many of the pressure points that lead to the crises in mid life crises.

In the middle of my busiest times, when I am frequently squeezed by the deadlines of commitment, I deliberately pause. I may take a stroll around the garden, cup of tea in hand, and let the pleasure of a hummingbird taking nectar from the orange blossoms expand my soul. Or I may take a walk around the block, even if I am out of town. It is by putting space in the rapid pace of our schedules that our minds are aerated, our thoughts ventilated, and our perspectives validated.

If I am too busy to smell the flowers, then I am *too* busy.

Few of us fulfill the "impossible dream" so blithely handed to us on our high school graduation cards. But there are possible dreams that we can fulfill at any age.

If we feel that life is passing us by, it may be a truism that needs dealing with. For many, life *is* passing them by. Daily we are handed a blank check that many of us never bother to fill in and cash.

On terminating a rollercoaster marriage that bumped its way through plummeting *downs* that never did pull *up*, a friend of mine said, "Now, I can travel and do some of the things I have always dreamed of doing."

It made me think. Was I being a hinderance to John in anything that he earnestly wanted to do in his lifetime? God forbid!

He was the facilitator of our family. Hardworking, sometimes to extremes—concerned and caring about our happiness—had we ever thought about the possibility of the family facilitating his heart's desire?

That night I suggested a long walk.

Rousseau said that he needed bodily motion to set his soul vibrating and give audacity to his thoughts. I have found walking good therapy to clear the cobwebs from the mind. Besides, one meets all sorts of interesting people on walks. People walking with people, people walking with dogs, people walking without dogs, and dogs walking without people.

The cadence of my short staccato step against his long stride broke a rhythm into the sporadic twitter of birds bedding down for the night. My hand held tightly onto his.

"Is there anything at all that you have really wanted to do in your life, like visit some place that you've always wanted to see, that you can't because of your responsibilities to me and the kids?" I asked.

"W-e-l-l," he said with a sly grin. "I guess there's always Bo Derek . . ."

"Seriously!" I insisted.

After a mile or two, probably concerned that I would refuse to turn about and retrace the route home until he shared his heart's desire, he confessed that he had always had a yen to visit Yugoslavia.

"It's said to be a beautiful country," he explained, "with its coastline on the Adriatic Sea. It's in Belgrade where the Sava River joins the Danube."

He could have knocked me over with a feather! Our roots in Scotland or Ireland, yes, but never in my wildest imagination would I have thought of Yugoslavia—I can hardly spell it, much less speak it!

"W-e-l-l," I stuttered, somewhat shaken, "let's go."

"You crazy or something?" he said. "With two kids in college and tuition costs rising?"

"Darling," I said, "I don't care if we have to sell all the furniture and mortgage the mortgage—you and I are going to Yugoslavia."

"When?" he teased.

"Before we hit our dotage, that's for sure!"

Some months back we had met an elderly couple at a business dinner. They had just returned from a trip to Europe.

"Go now, pay later, if you have to," they advised.

They had scrimped and saved for most of their lives, and then by the time they had enough money for their dream trip, they were not well enough to enjoy it.

So far the money has not come in, but the atlas has come out. We are setting Yugoslavia as a possible dream, and we are moving ahead on the *forward urge*, determined to get there.

When we are ninety-four, I want us to be able to smile at each other and say, "Hey—we made it to Yugoslavia!"

Knowing my husband, he will wink and say, "I've been thinking about Nicaragua . . ."

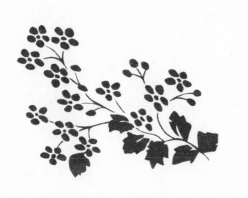

Grief Is a Love Word

When it comes to death, up until quite recently, I considered myself to be unflappable.

After all, I told myself, death should not be thought of as the last sleep, but rather as the last and final awakening—the laurel leaf in the crown of faith.

That is, until quite recently.

Recently, I discovered that when it comes to death—the fact—I am unflappable, but when it comes to dying—the act—I am more than flappable.

With all my spiritualizing, with all my theorizing, with all the platitudes, filed carefully through the years; with all my emotions neatly tagged and compartmentalized, with all my prerogatives and precautions analytically processed. . . . Silly me, I had not reckoned on the sting of hurt that peels them away like leaves on an artichoke, nibbled one by one, until all that is exposed is the heart, vulnerable, ready to be stripped and devoured.

I had not reckoned *grief.*

Grief is a love word. We do not grieve for those we do not love.

To love is to risk losing, but not to love is to have already lost. So we love, we lose, and we grieve.

We grieve not only for those we love and lose in death, but for those we love and lose who are not dead.

We grieve for things that could have been but aren't, and things that are but should not be.

Grief can be the friend who walks us through the sorrow and reaches for the joy that seeks us through the pain, or the enemy who stalks us in the shadows, and turns us from the promise of another day.

There is no quick fix for grief. It takes a working through. It sets its own pace and it will not be hurried; what is fast for one is slow for another. For those who grieve, time is not measured by minutes ticking off the hours, days and weeks, but by the counterpoint of heartache against heartease.

Alfred Lord Tennyson's childhood was so tragic and filled with such intense suffering that frequently as a young boy he would run into the churchyard and fling himself on the gravestones, longing for death.

The great joy of his life was his friendship with a college chum—a charming, brilliant, popular student at Cambridge, whom many scholars considered to be one of the finest and most gifted spirits of their day.

When that friend died, too young and too soon, he felt that all that was left for him was to curse God and die. Instead he "worked" his grief.

Tennyson moved the confusion, the pain, and the torturing sorrow of his loss, through hours of grief. Our legacy is *In Memoriam*, from which these stanzas are taken:

Forgive my grief for one removed,
   Thy creature, whom I found so fair,
   I trust he lives in Thee, and there
I find him worthier to be loved . . .

I sometimes hold it half a sin
   To put in words the grief I feel,
   For words, like Nature, half reveal
And half conceal the Soul within . . .

We had been through the war together, she and I.

There was many a day that she saw the hunger hollowing out my eyes, and she gave me her ration of a slice of bread. She patted me to sleep, singing quietly the songs we loved, "When Irish Eyes Are Smiling," "Peggy O'Neil," or "Alice Blue Gown."

Once in a while I would ask for the jolly upbeat of "McNamara's Band"—it took my mind off the cracked chilblains, the festering pussfilled sores on the knuckles of my hands and feet, and the cold that put nausea into the gnawing fear wrapped around my night.

As we shared a cramped corner in a dormitory with sixty-four other women, every blink of an eye, sniffle or sneeze, was amplified and hushed! I would sit bolt upright on my cot, like the prong of a comb broken to bend the wrong way, and study the sleeping figures, flat on their backs around me. They were cut from patterns of life ranging from the cream of the aristocracy to those of "questionable repute!"

Suddenly I would realize that other eyes were probably studying me, and I would slip back between the covers and pull them over my head like a shroud, a confused and frightened little girl.

More than many other things, our two and a half years of internment under the Japanese occupation of China taught us the value of privacy.

Mother wanted to live alone.

She had a tiny cottage not far from where we live in the hills of Sierra Madre. She planted an "English" garden, filled with larkspurs, hollyhocks, sweet William, and huge red and gold dahlias.

"Do come over," she would say, "they are bigger and better than ever this year!"

She said that every year, and indeed, they always seemed bigger and better than ever.

She dug beds of roses and bordered them with pansies, Johnny-jump-ups, and violets.

"Don't pick, just look!" she scolded the children as they passed on their way to school. For the tiny tots, she would go over and over the names of all the shrubs and flowers, as they pointed chubby little fingers and asked endlessly, "What's dat? And dat?"

She taught our own toddlers how to press leaves and flowers in waxed paper, between the pages of a "good fat book." She gave them slips of this and that in tiny pots and sent them home with dirt crusted deep underneath their fingernails.

"Mercy!" I would grumble, "I'll never get this clean."

The sirens screamed one morning. The paramedics called.

They had found her lying on her kitchen floor. The heart attack had come in predawn hours. Her bright copper tea kettle was topsy-turvy in the sink where she had dropped it, getting ready for a "wee drop" to woo the morning light.

"Will she pull through?" I asked the doctor.

Grim lines tightened grey around the corners of his mouth.

"He looks so tired," I thought, and I wondered how many sirens had screamed at him through that night.

His hand squeezed mine . . .

"Then teach me how to help her die," I whispered through a throat gone dry, and eyes swimming in a blur of tears.

Thank God for tears.

Our body needs our tears as much as our emotions need to have them flow. They lubricate our eyes and keep them moist; they cleanse and lift a piece of lint, or speck of dust; they wash away the fumes that smart and irritate.

Within each of us are reservoirs brim-full with tears.

Tears of joy and gratitude. Sentimental tears that well up when our hearts are touched—a petal hung with dew, the soft curve of a baby's cheek, or weepy, inexplicable tears that flow with a lovely piece of music.

Tears of frustration and anger. Tears of disappointment and hurt. Tears of regret. Then the sobbing, choking tears of grief.

Thank God for men strong enough to cry.

One man said, "Sometimes it's just not enough to

shake another man's hand firmly, look him in the eye, and nod. Sometimes it's not enough to put your arm around a woman, and pat her gently on the back while she cries for both of you."

Jesus wept—thank God.

The irregular bleep of the monitoring machine etched crazy patterns up and down the screen. Labored breathing beat the tempo, like a metronome, pacing a litany of benediction that made the bed an altar . . .

Inhale—Lord have mercy!
Exhale—Christ have mercy!
Inhale—Lord have mercy!

Grief squeezed me so that every bone felt crushed and words jumbled, inarticulate.

The cymbidium orchid grows from ugly bulbs and it sprouts plain tapered leaves. It does not bloom unless it is very tightly squeezed, clustered in a pot.

Once I put a cymbidium clump into the ground, thinking it needed space to stretch. It never flowered. It is only when squeezed almost to death that the matchless beauty of its stem buds six, seven, sometimes as many as eight pale, exquisite flowers . . . and under each a drop of honey-sweet nectar forms.

"So plant me in the soil of your strength, O Lord," I prayed. "Squeeze the grief in me, and from the ugly root of pain and sorrow grow something beautiful to bloom in joy."

Consecrated grief bears its own unique eternal bloom, and tears, like nectar, drop honey-sweet to God.

I sat for hours and rubbed circulation into ice cold feet. Just days before they had tingled on a freshly watered lawn. I tried to smooth away the bursts of blue and red veins that broke against the swelling skin.

I brushed hair damp with the struggle to survive, and spread lotion over lips parched dry. I quietly sang the songs we loved—those lilting Irish melodies. I patted her, as she had patted me, to ease the gnawing fear now wrapped around her night.

And when my prayers dried up, and my heart shriveled with denial, I read the Lamentations.

"The compassions of the Lord fail not, therefore have I hope."

I said them, like a rosary:

"It is of the Lord's mercies that we are not consumed ... *because His compassions fail not.*"

"They are new every morning; great is God's faithfulness ... *because His compassions fail not.*"

"The Lord is my portion says my soul; therefore I will hope in Him ... *because His compassions fail not.*"

"The Lord is good to them that wait for Him, to the soul that seeks Him ... *because His compassions fail not.*"

"The Lord drew near to me in the day that I called upon Him; he said, Fear not ... *because His compassions fail not.*"

"O Lord, you have pleaded the causes of my soul; you have redeemed my life ... because Your compassions fail not!"

Through those crucial weeks, I sat by my mother's

bed and stroked a thousand memories. They clogged my mind, and stumbled over each other pushing for recall.

I relived childhood adventures and told her stories of "remember when. . . ."

Tsingtao in the summer time. Enormous waves that tossed us up like corks. Tiger lilies growing wild along the cliffs and donkey rides trotting down the beach. I gave her visual images to conjure up familiar things and trip a switch to bring her back to consciousness.

I named the family names, and tasted once again our Chinese dinners at Sun Ya's with shark's fin soup, Peking duck, and the wailing music of the Sing-Song girls.

The angry words that clawed our past—resentments boiling hot, and ugly, ugly things. They all turned bittersweet, *because the compassions of the Lord fail not!*

She was a little sparrow, fallen, lying on her back with legs pulled up and eyes shut tight against the light. Jesus saw this sparrow fall—so did I. He threw his mantle over us and covered with his love, we warmed, and melted icy, ugly things.

I told her that I loved her, and I wondered if she heard.

The children didn't want to come.

We had nursed so many small furry creatures, swaddled in strips of towel, or cuddled in our arms, trying to tease life back into lifeless little bodies. Hamsters, rabbits, rats, kittens, dogs and guinea pigs too numerous to count.

From the time he was five, my son had learned to dig small graves, deep around the roots of the old oak tree in the upper terrace. There we committed back to the earth pets who had joyed and comforted our lives. We placed small rings of stones to mark the spots.

My daughter and I wept bitter tears the night we forgot to latch the coop and our hens fell prey to racoons. As one huddled, mortally wounded, we bent to our knees and stroked her ruffled feathers, "Oh Hilda, we're so sorry!" She peeped a pathetic little peep, as though to give us absolution, then keeled over—the next day she was dead.

Cha-Cha lapped up antifreeze. "So sweet, so good," she thought in her own doggy way, and one more friend returned as dust to dust.

The children came.

They learned the language of goodbye: the tender care that sits and holds a hand gone limp. They wet a cloth and wiped my Mother's brow and wet her lips with lemon swabs.

I thought about another swab—a sponge with vinegar . . . a hill called Golgotha and a mother standing there.

She could not reach to brush his hair, or stroke his hand—his hands were nailed to a cross. She could not put her mother's tender touch to wipe his brow.

She could not "work" her grief with acts of love. She stood and watched the blood and water flowing down. Her heart was squeezed to simply being there.

I wondered if a thousand memories clogged her mind. If thoughts went back to the babe in swaddling clothes, the visit to the Temple. I wondered if, standing there, she remembered, "I must be about my Father's business," and water changed to wine.

When he looked down at her . . . I wondered if the burden of her grief pierced a dagger through his heart more than the soldier's spear; and if to see the agony reflected in her eyes caused him pain far greater than the nails and crown of thorns.

The friends who stood with her to watch and wait. . . . For those who can do nothing but stand and watch and wait, their grief is caught for all eternity in the cluster at the cross!

For nights I lay across my mother's bed and pushed my body warmth against her legs, so she would know I was still there.

Days and nights mixed up and time stood still, until the mystery of that moment—the sun rose in my heart . . . my mother looked at me and smiled.

One day she won't, and I will burst my reservoir of tears.

My grief observed became my grief renewed.

How many weeks of intensive care spaced themselves through the years?

Life clung to life with tenacious arrogance. Brittle bones broke on brittle bones, fibrillations fluttered an already weakened heart and minor strokes frightened both of us. We called her our "resurrection lady." She bounced in and out of hospital like a yo-yo—I would put her in the arms of Jesus, convinced this was the end, and he would touch, then turn her back to me!

She was moved to the facilities of extended care.

Up and down the corridors, three by three, like wide-eyed pigeons tucked into roosts, small grey faces tufted with white peered out at me. They cooed little moans, or screamed at the predators of their night, waiting for those who never came.

A grief renewed for those who did not care. Poorer than the poor, they simply were not there.

Wheeled about in chairs, like gaily colored parakeets splashing red and green, or sunshine yellow plumage in their floral smocks, eager heads nodded acquiescence and dull eyes lit up to a word of kindness.

One man caught my arm each day, "Don't let me down," he begged, "please don't let me down!" I wondered how many people had let him down and dashed his hopes against a stoic silence.

A grief renewed for life, distilled to the essence of water sipped through a straw in a paper cup, a box of tissue, and the lifeline of a catheter processing its steady drip beside the bed.

The stored-up knowledge of the years translated to the intense concentration of stuttering to string together a simple sentence.

"Prophecies shall fail; tongues shall cease; knowledge shall vanish—love never fails" (1 Corinthians 13:8).

Love remained.

Strangers dressed in white became mother, father, child, and friend to those who had no mother, father, child or friend.

It fairly burst my heart! "Lord use your love flowing through my heart to be a rainbow, shining through their rain," I prayed. Once again I consecrated grief, and suddenly with my mother I had many other mothers and fathers up and down the hall.

A chocolate-covered mint, wafer-thin to freshen up a tired, tasteless mouth . . . . As eagerly as postulants, kneeling at a rail, they received a tender mercy. "This, too, we do in remembrance of you."

"My mother died so suddenly," Millie said, "I did not have the opportunity of caring and stroking from her the final pulse of life. But I determined to use my grief to do it for someone else." She does. Twice a week, and leaves her kiss, printed pale pink on each brow.

The griefs of guilt and regret are those with which we punish ourselves.

"If only I had . . ." or, "If only I hadn't . . ."

They flagellate our consciences and swill us in the limbo of our anxieties. These need a healing of our memories to move us out beyond circumstances over which we now have no control, and into affirmation of the present, over which we have a great deal of control. "What is, and what can be," rather than "what was."

Even as love initiates action, grief initiates action.

Her name was Sue.

She was a golden California girl. Blond hair bleached almost platinum by a scorching summer sun, her hazel eyes smoked blue in morning mists, green while surfing through the waves, and by candlelight flecked brown with the warmth of many autumn hues.

She was flippant, bursting with independence, anxious to stretch herself through the vulnerabilities of campus life, and yet a quiver, feather light, that wafted high or low, fanned by the breezes of self-doubt.

They had spent the evening tasting tea. Chamomile, Morning Thunder, Dynasty Green, and the Mixed Herbs of Sleepytime—but it was after midnight and they still were not sleepy.

The new semester had thrown them together; roommates in the hallowed halls of learning. After weeks of explosive tempers and seemingly endless hassles, they were modifying to each other and starting to build a mutual trust.

Lessons in learning were not as hard as lessons in living, or . . . lessons in loving!

Chris scanned the angles of the room, books were everywhere. Her eye sorted through the familiar clutter. Suddenly she saw it. Balanced precariously at the end of a shelf, like a sentry standing at attention, was an empty coke bottle. A slip of white, stained paper curled inside.

She stood and reached, "Hey, Sue, what's this?"

Sue barely raised her eyes. She turned and turned the small square box of tea. She gave a nervous little laugh. Sometimes we laugh because it hurts too much to cry.

Chris lifted the bottle towards the light, "September 22 . . . something pretty special, eh?"

The date lashed open wounds of memory. Sue bit her lip and with her knuckles clenching white, she crushed the paper box.

"That's all he bought me, one lousy bottle of coke!" The words scraped raw against each other— they had a bitter edge.

"I will never, ever forget . . . I sold my virginity for a bottle of coke."

She had carried the grief of her regret for over a year. Not only that, she had raised a monument to it. She put it on display to taunt and mock her. The empty coke bottle with its crumpled date jeered, "*I will never let you forget!*

"A good friend multiplies joy and divides grief," there are times of anguish when others help us to do that which we cannot, or will not do alone.

"One broken dream is not the end of dreaming," wrote Edgar A. Guest. Heaven reached down to Sue that night. With the help of Chris, she turned her grief over to the loving kindness of a God whose *compassions fail not*, and she made peace with herself. A moment's indiscretion that had destroyed her dreams of a love-fulfilled sexuality, rather than a one-night stand, had grown in her a bitter fruit from a bitter root. It could have colored relationships throughout her life. She dug it up and tossed it out.

Taking the empty coke bottle, the girls went outside. Under the stars, winking through palm fronds that etched a tapestry against the sky, they smashed it on a rock. It broke into a hundred pieces, glistening at their feet, and the soiled slip of paper was trodden underfoot.

Arm in arm they turned and walked from the night towards the new beginnings of another day.

Between the hours of two and three o'clock in the morning the body is at its lowest ebb, it is in its most vulnerable state.

For those who grieve for one they love who is not dead, life is suspended in a perpetual state of three o'clock in the morning.

That person might be living right beside us, and grief tugs at our heart for all the things we wish could be, but aren't.

Worse than the rejection of open hostility is the rejection coming through our intimacies. We yearn to reach out and hold and touch, to stroke and love. Instead, we find a wall of indifference and resistance that drowns us in the grief of shut-out love; the hurt of trying to be happy *in spite* of those we love instead of *because of* those we love.

If that one we love has left, we wake through many restless nights, remembering all that used to be. We wonder if they ever stir to think of us, or if in their hearts we are past remembering, while in our hearts they are past forgetting.

There is the grief of "letting go," to watch a child make his own seemingly irreversible mistakes. We fret over all the possibilities, and all the impossibilities. Whether they are well or ill; in pain or trouble;

out of money or in need of help . . . . We carry them, piggy-back on our prayers, out of sight, and strain like a tortoise looking up over his shell to see their faces.

"Faith is the bird that sings to greet the dawn while it is still dark."

If we take that Indian proverb, and through the dark night of our soul learn to sing its song of faith, we break the pain of heartache and stir the promise of the morning light.

Successful grief recognizes and is not reluctant to "feel" its varied agonies. It balks at all the old familiar places, winces at nostalgic scents, and lingers over mementos.

It gropes with aching arms, inching through the desolation, and moves towards the discovery of the reconstructed life.

I wrote a letter of consolation to a friend whose sister had recently died.

"I find myself laying cards and notes aside," she wrote back, "thinking, 'I'll send these down to Ann—she will love them,' and then stark reality hits, and I realize that I cannot call her on the phone, nor write to her. But then the blessed Holy Spirit reminds me that there is one thing I can still do with her, and that is to *praise God!*"

"The words of the Doxology, 'Praise Him all creatures here below, praise Him above ye heavenly host . . .' have new meaning as I realize that when we praise God we are united with those already with him, and we will all be praising him for eternity!"

Successful grief plants jonquils in the winter season of the heart and waits to see them burst to life with reassurance of the spring.

While successful grief does not deny or squelch itself, it does not hold itself hostage to love with the fear that to stop grieving might mean to stop loving. It does not stalk and haunt the past, captive in despair, but while treasuring the memories of yesterday, it looks to every new tomorrow as the promise of another day.

The essentials of the reconstructed life are something to do, something to hope for, and someone to love.

Parents who suffered the heart-tearing loss of a child formed a support group called Compassionate Friends. Knit together by an experience that can uniquely say, "I understand," they meet and talk through the hurts of their grief, then they reach out to others, perhaps in the middle of heartbreak, and offer themselves as a listening and a leaning post, to comfort and encourage.

Several years ago seven employees in a large Pasadena hospital met together and shared their mutual grief in the loss of their mates. "Half of me was gone," one said. "I felt as though I was seeing life through only one eye, and hopping on only one foot. My balance was out of whack!"

They decided to meet monthly to reinforce and encourage one another and to simply ease the loneliness by doing things together—to balance one another.

They call themselves *Patchwork*. I like the name. Patchwork takes the remnants of many pieces (our broken hearts), many colors (our varied experiences), and many different textures (our individual personalities), and stitches them all together in a brilliant and beautiful design, unattainable through any other means. In the same way, we patch and reconstruct our lives.

Each summer our family goes fishing in the high Sierras of California. I wait all year to feel that tug of trout on the end of my line, and I drool over the thought of a fish fry in the great outdoors.

How good it is to get away from the smog, the pressure points of the time zones in our lives, and to renew ourselves in the clear, crisp air of lakes, streams, and high plateaus. The Chinese call it the pause that lets the soul catch up with the body.

One of our traditions is to take the gondola ride up to the top of Mammoth mountain. The panorama is breathtaking. It is the top of the world—one step away from heaven.

But . . . for all its beauty, nothing grows on the top of Mammoth mountain. Fruit grows in the valley.

If we lived only on the mountain tops of life, our souls would be barren. It is in the deep and low places, often in the places hidden from everyone but God; it is in the valleys of our sorrows and our griefs that we cultivate . . . understanding, compassion, courage, sensitivity, sympathy, kindness, and all those tender mercies that form like drops of nectar, squeezed from the flowering of our lives.

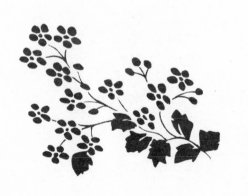

Is Your God a Day Late and a $ Short?

Is your God a day late and a $ short? Because mine frequently is, or so it seems.

Although the love of it may be the root of all evil, money keeps the wolf from the door, the bacon on the table, the gas tank filled, and the kids in college.

It is the push that comes to shove us out into the subway on a Monday morning, and the curve that grades the economy—usually by the length of the unemployment lines at one end, and the gold reserves in Fort Knox at the other.

Small may be beautiful, but less is generally not enough. Especially when that less won't pay the mortgage, or keep the lights turned on. One of the reasons we can't take it with us is that by the time we're ready to go, it has already gone—money, that is!

We may extol the virtues of poverty, but from a discreet distance while we pray it stays far away from us. Money may not be able to buy happiness, true; but, unfortunately, happiness cannot buy money. That is what keeps us looking up to God as the arbitrator of all our "haves," "have nots," and "would like to haves."

As one man told me, "I never pray better than when I have just come from making a bank deposit, nor with greater desperation than when I am going to see about a loan. Then I reach almost mystical heights of spiritual intensity and sincerity."

If things don't turn out the way we pray they should, we wag our finger and cluck our tongue at heaven, and sit down to analyze sixteen reasons why.

In our audacity, we put God on trial to defend why nice things happen to nasty people, and nasty things happen to nice people. When nice things happen to nice people, and nasty things happen to nasty people, we are willing to acquit him.

We are also willing to acquit him if the nasty people turn into nice people because of the nice things that have happened to them: but not if the nice people turn into nasty people because of the nasty things that have happened to them.

This leaves God in the middle of a muddle.

The fact of the matter is that when it comes to misfortune we ask, *"Why me, Lord?"* and when it comes to fortune we ask, *"Why not me, Lord?"*

While he was still in high school, my husband poured some of the hard-earned cash he made delivering the morning newspaper into a piece of waterfront property in an isolated spot several miles up the inlet from Vancouver, Canada. The access road was supposed to go in within a couple of years, at which time he predicted a development boom that would make him a fortune.

By the time we were married, some ten years later,

the property was still in its virgin state, well off the beaten path of civilization, with not a road nor development in sight. As an investment it had not done a thing except levy an annual tax on our stringent budget.

John thought I should take a look at it, so one drizzly Wednesday morning, almost a year to the date of our wedding, we rowed out from the dock at North Vancouver.

I have never been able to understand the rationale of a man who would spend hundreds of dollars on a flight north from California and then compromise to the thrift of a row boat ... rather than rent a motor boat, or, for that matter, hire a water taxi that was guaranteed to take us where we wanted to go, pronto, and then pick us up, hopefully in a couple of hours, which, was about the limit of my endurance to being soaking wet.

As I shivered in the stern of the little boat and felt the rain trickle rivulets down the collar of my windbreaker, I was torn between the exhilaration of the exquisite beauty of the Canadian Northwest and the physical discomfort that instantly programmed into my psyche a top priority for central heating and tea, served piping hot and preferably in a bone china cup. I decided there and then that when stretched beyond those two points, my commitment to love withers.

As his strong arms stroked a fast pace, in between huffs and puffs, John described our "dream house." His Pendleton shirt, faded jeans, and logger's boots displayed a physique in top condition. The fresh air, the rhythmic lap of the oars pulling against the water, and the fact that we were alone in the middle of nowhere stirred my primitive juices, and my emotions ran the gamut from lustful pride at being married to a bionic man, and sulky resentment at his attitude that compromised my comfort to a show of his strength.

We clambered onto the slippery bank and faced a steep cliff of insurmountable granite.

"Here it is, home," John beamed, "solid rock. The Bible says to build your house on rock!"

I leaned against the cold grey stone and watched the waves soak my shoes, my socks and the bottom of my slacks. Suddenly I knew the literal meaning of being caught between a rock and a hard place.

"Isn't this terrific?" he glowed.

"Yes," I lied.

The only fresh water was in a stream some three lots over. There was no sign of an access road, no potential electricity, and, what was worse, no sanitation. The dollars and cents value of an investment that he had been dangling before my eyes like a lucrative carrot disintegrated.

It took us over an hour to find a way up the cliff, then another to build a small fire and roast a pack of soggy wieners.

Six hours later, you never saw a woman so happy to get back to a hotel. I nearly kissed the floor as we fell in the door.

A few years later, we were offered quadruple what

John had paid for the lot. I felt it was an act of divine providence, and I groveled in gratitude. John snarled and wondered if we should hold on just a little while longer.

We decided to go to joint and individual prayer. To seek the guidance of God, to whom we had abandoned the direction of our lives, and to whom we had made a commitment of full surrender.

We tried to do everything right.

We searched the scriptures. We trusted in the Lord with all our hearts, and we sought not to lean to our own understanding. In all our ways we acknowledged him, and we expected that he would direct our path. (Proverbs 3:5).

We read James in several versions, and they all told us that if we lacked wisdom, we should ask God, and he would give it to us—liberally. *We did,* and expected that *he would.*

At the end of the week, we both felt an affirmation of the leading of the Holy Spirit. This we reinforced by a practical analysis of our circumstances. The car desperately needed replacing, raising children brought the stress of added financial demands, and the quality of our here and now could be much enhanced by a windfall profit.

God had obviously sent us some stupid buyer with more money than sense. Not feeling a bit sorry for him, but elated at our good fortune, we sold.

Two years later, the housing boom exploded across the North American continent—the lot was worth a hundredfold more; it would not only have bought us a new car, it would have paid off the mortgage on our home as well!

Our God was not a day late, but two years too early—and he was several thousand dollars short.

We felt shortchanged in the prayer line.

The fact that we had indeed made a fairly nice profit on an original small investment seemed irrelevant and trivial when compared to the enormous profit we could have made. We simmered with regret.

About the same time, a friend of ours was caught in between jobs. He had applied for the one he really wanted, out of state. Several months had passed and, despite many follow-through queries, he had not heard from the organization. Then, out of the blue, he was offered a job locally. He felt lukewarm towards it as it was a professional compromise. He had to decide whether to take it or not by the Monday, two weeks from date of the offer.

"My wife and I went to prayer," he said. "We were starting to crunch financially as our back-up reserves were literally being eaten up week by week. Like Gideon, we decided to lay out a fleece before the Lord, and seek his will through a sign."

So he would not misread the signs, Gideon opted for a double check-point: wet wool and dry ground the first night, dry wool and wet ground the second night.

"After putting through yet another query," our friend said, "if I still have no decision on the position I want by the deadline Monday, I will take the local job."

He activated prayer lines around his circle of friends. He asked for the moving of the will of God to guide and override any error in decision made either by organization management, or by himself.

Time passed. Nothing happened.

On the designated Monday, disappointed and disgruntled, but in obedient keeping with the covenant of his fleece, he accepted the local job. Tuesday morning the mail held a letter giving him the out-of-state position he had wanted so badly. His God was *exactly* a day late!

I wish I could say that the local job turned out for the best and all went well to affirm divine guidance, but it didn't. In order to keep the bread on the table he settled down in a business compromise that frustrated his professional goals for many years. Yet he believed, as heartily as Gideon, that he was moving under the authority of the sign of God's guidance.

Was his fleece that of a lesser God?

I have sat through so many prayer meetings where testimonies were shared of how this person asked for $400 and received $900 instead; or that person faith-promised $1,000 and was able to give $2,000 or more; and I have added my glory alleluia and amen to all the wonderful provisions of the Lord. But a part of me has winced.

Several years ago I tried to pull together a house of help for runaway kids in the canyon up the hill from where we live. They were smashed out on drugs, alcohol, or simply crumbling under the anguish of a wrong turn taken in the road map of their lives. For the most part they were not "bad" kids, just prodigals who had not returned home, and the tragedy was that in many cases they were "throw-away" kids and their parents did not want them home.

I asked God for $450 to confirm a lease. He gave me $120, and when I looked up at him startled with disappointment, he chastened my heart, "Before you ask for more, Fay, use what I have put in your hand."

I did, and when it was gone, another hundred dollars trickled in; and when that was gone and I once again offered God my empty hand, he showed me not more money, but talents programmed into that hand so that when donations dwindled creative stewardship could take over.

Together with other empty, willing hands, we worked out a source of long-term funding—a small thrift shop grew and over the years paid thousands of dollars towards the rent of that house of ministry.

We sometimes behave like the little kid who asked God to help him through a test, then sloughed off on his studies. When he got his final grade, he cocked a surprised eyebrow and said, "Thanks a lot, God, I flunked!"

God seldom does for us what he expects us to do for ourselves, or for him.

God is not hoodwinked—he also knows when we use prayer merely as an excuse for our own reluctance to become involved.

Since teaching me that his provision is frequently worked out through the availability of my own two hands, I study hands.

Large gnarled working hands, small trusting hands, garnished hands with long, painted finger nails, sticky chocolate-coated hands, stubby growing hands, sterile surgeon's hands, earth-soiled planting hands, artistic delicate hands, and trembling aged hands.

On my shelf are a pair of bookends—replicas of Albrecht Dürer's *Praying Hands*. These are the most celebrated hands in art.

I always thought they were the artist's conception of the hands of Jesus. But they are not—although, as a carpenter with rough "working hands" those of Jesus probably looked much like Dürer's painting.

Dürer and a young fellow artist, whom some sources name Hans, were struggling to make ends meet. They worked part-time to support themselves and studied art on the side. One day, frustrated by the sheer exhaustion of the effort, Hans proposed that he would work full time so Albrecht could study art full time. Then, after Albrecht had achieved success and sold some paintings, it would be a turn-about and he could support Hans while he studied art full time.

As Hans toiled long and hard as a laborer, Dürer's genius developed and emerged. Finally, the great day came when Albrecht had enough money jingling in his pockets from the sale of his work to reciprocate and support his friend. Hans quit his menial job and picked up his artist's brush—his hands had become calloused and his joints were enlarged and stiff. His fingers were twisted and ruined for the skill necessary to brush the artist's delicate strokes.

Albrecht Dürer was crushed with sorrow. He knew he could never return to Hans the skill he had sacrificed through his laboring hands, but he could give the world a tribute to the nobility of a friend's selfless love.

He painted the working hands, as he had so often seen them, lifted in prayer. He included the broken fingernails, the enlarged joints, and the heavy veins. Around the world the hands of his faithful intercessor and facilitator have become a symbol of prayerful, sacrificial love.

Daily I give my hands to God.

"Work through them, Lord," I pray. "Use them. Get them dirty when other hands may pull back from dirty jobs. Hold, touch, feel through them. Stroke, comfort, heal through them. Pray through them."

Some days he writes through them. On others he simply plucks flowers through them. He washes, scrubs, mends, or pulls weeds through them, and in their menial tasks they are still praying hands, serving him.

God does *not* "expect day labor, light denied."

He *is* God of the impossible; he *is* hope of the hopeless. When we are powerless to help ourselves, or when no one is able to help us, God moves his miracles through our lives.

The stars fill the African night with the brightness of endless galaxies visible in few other places in the world. As diamonds in the firmament they wink through the majesty of trillions of light years to aura the imagination of man and catch him in breathless wonder at the infinite power of creation.

"I stood on the verandah of the hospital," the doctor told me, "looking into the African night. I gripped the rail with both my hands as the tears poured down my cheeks. I searched the heavens to find the face of God."

In the telling of the memory, the tears once again spilled down his cheeks and he paused as words choked in his throat.

He had completed a surgery in the small mission station, and the man lay dying for lack of blood. Wedded to his calling with a passion that held in sacred trust the sanctity of God-given life, he was more than doctor, missionary, friend, or even saint. He was a scalpel curved against the palm of God.

"I have no blood," he cried. "You fed four thousand with seven loaves; you turned water into wine. . . . Fill this man's veins tonight!"

"Suddenly," he said, "I felt an arm around my shoulders—a heavy weighted arm that gripped me with a fierce strength that nearly spun me round about. Surprised, I looked behind me. There was no one there, yet I continued to feel that arm. A strange expectation filled my heart and my pulse quickened. Slowly I found myself walking back to surgery. There I saw my patient, with the rosy glow of life."

God took the miracle of that doctor's skill, the miracle of his heart's compassion, and the miracle of his faith in asking, to perform the miracle of his divine intervention.

"Not all my patients are so supernaturally saved,"

the doctor grinned, "but I never cease to feel that arm around my shoulders—his continual presence, that is my miracle!"

We are so programmed to the hype of the sensational that our spiritual eyes dim at the simplicity of the legacy that is our daily miracle.

The indwelling presence of the Holy Spirit, making intercession for us in all our infirmities; the intensity of the love of Jesus that gives and gives and gives; the mercy of his grace which promises to be our all sufficiency; and the awesome vulnerability of God, who laid the foundations of the earth and created light to break the darkness, in bending and limiting himself to our asking . . . the miracle of prayer.

R. A. Torrey said, "Prayer is the only omnipotence that God has granted to man—the power of prayer is the power of God.

Rule one of prayer is PRAY. Moment by moment, word by stumbling word, hesitantly or confidently, audibly or silently, God hears the whispers of our hearts. Sometimes it is a sigh—sometimes it is a scream.

Thinking about it is not praying; talking about it is not praying; reading about it is not praying; only praying is praying!

If we pray in faith, believing—good. If we pray, swimming in a sea of doubts, and fan a smoldering flax of hope—good.

I am embarrassed by the number of prayers I have falteringly, casually, flippantly, doubtingly, or even resentfully sent up to heaven, and in the unconditional love of his infinite mercy, looking through the frailty of my faith to the needs of my transparent heart, God has blessed those prayers.

So often I feel like the man who attended a Kathryn Kuhlman service. He watched with simmering doubt the crutches and wheel chairs set aside and radiant faces aglow with the healing power of God until he could bear it no longer. Putting his hand on a tumor the size of a walnut on his neck, he cried in desperation, "Hell, God—I need to be healed!" He felt the tumor leave, and the softness of his neck malleable to his hand.

Like the man, blind from birth, whom Jesus healed with clay moistened in spit (of all things!) ... "One thing I know," he said, "that whereas I was blind, now I see" (John 9:25).

We tremble in wonder.

Then I am amazed at the times I am spiritually tuned—I have confessed my sins, forgiven those who have trespassed against me, and prayed a prayer of faith expecting the dynamic of an immediate answer ... and I wait, and wait with no evident response.

It is our prerogative to ask; it is God's prerogative to answer. Jesus said, "*You* do the asking, *I* will do the answering." We resource the fullness of our opportunity, but dare not pit the perspective of our finite vision against the infinite wisdom of divinity, who works out his most perfect will in the lives of those who trust him. We rest in that trust and pray ... without ceasing!

The disciples asked, "Lord teach us how to pray."

176 / How to Do Everything Right & Live to Regret It

Jesus could so easily have given a six-part seminar on effective spiritual communication; or a ten-point outline on the helps and hazards of breaking through the human sound barrier to bend the ear of God.

He didn't.

Instead, he gave us the example of a prayer—two verses, some fifty-eight words short. They affect our lives and are the best of all possible places to start: "Our Father, who art in heaven . . ."

I like to pray, "*My* Father, who is in heaven . . ." or, when praying for my children, "Ian's Father, who is in heaven, teach him to hallow your name, bring your kingdom into life, give him yourself as his bread of life, and forgive him his sins . . ." and so forth.

Rule two of prayer is PRAY. When all nerve endings are short-circuiting, DON'T PANIC—PRAY! A friend of mine gives out little cards with that simple message.

After giving out hundreds of the cards on one particularly difficult day, she decided, "Prayer doesn't seem to be working, I think I'll try panic!"

She reversed her card to its blank side up on her refrigerator door, and she let loose. She snapped at those around her; she cried at her dilemmas; she groaned at the hurts that assailed her. She yelled and screamed and carried on.

Her husband came home, took one look, and said, "Well, you've finally gone bonkers!"

"It was the worst day of my life," she moaned. "Panic doesn't work, I tried it. Better stay with PRAY." She turned her message card back to its rightful position and ordered several hundred more.

Rule three of prayer is PRAY. It is not the position of the body but the condition of the heart that counts. We can stand on our heads and twiddle our toes and pray, and God will still hear us.

How lovely it is when our environment lends itself to prayer—those long walks in the woods, or sitting on a hillside with cool breezes caressing our hair. It is easy to feel the presence of God at times like those. I pray in the bathtub. Sometimes I shut my eyes and pretend that I am sitting on a hillside and I can almost feel the crisp breeze, only to realize that it is just the bath water getting cold and I had better shake a leg and flick a towel before I get pneumonia.

I pray when I am brushing my teeth. I have even prayed in the middle of making love—I thank God for kisses and that it was nice of him to program pleasure points into our bodies. He didn't have to!

I pray in the middle of a crowd when noise and clutter makes thinking hardly possible. I also pray in the quiet of the middle of the night when the silence amplifies every pounding thought.

The only *rule of prayer is* PRAY. Without circumventing scriptural directionals, encouragements, and admonitions (and there are many), the bottom line of prayer is to PRAY. When we do, the power of heaven picks up momentum to change our lives.

Much as we try to put him there, God is not on trial; the good news is that neither is man. Jesus Christ stood in the docket on our behalf.

If the answers to our prayers depended upon our

worth, they would never be answered—they would never even be heard. Through the righteousness of Christ, they are.

We tend to stroke *prayer* like a lucky rabbit's foot, and seek God's fleece rather than his face.

We try to manipulate his will to ours and sometimes call it faith. We push forward in the arrogance of our own stoic determination, limited by our finite vision, rather than pull back in the simple trust of his infinite plan.

We expect him to change the sovereignty of his omnipotent heart, instead of humbly asking him to give us a heart willing to be changed.

"Be still and know that I am God" (Psalm 46:10) means, "Relax, let God be God!"

I thank God for the prayers he has answered the way I prayed that he would.

I thank him, somewhat shamefully, for the prayers I prayed and then forgot all about; but he didn't, and in his lovingkindness he answered them anyway.

I also thank God for the prayers he didn't answer the way I prayed he would; I shudder to think of how some things in my life may have turned out if he had!

In the mystery of his timing, in the confusion where I do not understand—God is God. I will not diagnose him, I will not analyze him. I will obey him, I will adore him, and I will continue to lay my life before him.

The priorities of prayer are:

His Person—then his promise.
His Presence—then his provision
His Praise—then his power

This puts into perspective the "have," "have not," and "would like to have" of our life.

David Olson of World Vision writes, "God must have heard (and often turned down) millions of requests for ten speed bikes, nice weather, toothache relief, sexier figures, job promotions, and chances for a house in a prestigious neigborhood. Has He heard as many requests for a heart like Christ's, a mind like His, an eye for the lost, an ear to the needy, or ready hands?"

The intercourse of our spirit made one with his, prayer is the intimate communication of a love that should breathe through our every breath, pulse through our every heartbeat, and knit us to divinity.

When we delight ourselves in the Lord, through his *Person*, his *Presence*, and his *Praise* (Glory), we are enabled to say with Brother Lawrence:

"I know not what God purposes with me, or keeps me for; I am in a calm so great that I fear naught. What can I fear when I am with Him; and with Him, in His Presence, I hold myself the most I can. May *all things* Praise Him!"